Oral Treatment of Diabetes

(A Clinical and Experimental Review)

By

Werner Creutzfeldt, M.D.

Priv. Dozent for Internal Medicine
Department of Medicine,
University of Freiburg i. Br., Germany

and

Hans-Dieter Söling, M.D.

Department of Medicine,
University of Freiburg i. Br., Germany

Translated by

Cora Glees

Oxford

With 2 Figures

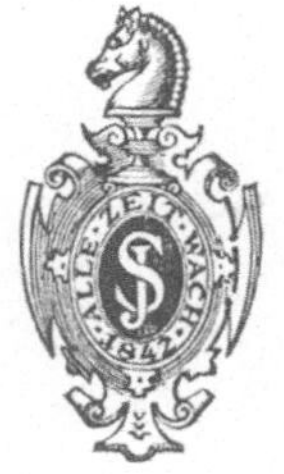

Springer-Verlag
Berlin · Göttingen · Heidelberg
1961

Revised English edition of a review, which appeared in Ergebnisse der inneren Medizin und Kinderheilkunde, Neue Folge, Band 15, Seite 1-213
(Springer-Verlag Berlin · Göttingen · Heidelberg)

Not in trade

ISBN 978-3-642-52693-0   ISBN 978-3-642-52692-3 (eBook)
DOI 10.1007/978-3-642-52692-3

Table of contents

Introduction

The problem of treating diabetes mellitus seemed to have been solved by the discovery of insulin and the production of purified crystalline insulin compounds whose time of effect can be varied by using different additions. Orally applicable substances for reducing the blood-sugar level have been searched for in order to free the diabetic from the necessity of daily injections.

There are also other reasons for this research. Pathophysiological investigations in diabetes mellitus have shown that metabolic errors are not always based on a simple insulin deficiency but that in many cases other insulin antagonistic factors play a part. For instance ,the concept of deficiency diabetes growth-onset type, usually found in juveniles and ectomorphs, was contrasted with the concept of hypertensive diabetes (R. SCHMIDT 1924, 1930) or „Gegenregulationsdiabetes" (BERTRAM) or „Überfunktionsdiabetes" (BARTELHEIMER 1940) or "Lipoplethoric-diabetes" (LAWRENCE) in which there is a positive correlation to the adipose hyperplastic habitus with hypertensive tendencies (BARTELHEIMER 1940, APPELS 1951). In this type of diabetes there is no ketosis tendency and a low insulin-glucose equivalent, i. e. relative insulin resistance (FALTA) due to a hormonal imbalance (too much blood-sugar-raising hormone is produced by the anterior pituitary lobe and the supra-renals and possibly also glucagon) or, to increased insulin degradation in the organism, especially the liver (insulinase system, MIRSKY 1949, 1956). Functional disorders of the liver (liver diabetes, NAUNYN) or of its enzymes and also of insulin inhibitors in the serum (BORNSTEIN and PARK, BORNSTEIN, 1953, BAIRD and BORNSTEIN) can also cause, pathogenetically, certain forms of diabetes. These still hypothetical conceptions are supported by research done on the insulin content of the blood plasma and the pancreas of human diabetic patients.

BORNSTEIN and LAWRENCE found only small amounts of insulin in the blood plasma, and WRENSHALL, BOGOCH and RITCHIE also WRENSHALL and HAMILTON the same in the pancreas of juvenile diabetics (growth-onset type, insulin deficiency diabetes). The plasma and pancreas of the older diabetics (maturity-onset type) was abundant in insulin, (approximately 50% of normal) this was independent of the length of illness. Because of this it is theoretically justifiable to search for remedies which will influence the contra-insular factors. Thus one would be able to attempt a more rational pathophysiological therapy for those diabetics who do not suffer from an absolute lack of insulin, rather than a symptomatic dosing of insulin.

It must be confessed that after 35 years of experience with insulin in the treatment of diabetes mellitus, it is still not possible to combat the secondary diseases (retinopathy, nephropathy, arterio-sclerosis, neuritis) using insulin alone. These appear as the life of the diabetic is lengthened due to insulin treatment. The research for substances exerting hypoglycaemic action should be carried out with the realisation that the best anti-diabetic drug is one which prevents the secondary diseases, and not only corrects the errors in carbohydrate metabolism. Many years of experience are needed to prove, in this respect, the efficiency of the drugs. It is of the utmost importance that all these preparations should have no harmful side-effects, even after many years of use; their exact mode of action must be clear. The correctly applied insulin therapy has hardly any harmful side-effects for the diabetic, besides hypoglycaemia, which shows again how necessary it is that the above mentioned criteria are fulfilled.

The unusually great number of publications on synthetic anti-diabetic drugs that appeared after the introduction of the sulphonylurea therapy in October 1955, shows the magnitude of medical research on the problem of diabetic therapy. The sulphonylurea bibliography consists of over 1300 publications. Added to this are increasing numbers of publications about the biguanides and other drugs with blood-sugar-depressing characteristics. Thus it is not possible to give exhaustive detailed references in this review. Also, as the clinical findings coincide this does not seem necessary. When possible, the first published information, especially on the systematic research of each specific question, is quoted. The question of priority cannot always be solved because the research work is carried on independently and simultaneously in different research groups and published at the same time. The references are detailed and complete only on the more controversial points (mode of action) and on special questions (side-effects). The different compounds are discussed in the order of their clinical significance.

Blood sugar lowering sulphonamide derivatives

A. Thiodiazole derivatives

SAVAGNONE (1941) published the first information, admittedly not heeded, on the blood-sugar-depressing properties of the sulphonamides in man. The same effect was observed in the rabbit, after dosing with a sulphonylurea derivative, (4 or 5 methyl-thioimidazole) in 1930 by RUIZ, SILVA, and LIBENSON. The real story of blood-sugar-lowering sulphonamides does not begin until 1942.

In 1942 JANBON, CHAPTAL, VEDEL and SCHAAP observed that 2-(p-amino-benzoylsulphonamido)-5-isopropyl-thiodiazole (VK 57, 2254 RP, IPTD), a syn-thetised sulphonamide made by VONKENNEL and KIMMIG, can cause serious hypoglycaemic conditions in patients in a poor general condition. Two patients died in hypoglycaemic shock. Further research on healthy subjects showed that the blood-sugar-lowering effect of this substance is parallel to the blood sulphonamide level (JABON, LAYERGES and METROPOLITANSKI). LOUBATIÈRES deserves the credit for immediately recognising the significance of this discovery. He did extensive experimental research on the mechanism of blood-sugar lowering by IPTD in dogs and rabbits. Already in 1946 the therapeutic possibilities arising from this discovery for the diabetic were discussed by him. The findings of LOUBATIÈRES deserve a special and detailed discussion, as he worked out the important experimental data, that are valid, even today, for the whole group of blood-sugar-lowering sulphonamide derivatives. This is often overlooked, especially in German papers.

I. Experiments

LOUBATIÈRES (a—e) found that IPTD caused reversible depressions of the blood-sugar level in dogs and rabbits that were parallel to the serum level of the sulphonamide. Repeatedly large doses caused severe glucopenic conditions in dogs. An IPTD intake of several days manifoldly increased the content of liver glycogen. IPTD was ineffective in pancreatectomised dogs and in those with idiohypophyseal diabetes. However, a definite effect on the blood sugar was proved in the 5/6—9/10 th partially pancreatectomised animals. In the averagely severe alloxan diabetes of the rabbit, IPTD suppressed glucosuria for the duration of medication, on deposing the drug, glucosuria recurred with equal severity. In cross-circulation experiments (connecting the pancreatic vein of a donor dog with the jugular vein of a recipient dog) IPTD caused a significant blood-sugar effect in the recipient dog.

LOUBATIÈRES deduced from his experiments that the insulin secretion of the β-cells was stimulated by IPTD.

Similar conclusions were reached by LA BARRE and REUSE after observing that IPTD depressed the blood-sugar level in cases of mild alloxan diabetes. Research on the relationship of the chemical structure to the blood-sugar-lowering characteristic, showed that the p-amino groups of the benzol ring are indespensible for the blood-sugar effect, while the aliphatic lateral chain of thiodiazole can be varied to a certain degree without loss of the hypoglycaemic effect (LOUBATIÈRES 1944 b, BOVET and DUBOST). Today we know (RUSCHIG et al. 1958 a and b) that the decrease in the blood-sugar level is not primarily determined by the sulphanilyl-rest of the thiodiazole group or of the sulphonylureas.

After several years of silence, the discussion was renewed on the mode of action of IPTD in 1954 and 1955. V. HOLT et al. described damaged α-cells, also a complete destruction of α-cells after IPTD application in the rabbit and rat (v. HOLT, KÖRNER and KÜHNAU 1954, 1955 a and b, v. HOLT and FERNER). The authors explained the hypoglycaemic action of sulphonamides in the normal animal as an uncompensated insulin effect after nesidiectomy. Total islet destruction was described in animals with alloxan diabetes. Here the absence of diabetic hyperglycaemia was explained by a defect in the production of glucagon, however it remains unclear why diabetic hyperglycaemia is found in pancreatectomised animals therefore also without insulin. It could be only partially proved that α-cell damage occurred after IPTD. CREUTZFELDT and TECKLENBORG (1955 a and b) found a moderate and very varied cell damage in guinea-pigs and rabbits in the form of plasma conglomerations, but never in the form of hydropic degeneration characteristic for $CoCl_2$ and synthalin. The number of α-cells was reduced only in one third of the cases. No parallelism was found between the degree of α-cell damage and the decrease in blood sugar. CHRISTOPHE, BELLENS, and GEPTS 1956 a found only a degranulation of the α-cells in rats after IPTD and no degenerative changes nor reduction in number, nesidiectomy was never observed. There was no definite blood-sugar-lowering effect in rats with full alloxan diabetes (CHRISTOPHE, BELLENS, and GEPTS 1956 a). Consequently, the decrease found regularly in the blood-sugar level after IPTD can hardly be explained by its inconstant, and only on very high dosage occurring α-cell damage.

After introducing the sulphonylureas into the diabetes therapy in Autumn 1955, research on IPTD was renewed to discover whether this sulphonamide has the same mode of action as the sulphonylureas. The results from this research confirmed the older findings. LOUBATIÈRES found new material for his theory that IPTD acts on the pancreas as an insulin stimulant. (LOUBATIÈRES 1955 a, LOUBATIÈRES, BOUYARD, FRUTEAU DE LACLOS 1955, LOUBATIÈRES, BOUYARD, FRUTEAU DE LACLOS and SASSINE 1956). The IPTD effect was reduced by simultaneously administering doses of anterior pituitary lobe extract in the dog. The blood-sugar-decreasing action was not weakened by successive extirpation of the supra-renals, thyroid, parathyroid glands, gonads and pituitary. However on pancreatectomy the effect was immediately annulled (LOUBATIÈRES, BOUYARD, FRUTEAU DE LACLOS, SASSINE 1956). The phenomenon of the "healing" of alloxan diabetes as described by LOUBATIÈRES was explained by a regeneration of β-cells in

1*

dogs observed for a length of time (LOUBATIÈRES, BOUYARD, FRUTEAU DE LACLOS 1958). After several days of IPTD dosing, a regular β-cell degranulation was described in rats (CREUTZFELDT, DETERING, and WELTE). Contrary to synthalin, IPTD leads to an increase of liver glycogen in dogs (LOUBATIÈRES 1946a) in rabbits (CREUTZFELDT and TECKLENBORG 1955a, BERINGER and KEIBL), and in rats (CREUTZFELDT and SÜTTERLE). In rats the liver glycogen decreases only on toxic doses (v. HOLT and KRÖNER 1955). Liver glycogen can still be mobilised by glucagon in rabbits under IPTD, but the blood-sugar rise is less than in the normal animal (CREUTZFELDT and TECKLENBORG 1955a). HOUSSAY and PENHOS observed that after IPTD administration adrenelectomised rats showed a significantly stronger blood-sugar-decreasing effect, while hypophysectomised rats displayed the same effect as found in the normal animal. Thus they emphasise a difference between the insulin and IPTD effect (animals without pituitary being highly insulin sensitive). IPTD increases and prolongs the insulin effect in dogs without pancreas or viscera, therefore a certain amount of circulating insulin is necessary for the action of IPTD, not however intact β-cells (LOUBATIÈRES, BOUYARD, FRUTEAU DE LACLOS, SASSINE and ALRIC 1956, HOUSSAY, PENHOS, URGOTTI, TEODOSIO, APELBAUM and BOWKETT 1957).

As all these results correspond to those found after administration of sulphonylureas, which will be discussed later, the same mode of action cannot be doubted. The above mentioned α-cell changes after IPTD first described by v. HOLT and recently confirmed by KRACHT (1959) in the rat, gave rise to divergent opinions. This question must be left open despite the fact that no α-cell damage was found after IPTD administration in several histological investigations (BENCOSME, MARIZ and FREI; DE BASTIANI and GRANATA; MIYAKE also LUNDBAEK and NIELSEN). Also VUYLSTEKE and DE DUVE were unable to confirm the decrease in pancreatic glucagon after IPDT described by v. HOLT, KRÖNER and KÜHNAU (1956a). One must show discretion when trying to separate IPTD as an α-cyto-toxic substance from the sulphonylureas, as all other experimental data corresponds to that of the sulphonylureas. We believe that the inconsistent α-cell damage is only a side-effect of IPTD. It does not explain either the mechanism of hypoglycaemic activity, or the part played by the α-cells in keeping the blood sugar static, or the cause of diabetic hyperglycaemia. This is demonstrated by the ineffectiveness of IPTD and other thiodiazol derivatives in severe alloxan diabetes (CHEN, ANDERSON and MAZE 1946, LA BARRE and REUSE 1947; CHRISTOPHE,

Table 1

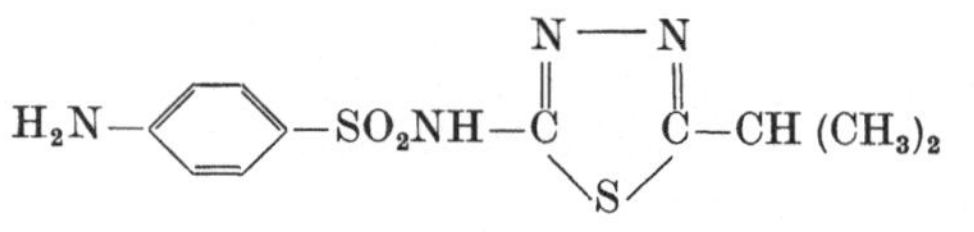

$$H_2N-\langle\ \rangle-SO_2NH-\underset{\displaystyle \diagdown_{S}\diagup}{\overset{\displaystyle \overset{N-N}{\underset{\parallel\quad\parallel}{C\qquad C}}}{}}-CH(CH_3)_2$$

IPTD

$$H_2N-\langle\ \rangle-SO_2NH-\underset{\displaystyle \diagdown_{O}}{\overset{\displaystyle \overset{HN-CH_2}{\underset{|\qquad |}{C\qquad CH_2}}}{}}-CH_2CH_3$$

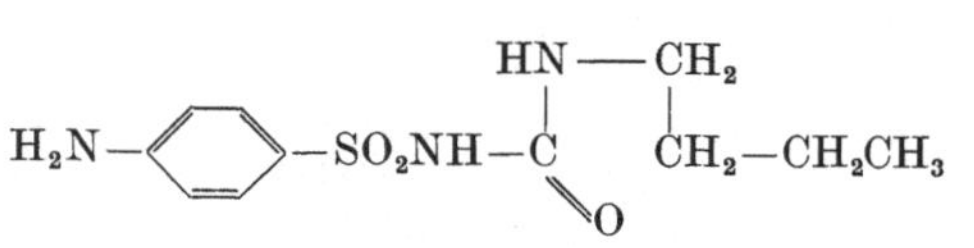

BZ 55

BELLENS and GEPTS 1956a, LOUBATIÈRES, BOUYARD, FRUTEAU DE LACLOS and SASSINE 1957), where only the β-cells and not the α-cells are reduced or missing. IPTD and the sulphonylureas are very similar in structure as shown when drawing BZ 55 in the form used by McLAMORE et al. (1959) (comp. Tab. 1).

II. Clinical experience with thiodiazole derivatives

Shortly after the first reports of the successful treatment of human diabetes with sulphonylureas, papers appeared on the success IPTD had in the diabetes therapy (LOUBATIÈRES 1955a and b, LOUBATIÈRES, BOUYARD and FRUTEAU DE LACLOS 1956, LOUBATIÈRES 1957, AZERAD 1956, UREY et al.). Therapeutic success was achieved in the same group of patients that also reacted to sulphonylurea therapy (see below) ("sthenic" patients whose diabetes appeared only after the 45th year of life and whose insulin requirements were not more than 20—30 U/day). In humans the dose was only 1/10th to 1/20th of the amount of IPTD given in the animal experiments. After this success IPTD was of equal clinical value as the sulphonylureas, and the experimental research carried out with IPTD can be used as a model for the investigations into the mode of action of these compounds.

LOUBATIÈRES (1957) states that IPTD is slightly less effective than the well known sulphonylureas. However there is no comparative systematic research on this question. Therefore the results from comparative investigations we carried out in 1956 on IPTD and D 860 will be mentioned. We treated 21 unselected diabetics first with IPTD for 6 days (3 g/day), and after a 3 day pause the same patients with D 860 (3 g/day) for 6 days. There was *no* effect with IPTD in 12 cases or with D 860 in 8 patients. An *insufficient* effect occurred 3 times with IPTD and once with D 860. IPTD had a *good* effect in 6 of the diabetics while D 860 with 12. Thus IPTD is less efficient than D 860 using the same dosage, but had a good effect on the glucosuria and hyperglycaemia of several diabetics. According to these experiments there is no fundamental difference between both substances. Possibly higher doses of IPTD would have the same metabolic effect. Despite the fact that our IPTD patients showed no side-effects during our short observation time, we decided not to increase the dose or lengthen the treatment as according to our animal experiments (rabbits and rats) IPTD is more toxic than D 860. We do not know of any publications of systematic research on the toxicity of the thiodiazol derivatives.

The p-aminobenzoylsulphamido-tertiobutyl-thiodiazol derivative (2259 RP) is said to have the same effectiveness as D 860 and BZ 55 (LOUBATIÈRES 1957). This preparation is on the French market as Glipasol. The therapeutical indications are the same as for the sulphonylureas. UHRY et al. treated 35 diabetics with 2259 RP and thought this substance even more effective than the sulphonylureas. An allergic erythema was seen as side-effect. Liver function was not investigated. Thus the following publication of DAVIS, KERR and BOGOCH (1959) is of interest: definite signs of liver damage were observed in 17 of 31 patients after 8—50 days of treatment with 2259 RP; 5 patients with jaundice were liver biopsied and focal necrosis and periportal infiltrations were seen. The authors warn against the use of this substance.

B. Sulphonylureas

Substances from the sulphonylurea group are of the greatest practical significance as oral anti-diabetic drugs (comp. Table 7, p. 10). Their blood-sugar-lowering characteristic was first discovered in 1951, in N_1-sulphanilyl-N_2-isopropyl-carbamide synthetised by HAAK, known as Loranil, (Firma Heyden, Dresden). KLEINSORGE (1956a and b) reported that he did some experimental and clinical research already in 1951—1952 with Loranil and the similar N_1-sulphanilyl-N_2-butylcarbamide on the bacteriostatic and blood-sugar-lowering properties; also on the blood and tissue levels and the excretion of this compound, both in man and in animals. A distinct potentiation of the insulin effect was seen in most cases of non-selected diabetics who retained their individual insulin doses (KLEINSORGE 1956a, BARTH and KLEINSORGE). A systematic diabetic therapy was not tried owing to the possibility of toxic damage. The use of the drug in bacteriostatic therapy was not advised, owing to the dangerous hyperglycaemias that were observed. This early research was not published until 1955 by FRANKE and FUCHS, who reported on the first successful systematic treatment of diabetes mellitus with BZ 55. Shortly before this ACHELIS, HAACK, and HARDEBECK described a first account of the chemistry, pharmacology and the clinical significance of BZ 55 during the 22nd meeting of the German pharmacological society.

One must merit LOUBATIÈRES with the first systematic research on the blood-sugar-lowering sulphonamides, while FRANKE and FUCHS were the founders of a diabetes therapy using the sulphonamide derivatives. They were primarily concerned with the practical question and only secondarily with research on the mechanism of action. The reverberation shown by a flood of publications and later through the international press following their report was increased by a simultaneous publication of BERTRAM, BENDTFELD and OTTO (1955) (before the early death of FRANK the manufactures had given the preparation to BERTRAM for continuing the investigations). Only a part of the further research was on BZ 55. It had meanwhile been proved that the hypoglycaemic activity was not correlated to the sulphanilyl group but is also a characteristic of N-[4-methylbenzoyl-sulphonyl]-N'-butylcarbamide (D 860) (EHRHARDT 1956). As D 860 did not only have no bacteriostatic properties but also the least side-effects, it became the most used sulphonylurea especially in the Anglo-American countries. This is seen in the large number of experimental and clinical publications on D 860. Later other compounds were used in the diabetes therapy (comp. Table 7). These seemed to be more effective but were also more toxic. This is so in the case of chlorpropamide and metahexamide. Therefore today after 4 years of experience with sulphonyl-ureas it is retrospectively fortunate for the clinic that BZ 55 and especially D 860 came into use as harmless oral antidiabetic drugs. Thus the great experiment started in 1955 to which authors like LOUBATIÈRES and KLEINSORGE could reach no decision, ended with impunity for the diabetic. Simultaneously diabetic research was stimulated and developed to a surprising extent.

In the following BZ 55 and D 860 will first be described. Metahexamide will be separately discussed because chlorpropamide is not on the market in Europe and metahexamide has been withdrawn in most countries owing to its side-effects. A review of the complete group of drugs is found in the following chapter.

I. Constitution and activity

There is hardly another pharmacologically active compound that has been subjected to similar exhaustive investigations of the relationship between constitution and effectiveness as have the sulphonylureas. The following account is from papers by HAAK (1958), RUSCHIG et al. (1958a and b), also by McLAMORE et al. They investigated more than 850 prepared compounds. Primarily, the blood-sugar-decreasing effect was studied in most substances; secondarily only, they considered toxicity and other pharmacological properties. Many blood-sugar-lowering compounds could however already be discarded on orientation examination.

Discrimination was made more difficult because the effectiveness varied in the different species. Some substances had in dogs a good, in rabbits a bad effect and vise versa. This is due to a different resorption, distribution, degradation and excretion in the organism; these factors are only known for a few compounds.

a) Sulphonylureas

The compounds from the sulphonylurea chain are characterised in the following general formula as doubly substituted sulphonylureas:

$$R_1-SO_2 \cdot NH \cdot CO \cdot NH-R_2$$

R_1 must be a rest with more than two C-atoms, and R_2 with more than one C-atom, so that the blood sugar lowering effect may be maintained. Apart from this, both rests can be varied within certain limits.

R_1

The following rule was worked out for R_1 where R_2 was generally a n-butyl rest of which was taken no notice.

1. A non-substituted, or a once, twice, or three times substituted *phenyl rest* is effective if the substituents are alkyl- or alkoxy rests with one to six C-atoms; also effective are the sulphonylureas in which the R_1 in the benzol ring is substituted by a halogen. On introducing a p-amino group, the blood-sugar-decreasing effect and the bacteriostatic action of the sulphanilyl group remains. The benzol ring can also be substituted with alkyl- and alkoxy rests *plus* halogen or combined with an amino group. The introduction of halogens in the lateral chain increases the toxicity. In Table 2 are shown the characteristic compounds of this kind.

Table 2

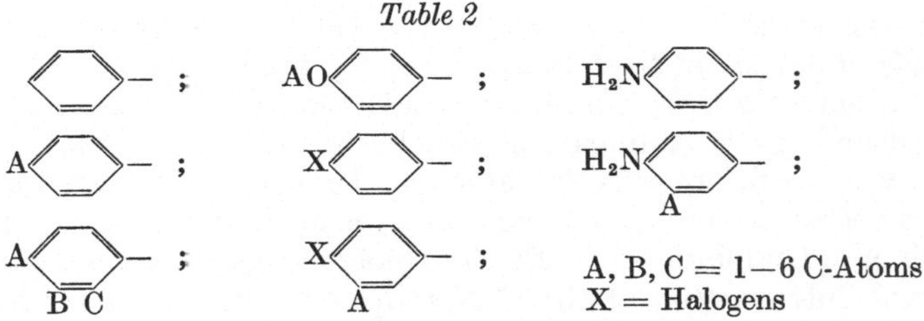

However, a substituted phenyl rest with a hydroxyl group, or carboxyl rest, or their esters or amides is *ineffective*; the blood-sugar-decreasing action is eliminated on introducing a NO_2 group (s. also Table 3).

Table 3

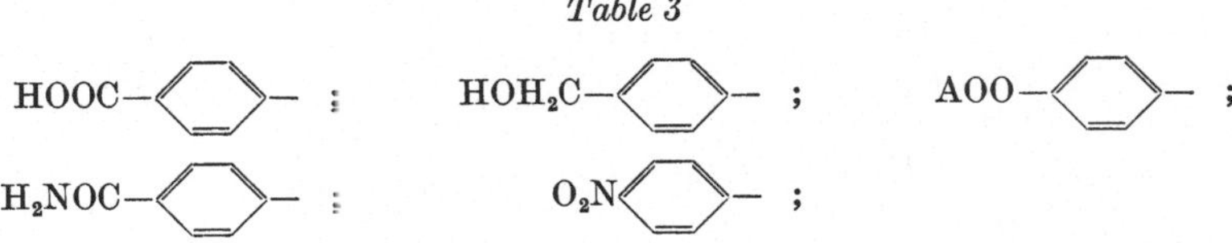

2. In the place of the various substituted phenyl rests mentioned above, *aliphatic* and *cyclophatic rests* as R_1 were inserted and investigated. In order to attain a decrease in the blood sugar, these rests had to have at least 2, and not more than 6—8 C-atoms.

Phenylalkyles are effective as rests if the alkyl part contains 2—4 C-atoms. Phenylalkyl ethers are less effective and phenylmethane sulphonylureas are ineffectual (s. Table 4).

Table 4

3. Sulphonylureas with *different cyclic systems* for R_1 are effective e.g. naphthaline, tetralin, diphenyl and diphenylether sulphonylureas, but not anthrachinon-sulphonylureas and the related compounds (s. Table 5).

Table 5

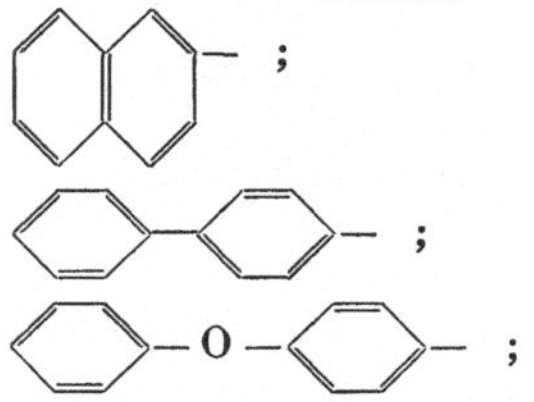

4. No rule could be made for the use of different *heterocycles* as R_1. While e.g. benzthiazol-sulphonylureas or thiophene sulphonylureas are blood-sugar-lowering, others e.g. 4-phenylthiazol-sulphonylureas are ineffectual.

R_2

In the discussion of the R_2 component, a p-tolyl rest will be generally inserted for R_2.

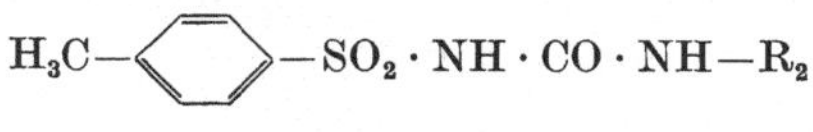

$$H_3C-\langle\ \rangle-SO_2\cdot NH\cdot CO\cdot NH-R_2$$

1. The best effects are found with the p-tolyl-sulphonylureas with *aliphatic and cycloaliphatic rests* of 3—6 C-atoms for R_2; the effect commences with 2 but decreases with more than 7, and ceases with 12 C-atoms. The rests can be differently branched and single conjugations can be present. The cycloaliphates, cyclopropyl to cyclohexyl, are effective as rests. Toxicity is increased and the blood sugar effect decreased on introducing a halogen as R_2. If a hydrogen is replaced by sulphhydril or a disulphide, or if ether or thioether inserted, action is unimpaired. However, the introduction of the OH-group, or a base or ester in R_2, renders sulphonylureas useless (s. Table 6).

Table 6

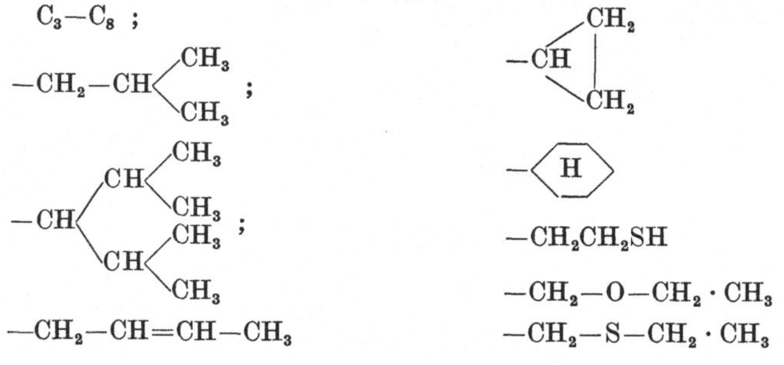

2. The use of *aromatic* or *heterocyclic compounds* as R_2 often leads to more effectual and also to more toxic substances. The investigated phenyl, p-tolyl-p-methoxyphenyl, p-dimethylanilide-sulphonylureas, as substituted benzole representatives, were less effective and less compatible than those compounds mentioned above. Better effect and compatibility was found on introducing aryl-alkyl rests, contrary to aryloxyl-alkyl rests as R_2.

3. A special form of p-tolyl-sulphonylureas compounds shall be listed that are conjugatedly substituted by short aliphatic rests at N':

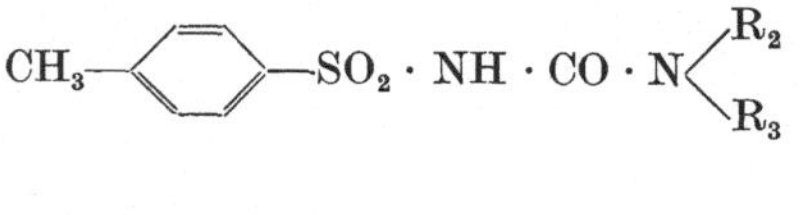

$$CH_3-\langle\ \rangle-SO_2\cdot NH\cdot CO\cdot N\langle {}^{R_2}_{R_3} \qquad R_2 \text{ and } R_3: CH_3 \text{ to } C_4H_9$$

b) N-sulphonyl-N'acylureas

These can be described as a special sub group of sulphonylureas with the general formula:

$$R_1—SO_2 \cdot NH \cdot CO \cdot NH \cdot CO—R_2$$

The influence of the rests R_1 and R_2 on the blood-sugar effect of the substances is thus similar as in the sulphonylureas. The structure of R_2 exerts an especially strong influence.

c) Sulphonylurethane

The urea can be substituted by other derivatives of carbamic acid and thio-carbamic acid. Thus certain *sulphonylurethanes* were found to be blood-sugar lowering having the general formula:

$$R_1—SO_2 \cdot NH \cdot CO \cdot O—R_2$$

R_1 and R_2 also had in this case similar influence on the effect as in the sulphonyl-ureas.

d) 2-sulphonamido-1,3,4-thiodiazoles

The carbamic acid trunk can also be built into cyclic compounds. Known since 1942, 2-(p-amino-benzoylsulphonamido)-5-isopropyl-thiodiazole called IPTD, is a typical representative of this class (comp. p. 2).

$$R_1—SO_2 \cdot NH—C \overset{N—N}{\underset{S}{}} C—R_2$$

The same rules apply for the substitution of R_1 and R_2 as mentioned for the sulphonylureas.

e) Sulphonylthioureas

The sulphonylthioureas $(R_1—SO_2—NH—CS—NH—R_2)$ are ineffectual (RUSHING et al.), however according to McLAMORE et al., also ZAWACKI and JUNG they are blood-sugar active. The maximal blood-sugar-lowering effect of the thiourea derivative of BZ 55 is 3/4 that of the carbamide compounds, while in the thiourea derivative of D 860, it is half that of the carbamide compounds (ZA-WACKI and JUNG).

f) Ineffective sulphonylureas and their derivatives

Other substances, similar in structure or related to the sulphonylureas, were blood sugar inactive. Every further change in the core of the compound led to ineffectiveness. The following compounds had no effect:

$$R_1 — CO—NH—CO—NH — R_2$$
$$R_1 — SO_2—CH_2—CO—NH — R_2$$
$$R_1 — SO_2—NH—CO—CH_2 — R_2$$
$$R_1 — SO_2—NH—SO—NH — R_2$$
$$R_1 — SO_2—N=C—NH—R_2$$
$$\underset{NH_2}{\mid}$$

Table 7

Abbreviation	Formula and chemical description	Generic name	Trade name
IPTD, 2254 RP	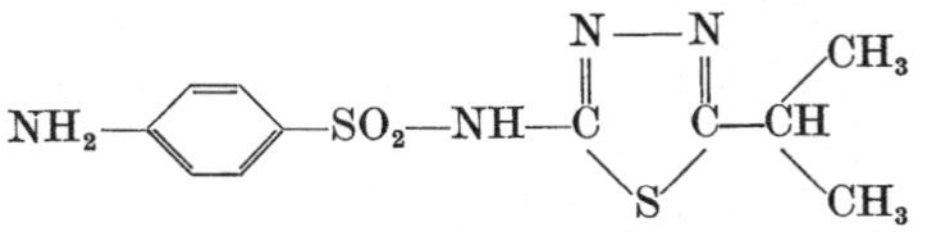 NH_2—〈 〉—SO_2—NH—C(=N—N)—S—C(CH_3)—CH(CH_3)_2 thiodiazole ring 2-(p-aminobenzoylsulfamido)-5-isopropyl-thiodiazole	—	—
2259 RP	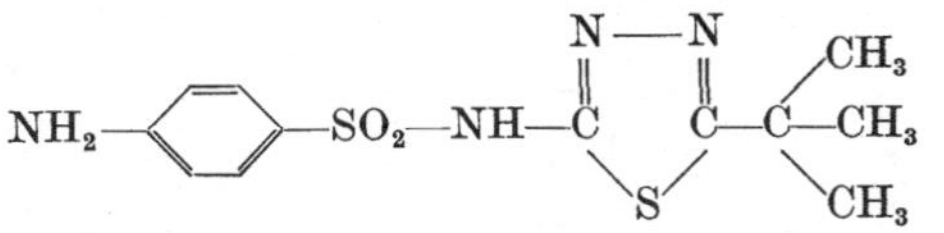 NH_2—〈 〉—SO_2—NH—C(=N—N)—S—C—C(CH_3)_3 thiodiazole ring 2-(p-aminobenzoylsulfamido)-5 tertio-butyl-thiodiazole	Glybu-thiazole	Glipasol(Rhône-Poulenc, Paris, France)
BZ 55	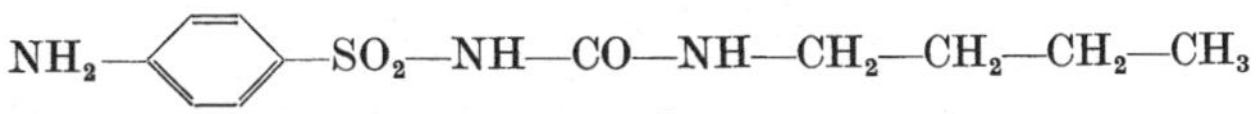 NH_2—〈 〉—SO_2—NH—CO—NH—CH_2—CH_2—CH_2—CH_3 N_1-sulphanilyl-N_2-butyl-carbamide	Carbut-amide	Nadisan(C.F.Boehringer u.Söhne,Mannheim,Germany) Invenol (Farbwerke Hoechst AG., Frankfurt/M.-Höchst, Germany) Oranil (VEB Chem. Fabrik v. Heyden, Radebeul/Dresden, Germany) Alentin (Orion, Finland) Glucidoral (Les Laboratoires Servier, France) Inbuton (Vitrum, Norway) Talanton (N. V. Organon, Oss/Holland)
D 860 U 2043	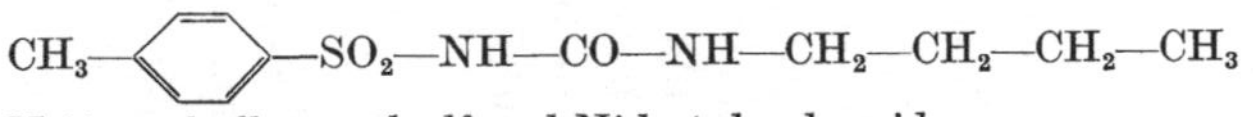 CH_3—〈 〉—SO_2—NH—CO—NH—CH_2—CH_2—CH_2—CH_3 N-(4-methylbenzoylsulfonyl-N′-butylcarbamide	Tolbut-amide	Rastinon (Farbwerke Hoechst AG., Frankfurt/M.-Höchst, Germany) Artosin(C.F.Boehringer u.Söhne,Mannheim,Germany) Orabet (VEB Chem. Fabrik v. Heyden, Radebeul/Dresden Germany) Orinase (The Upjohn Comp., Kalamazoo, Mich./USA) Dolipol (U.C.C., France) Areosal (Lundbaek u. Co., Kopenhagen/Denmark)

Table 7 (Continued)

Abbreviation	Formula and chemical description	Generic name	Trade name
K 386 D 970	CH_3—[benzene]—SO_2—NH—CO—NH—CH(CH_2—CH_2 / CH_2—CH_2)CH_2 1-cyclohexyl-3-p-tolylsulphonyl-carbamide bzw. N-(4-methylbenzoylsulphonyl)-N-cyclohexyl-carbamide	—	Diaboral (Carlo Erba, Italy)
P 607 D 810	Cl—[benzene]—SO_2—NH—CO—NH—CH_2—CH_2—CH_3 N-propyl-3-p-chlor-benzoylsulphonyl-carbamide bzw. N-(p-chlorbenzoylsulphonyl)-N'-propylcarbamide	Chlor-prop-amide	Diabenese (Chaz. Pfizer u. Co., Brooklyn 6, N.Y./USA)
WP 40 D 301	CH_3—[benzene, NH_2]—SO_2—NH—CO—NH—CH(CH_2—CH_2 / CH_2—CH_2)CH_2 N-(3-amino-4-methyl-benzoylsulphonyl)-N'-cyclohexylcarbamide	Metahex-amide	

II. Animal experiments with BZ 55 and D 860

a) Pharmacology and toxicity

1. Methods for determining in blood and urine

BZ 55 can be determined in serum and urine with the method of BRATTON and MARSHALL (1939) or by modification of this method (HÄUSSLER 1956, MOSS 1957); because as a purified sulphonamide it shows diazotisation on addition of a coupling reagent. These conditions are not fulfilled for D 860. Therefore new methods were worked out (SPINGLER 1957, FORIST, MILLER, KRAKE and STRUCK 1957). FORIST's method (transforming D 860 through amylacetate to butylamine, the reaction with dinitrofluorbenzole, photometric determination of yellow dinitraniline derivative) is reliable in serum and urine according to numerous authors and own estimations.

2. Absorption from the intestine

The question of absorbability is of great practical importance since medications are given orally. BZ 55 and D 860 are relatively badly soluble in water, but usually form soluble alkaline salts. Thus, the pure substances are hardly absorbed in rodents as they have little intestinal alkali, but are easily absorbed in the presence of bicarbonate or as sodium salt (D 860: SCHOLZ and BÄNDER 1956, BÄNDER, HÄUSSLER and SCHOLZ 1957; BZ 55: M. A. ROOT 1957). This factor plays no part in carnivorous animals or humans as both have sufficient intestinal alkali (SCHOLZ and BÄNDER, M. A. ROOT 1957a). Absorption from the intestine is complete in dogs and in rats and rabbits on sufficient alkali intake as found in research done with ^{35}S labelled D 860 (BÄNDER and SCHOLZ, MILLER, KRAKE, VAN DER BROOK and REINEKE 1957). Both D 860 and BZ 55 are excreted through the gall bladder, but cannot be proved present in the faeces. They travel via the enterohepatic circulation (BÄNDER and SCHOLZ, PELLEGRINI 1956, QUATTRIN, JACONO and BRANCACCIO, SÜDHOF et al. 1958).

3. Distribution in the organism, tissue and protein bond

WICK, BRITTON and GRABOWSKI (1956) using eviscerated and nephrectomised rabbits, confirmed that D 860 was distributed only in the extracellular space. Correspondingly BÄNDER and SCHOLZ (1956) found ^{35}S labelled D 860 in the blood, bile and in the urine. There was no concentration in any organ; thus, the substances are able to invade liver cell since they were found in the bile. GUGLIELMO and ZUCCONI found ^{35}S labelled BZ 55 in the urine, also in noticeably high concentrations in the liver of rabbits (3—6 hrs. after a single injection, 10 times more concentrated than in other organs and in the blood). The detailed investigations of QUATTRIN, JACONO and BRANCACCIO (1957) show that BZ 55 has a slightly larger *distribution space* in rabbits and guinea-pigs as shown by the relatively high concentrations found in the organs (compare also KLEINSORGE, 1956a, KUETHER et al. 1956, STUHLFAUTH et al. 1960). Also in man, the distribution space for BZ 55 was defined as twice that of D 860 (STOWERS, MAHLER and HUNTER 1958). Approximately 50—60% of BZ 55 determined in the plasma is bound to protein both in the rabbit and man (QUATTRIN, JACONO and BRANCACCIO 1957). In the rabbit, D 860 is bound to the serum albumin to about 40—50% (WITTENHAGEN, MOHNIKE and LANGENBECK). Nothing is known about the firmness of this bond. Probably this is not significant owing to the short half-life time of D 860.

4. Degradation and excretion

BZ 55 and D 860 are degraded in the organism to substances that have no hypoglycaemic activity. BZ 55 is acetylised (ACHELIS and HARDEBECK, M. A. ROOT 1957), but great quantitative differences are found in the various species. Thus the conjugated portion is high in rabbit's serum but low in the dog and monkey (M. A. ROOT 1957). In man BZ 55 is mostly found as free sulphonamide in the serum (FRANK and FUCHS, ACHELIS and HARDEBECK, KLAUS and STRIPECKE). D 860 is carboxylised in the human, in the rabbit, and also in the guinea-pig and rat (WITTENHAGEN and MOHNIKE, DORFMÜLLER 1956a, LOUIS et al., WITTENHAGEN, MOHNIKE and LANGENBECK). The resulting carbonic acid is said to have a slight blood-sugar-raising effect (ADAMI, LARDARUCCIO and CARDANI). One exception is found in the dog. Here the n-butyl-group of D 860 is split off in the organism, the degradation product being p-tolylsulphonylurea and p-tolyl-sulphamide (MOHNIKE, WITTENHAGEN and LANGENBECK 1958, WITTENHAGEN, MOHNIKE and LANGENBECK).

In the rat, D 860 is said to be conjugated with an organic base (MILLER, KRAKE, VAN DER BROOK and REINECKE 1957). WITTENHAGEN, MOHNIKE and LANGENBECK believe, however, that the not identifiable compounds found by MILLER et al. are hydroxymethyl compounds (an intermediate product of the oxidation of D 860 to carbonic acid) and free D 860. The oxidation of D 860 takes place in the liver and kidney, not in the muscle tissue, as shown on organ slices of the rat by WITTENHAGEN, MOHNIKE and LANGENBECK. Altered and un-altered sulphonylureas are entirely excreted through the kidneys (BÄNDER,

SCHOLZ 1956, GUGLIELMI and ZUCCONI, MOHNIKE and WITTENHAGEN 1957, QUTTRIN, JACONO and BRANCACCIO 1957, LEE, ANDERSON and CHEN). The relationship between unaltered, conjugated, and degraded portions differs considerably in the individual species, and the same is partially true for the rate of elimination. BZ 55 is more slowly eliminated, as it is acetylised in the organism than D 860 that is carboxylised to carbonic acid in many species. In the dog the excretion of D 860 is delayed because the degradation mechanism here is different (MOHNIKE, WITTENHAGEN and LANGENBECK 1958, BÄNDER, HÄUSLER and ZCHOLZ 1957). The clearance of BZ 55 in the dog is 2.9 ml/min/m² at different plasma levels, and the tubular reabsorption 96% (LEE, ANDERSON and CHEN). The same authors state that BZ 55 in the dog leads to a slight decrease in the maximal reabsorption of glucose (TM_G) of 6%, while the glomerular filtration rate is not influenced. PETROVIC, PILGRIM and SÜDHOF, however, found a significant decrease in TM_G of 36% in canine experiments. Their experimental results appeared to be more exact than those of LEE et al., as they investigated the influence of BZ 55 on TM_G in the same animals before and after treatment. Whether these results are significant in the lowering of the renal threshold for glucose in man is doubtful and will be discussed later. A decrease in TM_G of 10% was observed after insulin dosage (SHANNON et al., 1941).

5. *Plasma level and blood-sugar lowering (relationship of dose and effect)*

The relationship of dose and effect was carefully studied for BZ 55 by ACHELIS and HARDBECK, MOHNIKE and HAGEMANN also M. A. ROOT (1957); and for D 860 by BÄNDER, HÄUSSLER, and SCHOLZ, DULIN, MORLEY, and NEZAMIS, HASSELBLATT, and BASTIAN, also HASSELBLATT and BLUDAU. A good correlation is always found between plasma level and orally or intravenously given sulphonylureas. A blood sugar decrease commences at a plasma level of 10—20 mg-%. There was within a limited range a positive dose-effect relationship (50—250 mg/kg i.v.) for BZ 55 in the rabbit. Higher doses led to blood sugar increase and smaller doses were ineffective (ACHELIS and HARDEBECK, MOHNIKE and HAGEMANN, and M. A. ROOT). ROOT (1957) found also in rats an increase in the blood-sugar-lowering effect on dosing 50—150 mg/kg orally. 1000 mg/kg were considerably less effective. The decrease in the blood-sugar effect on higher doses is traced back to toxic side-effects and stimulation of the adrenergic system. In the dog, blood sugar is only slightly depressed with 400 mg/kg (M. A. ROOT). The duration of the blood-sugar effect depends on the rate of acetylisation and excretion. Rabbits acetylise faster than dogs and therefore display a blood-sugar decrease of shorter duration. There is also only a good dose-effect relationship for D 860 within certain limits, differing according to species. In the dog it lies between 5—100 mg/kg (BÄNDER, HÄUSSLER and SCHOLZ), in the rabbit between 50—500 mg on a single dose given orally (BÄNDER, HÄUSSLER and SCHOLZ), between 6—72 mg/kg/hr on i.v. permanent drip infusion (HASSELBLATT and BLUDAU); in the rat, between 100 and 250 mg/kg D 860 given orally (DULIN, MORELEY, and NEZAMIS 1956), and in the mouse there is a straight line dose-effect curve between 250 mg/kg and 500 mg/kg s.c. measured by the number of convulsant animals (HASSELBLATT and BASTIAN 1958). If the respective dose is exceeded, there is a decrease in the blood-sugar-lowering effect; in the toxic ranges as also with BZ 55, a blood sugar raising. The duration of blood-sugar effect again depends on the rate of elimination. In the dog it is significantly delayed because the degradation mechanism is different in this species (see this page above). The plasma half-life time for D 860 is 5 hrs for the rabbit, but 24 hrs for the dog.

6. Bacteriostatic characteristics

BZ 55 and D 860 are completely different in regard to their bacteriostatic properties. BZ 55 is effective in vitro and vivo against gram-positive and gram-negative microorganisms (ACHELIS and HARDEBECK, ORTEL and MOHNIKE, LEWIS). It is especially active against dysentery, enteritis and coli bacteria (ORTEL and MOHNIKE). D 860 has only a slight, therapeutically meaningless effect on gram-positive and gram-negative germs (streptococci, staphylococci, aerobic spores) (ORTEL and MOHNIKE, LEWIS). Carboxylised D 860 and acetylised BZ 55 are without bacteriostatic effect. The tetracycline effect is not influenced by simultaneous administration of D 860 to infected mice (LEWIS).

7. Toxicity in animals

α) Acute toxicity. A difference must be made when discussing acute toxicity of sulphonylureas between the genuine toxic effects and the hypoglycaemic reactions which are not actually toxic because the specific pharmacological effect of these substances lies in lowering the blood-sugar level. Genuine hypoglycaemic convulsions on increasing the sulphonylurea doses are unusual.

Hypoglycaemic convulsions were described in normal animals (rabbits) on oral (not i.v.) doses of BZ 55 (ACHELIS and HARDEBECK, M. A. ROOT 1957), also after orally given doses (CREUTZFELDT and FINTER) and subcutaneously (BERTHET, SUTHERLAND and MAKMANN) given D 860 in rabbits and on subcutaneous doses of D 860 in mice (HASSELBLATT and BASTIAN). They were checked by administration of glucose. As mentioned on p. 13, when exceeding a certain limited dose there is, in most species, a strong adrenergic counter-regulation. This counteracts the blood-sugar decrease and there is no hypoglycaemic shock. In adrenalectomised rats, dogs, cats and toads, both BZ 55 and D 860 in relatively low doses cause hypoglycaemic shocks (DULIN, MORLEY and NEZAMIS, HOUSSAY and PENHOS, HOUSSAY, PENHOS, TEODOSIO, BOWKETT and APELBAUM, GORDON, BUSE and LUKENS). As the sulphonylureas, contrary to insulin, do not cause a reduction in liver glycogen but an increase, epinephrine probably has less effect in the liver and more in the periphery (activating muscle phosphorylase). The adrenergic counter-regulation is probably not only caused by the blood-sugar decrease, since a high dose of insulin causes hypoglycaemic shocks even in intact animals. It is more likely, according to pharmacological and morphological investigations, that D 860 acts directly on the adrenal medulla (BÄNDER 1958). Toxic doses certainly also cause cerebral reactions. Thus, convulsions are caused in acute toxic experiments where blood sugar is increased or normal (SCHOLZ and BÄNDER, MOHNIKE and HAGEMANN 1956, ANDERSON, WORTH and HARRIS). For the rest, toxic symptoms occurring after BZ 55 and D 860 are atypical. Death is due to paralysis of the respiratory and/or, circulatory centre. The effect of high doses of D 860 on the neuromotor function of the cat was especially analysed (GERSTENBERG, HASSELBLATT, and SCHMIDT), and a direct effect on the spinal cord was found.

The DL 50 of BZ 55 for the mouse is i.v. 1.9 g/kg, i.p. 2.1 g/kg, s.c. 2.6 g/kg and orally 3,5 g/kg; and for the rat i.v. 1.0 g/kg and orally 10.3 g/kg (ANDERSON, WORTH, and HARRIS). The DL 50 of D 860 is for the mouse i.v. 0.6 g/kg, s.c. 0.75 g/kg, orally 2.5 g/kg; for the rat, orally 4.0 g/kg (SCHOLZ and BÄNDER). No specific changes were found on histologically examining acutely poisoned animals.

β) Chronic toxicity. Experiments on chronic toxicity were made on rats, rabbits, dogs, and monkeys. Here ten times the daily human dose was given for four months (ACHELIS and HARDEBECK, V. HOLT, KRACHT, KRÖNER, and V. HOLT

1956, Kracht, v. Holt, and v. Holt, Anderson, Worth, and Harris; Scholz and Bänder, Creutzfeldt and Finter 1956, Creutzfeldt, Detering, and Welte; Bänder, Häussler and Scholz, Bänder 1959). Only very high doses retarded growth or caused weight loss. The changes in the islets of the pancreas and the glucose tolerance will be discussed in the chapter on the mode of action (comp. p. 29 and 37). Here are mentioned only a few organic changes observed in the chronic animal experiments having no relation to the mode of action.

Liver. In most chronic experiments with BZ 55 and D 860, no morphological changes were observed. Only on higher dosage (1 g/kg D 860 in rats, Scholz and Bänder, Bänder 1959 also rabbits Creutzfeldt and Finter 1959) there appeared a slight fatty degeneration of the liver. Kracht, v. Holt and v. Holt saw these moderate to severe fatty degenerations in feeding experiments in rats with BZ 55 after 4—7 months already with doses of under 0.3 g/kg, but they showed no further augmentation. Knick (1958) reported liver damage after feeding 500 mg/kg D 860 in rats, but could not reproduce these changes in a new experimental series (Knick 1959). The dog is an exception. Thus a decrease in bromsulphonephthaleine clearance after D 860 was observed in the dog (Purnell et al., Elrick and Purnell). Sirek, Logothetopoulos, and Best found an enlarged liver and liver cell changes in normal dogs (cytoplasmatic enclosures and gall bladder thrombi) after chronic treatment with only 30 mg/kg D 860. These observations are contradicted by Bänder and Scholz and Bänder (1959). The authors agree, however, that pancreatectomised dogs scarcely tolerate the sulphonylureas for which liver damage could be responsible. Campbell and Lazidins 1956, Schambye (1957), Sirek and Best (1957), Ricketts, Wildberger and Schmid (1957), Sirek, Sirek, Hanus, Monkhouse, and Best (1959) found, after prolonged dosing with BZ 55 and D 860 in dogs without pancreas, fatty liver degeneration, jaundice, pathological bromsulphonephthaleine retention, reduced prothrombin and albumin synthesis. A few animals died from haemorrhages. These changes occurred despite simultaneous insulin administration. As explanation for this conspicuous behaviour, it must first be mentioned that the liver of a pancreatectomised dog is no longer normal. This does not explain however the above values found in the liver of normal dogs. It is therefore possible that also toxic metabolites appear during sulphonylurea degradation in the dog. According to Mohnike, Wittenhagen, and Langenbeck, D 860 metabolism is different in the dog than in man and other species. The influence of BZ 55 and D 860 on experimental liver damage is discussed on p. 84.

Kidney. No morphological kidney changes were observed after administration of BZ 55 and D 860 by most research workers. After high doses of D 860 (Creutzfeldt and Finter 1956) and BZ 55 (Mohnike and Hagemann), isolated tubular damage was found in the rabbit. Kracht, v. Holt, and v. Holt (1957) saw after 7 months of BZ 55 administration, large, coarse, brown crystals in the vacuoles and epithelia of the proximal convoluted tubules in rats. Schambye (1957) described marked degenerative kidney changes after BZ 55 and D 860.

Thyroid. Long-term treatment with high BZ 55 doses (Achelis and Hardebeck, Kracht and Rausch-Stroomann 1956, Kuusisto and Antila 1956, Kracht, v. Holt, and v. Holt 1957, Brown and Solomon 1958) and D 860 (Miller, Dulin 1956, Creutzfeldt, Detering, and Welte 1957) led to an enlargement and morphological activation of the thyroid in rats and dogs. The effect corresponds to that of mild thyreostatica of the thiouracil type (Brown and Solomon), and is stronger with BZ 55 than D 860. Therefore, after a 2—3-week D 860 treatment, thyroid weight is still normal (Logothetopoulos and Salter, Antila, Kuusisto, and Härtel). This is confirmed by determining the [131]J uptake and the protein bound iodine (KUUSISTO and ANTILA, BROWN and SOLOMON). Goitre development is prevented by administration of iodine (BROWN and SOLOMON). The observed serum cholesterol rise in rats after sulphonylurea administration (HÄRTEL and ANTILA 1956) is traced back to its thyreostatic effect (HÄRTEL 1958). The normal therapeutic doses in man have no significant influence on the thyroid (McGAVACK et al. 1957, s. p. 72).

Pituitary. No changes were generally found in the pituitary. KRACHT, V. HOLT, and V. HOLT (1957) found in rats after BZ 55 administration for 7 months, countless vacuolised polygonal β-cells (so called thyreoidectomised cells) as could be expected by the clear thyreostatic effect of BZ 55 in rats. The other cells of the pituitary were normal.

Adrenal cortex. Commencing BZ 55 therapy, slight activity is seen in the adrenal cortex (KRACHT and RAUSCH-STROOMANN). Later the histological picture is normalised and finally replaced by a slight involution and narrowing of the cortex (KRACHT, V. HOLT, and V. HOLT).

Adrenal medulla. After single application of D 860 (CREUTZFELDT and FINTER 1956, BÄNDER 1958) and BZ 55 (GEPTS, CHRISTOPHE and BELLENS 1956b, KRACHT, V. HOLT, and V. HOLT) in rabbits, rats and mice, degranulation and vacuolisation of the epinephrine producing cells, and partially also of the arterenol (nor-epinephrine) producing cells of the supra-renal medulla is found after 6—12 hrs. The extent of these changes is parallel to the blood sugar decrease and can therefore be indicated as being the same as after insulin and guanidine derivatives (CREUTZFELDT and FINTER 1956). According to BÄNDER (1958), the first cell changes in the rabbit are already found 20 minutes after administration of D 860—long before the beginning of the blood-sugar decrease. Therefore it is possible that D 860 acts directly on the medullary cells. Contrary to this are the observations of GONNARD, PELOU, and NGUYEN PHILIPPON, who found a stronger decrease of the adrenal catecholamine content through insulin than by BZ 55. In chronic experiments the adrenal medulla appeared normal.

Gonads and pregnancy. KRACHT, V. HOLT, and V. HOLT saw on 7 monthly BZ 55 administration in rats, a commencing atrophy of the seminal vesicles. After dosing for one year, KRACHT (1957) observed a severe testicular atrophy, primarily tubular in origin, secondarily affecting the Leydig cells. PINTO and NALLAR saw nidation disturbances in rats if BZ 55 (250 mg/kg) was given from the first day of pregnancy; similar changes for D 860 were not described. Only MANCINI et al. (1958) found, after very high D 860 doses (1—3 g/kg), severe morphological testicular changes in rats. These also appeared on insulin injections (50—400 U/kg) and were less severe on simultaneous glucose administration. However, D 860 and insulin were administered in unusually large doses. BÄNDER and SCHOLZ (1956) could not prove a change in the number of young rats using D 860 in generation experiments. TUCHMANN-DUPLESSIS and MERCIER-PAROT (1958, 1959a and b) also DE MEYER and ISAAC-MATHY (1958) observed, after administering BZ 55 to rats in the first 12 days of pregnancy, increased abortions and anomalities. 25% of the living young were deformed after high doses (600—900 mg/kg). The eyes were primarily damaged. Insulin produced no anomalities, therefore the blood-sugar decrease was not to blame. Non-blood-sugar-lowering sulphonamides of the same doses had no teratogenous characteristics (DE MEYER and ISAAC-MATHY). Other blood-sugar-decreasing sulphonamides were also tested. It was found that after D 860, only 2% of the young were deformed, while after p-amino-benzoyl-sulphamido-tertio-butyl-thiodiazol (2259 RP) no deformities appeared (TUCHMANN-DUPLESSIS and MERCIER-PAROT 1959b). Therefore, it appears that especially in high doses, BZ 55 has teratogenous characteristics. In this connection it must be mentioned that BZ 55 inhibits the growth of various transplantation tumours in animals. This cannot be explained by the blood sugar decrease alone, as long-acting insulin produces no similar effect (KUNZ 1957). D 860 in high doses (1—2 g/kg) blocks mitosis in the metaphase in the crypts of Lieberkühn in rats and inhibits the growth of the roots of V. Faba already on addition of 27 mg-% D 860 to the water (GERSCHENFELD and SOLARI 1957a and b).

8. Incompatibility and the influence of other drugs on the mode of action

In the pharmacological test, D 860 does not influence the action of acetylcholine, histamine, barium chloride, and papaverine on the intestine. The uterine reaction to histamine and ergotamine and the adrenaline contraction of the seminal vesicles, remains also unchanged by D 860 (SCHOLZ and BÄNDER 1956). STEWART (1957b) found antagonistic action between BZ 55 and D 860 and the oxytocin effect on the isolated uterus of the rat. Also the antidiuretic effect of adiuretin is abolished by D 860 and BZ 55 in the rat (STEWART 1957b). The after-effect of evipane anaesthesia is lengthened by 60% in rats previously treated with D 860 (BÄNDER and SCHOLZ 1956). Daily BZ 55 treatment in dogs had no influence on the disappearance rate of i.v. administered ethanol. There was no significant difference in the acetaldehyde and pyruvic acid level in the blood after ethanol doses with or without previous BZ 55 treatment (FORNEY and HULPIEU). However the blood-acetaldehyde level was slightly raised and the pyruvic-acid level lowered. CZYZYK and MOHNIKE (1957) made similar observations in rabbits premedicated with BZ 55 and D 860. Ethanol and acetaldehyde were significantly increased in the blood only in one animal with an unusually high blood-sulphonamide level (100 mg-%). These animal experiments show that the effect of sulphonylureas on the alcohol dehydrogenase in vivo is slight; therefore there is no "antabuse effect" (findings in man s. p. 73). The influence on blood the sugar decrease, after sulphonylurea doses by other drugs, has not been sufficiently investigated. Diethylbarbituric acid (Veronal) and chlorpromazine (Megaphen) inhibit the blood sugar decrease following D 860 application while the insulin hypoglycaemia is not influenced by the same drugs (HASSELBLATT and SCHUSTER). Only hypotheses exist as to the nature of this inhibitary action; these are mentioned in the discussion on the mode of action of sulphonylureas (comp. p. 40). Also unclear is the potentiating effect that a previous treatment with thyroxine (HASSELBLATT and BASTIAN, CREUTZFELDT and FINTER 1959) and STH (PASCHKIS, RUPP and JASOVSKY) has on the D 860 hypoglycaemia in the rat. The weakening of a D 860 hypoglycaemia through glucocorticoide premedication in the rat (PASCHKIS, RUPP, and JASOVSKY) and in rabbits (LAZARUS and VOLK 1958) can be satisfactorily explained by a strain on the β-cells in the sense of a steroide diabetes (s. p. 26). Rabbits premedicated with dihydroergotamine show a stronger blood-sugar decrease caused by blocking epinephrine secretion after D 860 similar to adrenalectomised animals (BÄNDER, HÄUSSLER, and SCHOLZ).

b) Mode of action

1. Research in vitro

The countless experimental investigations on the mechanism of action have shown some organs, or organ systems, to be mainly affected; others are exempted. Thus was not to be expected that the problems could be completely solved by research done in vitro. As functional organic change under influence of drugs most probably has a nervous or biochemical origin, the effects in vitro will be discussed first. On one hand, if these satisfactorily explain the phenomena observed in vivo depends on the conditions of concentration and milieu found at the site of effect. This has been little investigated for the different organs and cell fractions. On the other hand, a finding observed in vitro can only be seen as physiologically relevant, if in vivo in the intact animal, or if in diverse exstirpation experiments actual, corresponding changes in the glucose metabolism are found. If this is not the case, one can consider there to be an unspecific effect on the enzymes in vitro. Therefore we will first discuss the findings and form no extravagant conclusions. Finally in enzymatic research on organs of in-vivo treated animals, the conditions of premedication must be taken into consideration in order that direct, from secondary effects, may be separated.

α) **Muscle tissue.** The findings of several authors are contradictory. An increase in glucose uptake by the diaphragm in normal rats through sulphonylureas (concentration under 50 mg-%) was observed by CANAL, GARATTINI, and TESSARI; MOHNIKE, KNITSCH, BOSER, and WERNER; PLETSCHER and GEY; LUNDBAEK, NIELSEN, and RAFAELSEN also RAFAELSEN. RAFAELSEN and LUNDBAEK found the same with BZ 55 also by the diaphragm of alloxanised rats. CLARKE et al., FRY and WRIGHT found no increased glucose uptake by the rat diaphragm in vitro with sulphonylureas. The insulin effect in vitro was not increased by D 860 (CAHILL, HASTINGS, and ASHMORE). The glucose uptake by the diaphragms of rats premedicated with sulphonylureas was not increased in the experiments of RECANT, FISCHER, also FRY and WRIGHT. ORTIGOSA, GARCIA-FERNANDES, and R.-CANDELA, however, found increased glucose uptake in the same experiments. Remarkable is that all research workers found no glycogen increase, typical for the insulin effect, in incubated rat diaphragms under sulphonylureas even when a decrease in the glucose concentration was proved (CLARKE et al., v. HOLT, v. HOLT, KRÖNER 1956, FIELD and WOODSON; PLETSCHER and GEY; MOHNIKE, KNITSCH, BOSER, and WERNER; LUNDBAEK, NIELSEN, and RAFAELSEN, RAFAELSEN). GARATTINI, PAOLETTI, and TESSARI only found an increased ^{14}C activity glycogen of the diaphragm after incubating the diaphragms of normal or insulin treated alloxan-diabetic rats (not however in untreated diabetic rats) with ^{14}C labelled glucose. This phenomenon could only be explained by increased glucose oxidation through the diaphragm. The O_2 consumption rose accordingly (MOHNIKE, KNITSCH, BOSER, and WERNER, PLETSCHER and GEY), also the CO_2 production from ^{14}C glucose (PLETSCHER and GEY; GARATTINI, PAOLETTI and TESSARI) when incubating the rat's diaphragm and adding D 860 and BZ 55 (under 50 mg-%). Also in the isolated frog muscle, O_2 consumption was increased by D 860 owing to the oxidation of excess lactic acid (GOURLY and DODD). Curiously, BZ 55 almost inhibited the O_2 consumption in the frog muscle, this being similar to sulphanilamide. GOURLY examined further sulphonylureas with various p-substitutents in the benzol ring and found different effects on the O_2 consumption. As the sulphonylurea concentration of 200 mg-% was unusually high, it can be discussed in how far the phenomenon is unspecific. The concentrations of sulphonylureas, in the medium of the above cited incubation experiments, were between 0.5 and 50 mg-% ($2 \times 10^{-5} - 2 \times 10^{-3}$ mol/l). Even though the best results were achieved with relatively high concentrations (30—50 mg-%), significant results with regard to glucose uptake (MOHNIKE, KNITSCH, BOSER, and WERNER; PLETSCHER and GEY; RAFAELSEN) and the O_2 consumption (PLETSCHER and GEY, RAFAELSEN) were gained with physiological concentrations (under 20 mg-%). Finally cristalline muscle phosphorylase was not affected by D 860 concentrations under 50 mg-% (MOHNIKE, KNITSCH, BOSER, and WERNER, KNITSCH 1957). For effects of D 860 on the isolated heart-lung preparation see p. 23.

β) **Adipose tissue.** RENOLD et al. (1959) investigated glucose metabolism of isolated adipose tissue in the rat in the presence of D 860. The CO_2 production from completely ^{14}C labelled glucose was increased when 80 mg-% D 860 were added to the medium, while the fatty acid synthesis simultaneously decreased. This unusual constellation was found in spite of the fact that D 860 stimulates the pentose phosphate cycle, as was shown by research done with glucose-1-^{14}C and glucose-6-^{14}C. Chlorpropamide had the same effect as D 860. R-CANDELA and LOPEZ-QUIJADA found an increase in the glucose uptake and an increase as well in the synthesis of glycogen by the epididymal fat pad after addition of D 860 in a concentration as small as 2.5 mg-%. However, DITSCHUNEIT, PFEIFFER, and ROSSENBECK were not able to detect any influence of 20 and 200 mg-% of D 860 in the medium on the glucose uptake or oxidation of C-1-labelled glucose by the epididymal fat pad in vitro. Chlorpropamide increased the glucose uptake but not the oxidation of glucose-1-^{14}C.

Following research on the effects of sulphonylureas on the adipose tissue in vitro had negative results (the authors did not work with ^{14}C labelled glucose). KRAHL (1957) failed to find a stronger glucose uptake of the adipose tissue in the presence of BZ 55. Also KNITSCH and MOHNIKE (1958) found after incubation of adipose kidney tissue with 15 mg-% BZ 55 in the medium, no increase in glucose consumption and no glycogen increase in the rat. In vivo, they saw an increase of glycogen in kidney and testicular adipose tissue in rats after BZ 55 premedication. HUMBEL, STAUB and FROESCH saw no effect of BZ 55 on the glucose uptake and on the R.Q. of the incubated epididymal fat pad in the rat.

PROD'F OM and PLATTNER (1957) described isotope experiments in vivo where a decreased lipogenesis occurred in the adipose tissue of mice; they had been premedicated with BZ 55. ASHMORE, CAHILL, EARLE, and ZOTTU however, saw in rats premedicated with D 860 no decrease in ^{14}C incorporation in the fatty acids of peripheral tissue.

γ) **Liver tissue.** The research on the influence of liver enzymes by sulphonylureas is manifold. Partially, sulphonylureas were added to the medium, and sometimes the livers of premedicated animals were used; some of the research workers used homogenates and other liver slices. Many results were only obtained when using unusually high sulphonylureas concentrations so that their value is questionable. KUETHER et al. (1956) determined the sulphonylurea concentration in various fractions of liver tissue four hours after dosing with 100 mg/kg BZ 55 and found remarkably low values that had no influence on the enzymes in vitro. Against this can be said that the measured sulphonylurea concentration in different cell fractions indicates nothing about its concentration at the enzyme molecule. This can be significantly higher. It is possible that the conjugation of the substance which is crucial for the effect occurs in vivo with the enzyme; in vitro, it is resolved through dissociation. STUHLFAUTH et al. who generally found higher tissue concentrations than KUETHER proved that BZ 55 was firmly bound to the liver mitochondria and only freed on their destruction.

Glycogenolysis. Spontaneous glucose libertation from the liver slices of rats premedicated with sulphonylurea is reduced (TYBERGHEIN, HALSEY, and WILLIAMS, RECANT and FISCHER). Liver slices of untreated rats show reduced glucose libertation if the sulphonylurea concentration in the medium is 25 mg-% and more (CLARKE et al.). In other investigations the concentration had to be higher (MOHNIKE and KNITSCH 1956, BERTHET, SUTHERLAND and MAKMAN). VAUGHAN (1956, 1957) failed to find an effect of D 860 on the spontaneous glucose release of liver slices at a concentration of 150 mg-%. However, they observed an impressive inhibition of the glucose release by epinephrine and glucagon when the D 860 concentration was 15—150 mg-%. This was also found by BERTHET, SUTHERLAND and MAKMAN and is probably caused by inhibition of phosphorylase reactivation through epinephrine and glucagon. On the other hand, this reaction was also inhibited by non-blood-sugar-decreasing sulphonylureas and sulphonamide derivatives (e. g. gantrisin) in the same concentrations (100 mg-%) (BERTHET, SUTHERLAND, and MAKMAN). Against the physiological importance of the findings of VAUGHAN speak the results of MILLER, SOKAL and SARCIONE at the isolated perfused rat liver. In the experiments of these authors high concentrations of D 860 (20—30 mg-%) in the perfusing blood maintained before and during administration of glucagon, failed to inhibit the glycogenolytic action of the latter agent.

Glucose-6-phosphatase-activity. Glucose-6-phosphatase activity in liver homogenates or microsome preparations decreases on D 860 and BZ 55 addition (MOHNIKE and KNITSCH 1956 b, KNITSCH 1957, MOHNIKE, KNITSCH, BOSER, and WERNER, BERTHET, SUTHERLAND, and MAKMAN, ASHMORE, CAHILL, and HASTINGS, KUETHER et al., WEBER and CANTERO, SUMM and WALLENFELS). In most investigations inhibition occurred in concentrations from 100 mg-% of 20% and more. Only MOHNIKE and KNITSCH also WEBER and CANTERO saw corresponding effects already with 50 mg-% D 860. Most authors therefore doubt that the effect on glucose-6-phosphatase is important for the mode of action, especially as non-blood-sugar-decreasing sulphonylureas and other sulphonamides also inhibit this enzyme (BERTHET, SUTHERLAND, and MAKMAN, ASHMORE, CAHILL, and HASTINGS).

The inhibition of glucose-6-phosphatase can be proved to the same extent in liver extracts from animals with alloxan diabetes (KNITSCH and MOHNIKE 1956, KNITSCH 1957), these animals have an elevated glucose-6-phosphatase activity as was shown by ASHMORE, HASTINGS, NESBETT, and RENOLD. The behaviour of glucose-6-phosphatase activity in the liver of sulphonylurea premedicated animals is especially interesting. An average decrease in activity of 20% was found in this case (HAWKINS, ASHWORTH, and HAIST, ASHMORE, CAHILL, an HASTINGS; TYBERGHEIN, HALSEY, and WILLIAMS; HAWKINS and HAIST; SUMM also WALLENFELS, SUMM, and CREUTZFELDT; LINKE, RIEDERLE, and SCHULZ). It is however important that the decrease in activity after sulphonylurea doses in vivo was not demonstratable within the first five hours despite a blood sugar decrease (ASHMORE, CAHILL, and HASTINGS, FRY and WRIGHT, SUMM also LINKE, RIEDERLE, and SCHULZ), therefore, it does not explain the acute decrease in blood sugar. There is no inhibition of glucose-6-phosphatase activity after sulphonylurea doses in vivo in alloxan-diabetic rats; whereas insulin normalises the increased glucose-6-phosphatase values (HAWKINS and HAIST, LINKE, RIEDERLE, and SCHULZ). It is therefore probable that glucose-6-phosphatase in vivo is not directly influenced by sulphonylureas, but by endogenous insulin.

Gluconeogenesis. BORNSTEIN (1957) described activity inhibition of 30% of alanine transaminase prepared from rat livers by BZ 55 and D 860 in vitro, but only at 100 mg-% sulphonylurea concentration. In vivo inhibition of liver alanine transaminase can first be proved 24 hrs after sulphonylurea administration (ZACCO, LEONARDI, and NERINI). According to recent investigations of DOWNIE, BORNSTEIN, and BREIDAHL, the described phenomena are only due to a simulated enzyme inhibition, therefore not to a diminished production of keto acids, but to an acceleration of substrate oxidation in the Krebs cycle. Accelerated oxidation of α-keto-glutarate can already be found with a sulphonylurea concentration of 30 mg-% and also causes a reduction in gluconeogenesis.

Ketogenesis. RENOLD et al. (1959) (see also BOSHELL et al.) showed that ketogenesis in liver slices of normal, 48 hrs fasting, alloxan-diabetic, and pancreatectomised rats was considerably inhibited by D 860. Inhibition of 30% was already caused by a concentration of 20 mg-% D 860. High insulin doses (0.1 U/ml) are ineffective in vitro. Also other sulphonamides have only a minimal effect on ketogenesis in vitro. Therefore, a direct sulphonylurea effect must be present. This could be explained by increased supply of oxalo acetic acid by activation of the CO_2 fixation through the way found by UTTER (SUMM, CREUTZFELDT, and WALLENFELS).

Glycolysis. LAMPRECHT and TRAUTSCHOLD (1958) found in the so-called "hunger diabetes" (starvation diabetes) a triose-phosphate block appearing after glucose loading (which was eliminated momentarily with high insulin doses of 5 U). Further research work of LAMPRECHT and TRAUTSCHOLD (1958 b) showed that starving rats given BZ 55 for several days displayed a weak but similar effect. The best effect was however gained with BZ 55 plus 1/50 of the effective insulin doses (0.1 U). Thus sulphonylurea increases the glycolytic glucose turnover where small exogenous insulin amounts have a strong potentiating effect.

Complex influencing of countless enzymatic reactions. WALLENFELS and SUMM also WALLENFELS, SUMM, and CREUTZFELDT (see also SUMM) found the activity of a larger number of pyridine nucleotide dependent liver dehydrogenases to be influenced in vitro by sulphonylureas—partly activited, partly inhibited. The effects were achieved in liver homogenates and in solutions of some pure crystalline enzymes or enzymes existing in highly purified form with D 860 concentrations from 30 mg-%. It was found that the coenzyme concentrations were important. Therefore, the sulphonylureas under these experimental conditions could compete with a coenzyme for the active place at the enzyme protein. Added to this direct effect, there is another change after premedicating the animals in vivo probably caused by adaptation in concentration of the single enzymes. From the complex enzyme activity changes result alterations in the actual concentration of numerous substrate systems which are in an (enzymically regulated) steady-state equilibrium with glucose. Thus not the absolute value of enzyme inhibition is significant for the effect on liver metabolism, but the resultants of equilibrium changes of many reactions. WEBER and CANTERO reached the same experimental conclusion. Important is the fact that the same metabolic changes occur also in other organs (e.g. islet system) and cause those changes there which are necessary for the mechanism of action of sulphonylureas (WALLENFELLS, SUMM and CREUTZFELDT, RENOLD et al. 1959, SUMM, CREUTZFELDT and WALLENFELS (comp. p. 39)].

δ) Insulinasesystem. Under normal conditions insulin is destroyed by insulinase which is found in various tissues, especially in the liver (MIRSKY 1956). This enzyme system is not specific for insulin, but according to MIRSKY plays a part in the pathogenesis of some forms of diabetes. MIRSKY, PERISUTTI, and DIENGOTT (1956) described a non-competitive inhibition of liver insulinase in vitro on addition of D 860 in animals premedicated with sulphonylureas. VAUGHAN (1956) missed an inhibition of insulinase activity in vitro in experiments with a concentration range of 10—80 mg-%. WILLIAMS and TUCKER; BERSON et al., also STRÄSSLE and PLETSCHER first observed a noticeable inhibition of insulinase activity from 100 mg-% D 860 and 250 mg-% BZ 55 in the medium. Also glucagon and ACTH degradation is inhibited at the same sulphonylurea concentrations. According to STRÄSSLE and PLETSCHER the insulinase inhibition through sulphonylureas is only non-competitive with low insulin concentrations; with high insulin concentrations (not present in the organism), it has competitive nature. Their investigations showed that sulphonylureas inhibit mainly the enzymically active fraction of insulinase; they have no effect on the splitting of insulin through glutathion. Most research workers agree that because of the sulphonylurea concentration necessary in vitro for insulinase inhibition (ten times higher than the average plasma level), it is unlikely that insulinase inhibition is important for the sulphonylurea mode of action. For Cox, HENLEY, and WILLIAMS; WILLIAMS and TUCKER; BERSON et al. also MORTIMORE et al., contrary to MIRSKY, saw no effect on the insulinase activity and insulin degradation in animals premedicated with sulphonylureas.

MIRSKY, PERISUTTI, and GITELSON (1957) argued that in their experiments using [131]J-labelle dinsulin, the splitting of I^{131} from insulin is mainly procured by the heat stable insulinase factor. The authors deduced from this that at least the prolongation of hypoglycaemia, which is practically uninfluenced by sulphonylureas, is the consequence of delayed endogenous insulin degradation (while the initial sugar decrease is brought about by insulin release from the β-cells).

ε) **Insulin aggregation in vitro.** Insulin shows strong aggregation in the presence of zinc ions. E.g. in a 1% insulin solution in the presence of 1% zinc, particles are aggregated with a molecular weight of over 200,000 (FREDERICQ 1956). If the zinc ion concentration is increased, the aggregation is so strong that insulin precipitates. The ratio of zinc to insulin in the Brockmann's bodies is 3.3 (MASKE, MUNK, HOMAN, and MATTHIJSEN).

WALLENFELS, BURCHARD, and SUND now found that addition of BZ 55 in vitro (500 mg-%) prevents insulin precipitation in the presence of zinc. If the zinc concentration was increased (more than one zinc molecule to one insulin molecule, M.W. 5777), insulin was precipitated even in the presence of BZ 55. On investigating the aggregation with aid of light dispersion, it was seen in a zinc: insulin ratio of 0.67 that the insulin particles consisted of 5.2×10^4 monomeres (M.W. of single monomeres 5777). In the presence of BZ 55 the particles only contain 12 monomeres (M.W. 80,000). The significance of these in vitro investigations of WALLENFELS, BURCHARD ,and SUND will be discussed later (p. 39). The authors also found a decomposition of glutamic-acid dehydrogenase through BZ 55 and D 860 but not through other sulphonamides.

ζ) **Respiratory activity of kidney slices and dopadecarboxylase.** FREINKEL and INGBAR found in the kidney slices in rabbits in Warburg's apparatus a reduction in O_2 consumption of about 50% on addition of D 860 (130 mg-%). Besides this the water content of the incubated slices increased greatly in the presence of D 860, while the oxidation of ^{14}C-labelled glucose was not increased or incorporated in tissue lipids. The blood-sugar ineffective carbonic acid of D 860 was in every way only 1/5 th as active as D 860. The authors discussed with discretion, because of the high concentrations used, the possibility of a localised Pasteur effect, valid for different tissues or an unspecific toxic effect.

GONNARD et al. (1959) observed in kidney extracts, using a BZ 55 concentration of 250 mg-%, an inhibition of the dopadecarboxylase. This they believed significant for the reduced catecholamine content of the supra-renals after BZ 55 treatment. Thus this reduction was not the result of epinephrine release but of a reduced catecholamine synthesis.

2. Effect in the eviscerated, decerebrated and diabetic animal

α) **Eviscerated and decerebrated animal.** Cox, HENLEY and WILLIAMS (1956) saw a blood-sugar-decreasing effect with D 860 in eviscerated rats (functional elimination of liver, intestinal tract, and pancreas was performed by ligature). LANG and SHERRY were not able to confirm this in totally eviscerated rats injected with glucose. HOUSSAY, PENHOS, URGOITI, TEODOSIO, APELBAUM, and BOWKETT were also unable to find a blood-sugar-lowering effect of D 860 in totally eviscerated dogs, they could achieve, however, a depression of the blood sugar by

D 860 in presence of a constant insulin infusion. Fritz, Morton, Weinstein, and Levine (1956) examined utilization of glucose and the distribution of galactose in eviscerated dogs with and without insulin; Wick, Britton, and Grabowski examined the oxidation of ^{14}C glucose as well as the transfer of glucose in eviscerated rabbits with and without insulin. Both these research teams noted the absence of any effects of sulphonylureas and rejected any peripheral effects in vivo. The same has been reported by Dulin and Johnston (1957) for the eviscerated rat infused with glucose and insulin; no lowering of blood sugar was obtained with D 860. Creutzfeldt, Deuticke and Söling saw in eviscerated nephrectomised rats constantly infused with glucose no blood-sugar decrease after D 860 but found a significant potentiation of the insulin effect through this sulphonylurea. Only in the pancreatectomised and hepatectomised chicken did D 860 lower the blood sugar (Hazelwood). The cause of these interesting findings is not known. Khachachirian and Badeer investigated the glucose uptake from the peripheral blood in denervated heartlung preparations (dog). They found a significantly increased glucose uptake after adding D 860 (50—100 mg-%). 25 mg-% D 860 in the peripheral blood had no effect.

Decerebration does not abolish the blood-sugar decrease following D 860; on the contrary, decerebrated rabbits show an enhanced blood-sugar depression, therefore similar to adrenalectomised animals (Bänder, Häussler, and Scholz). After vagotomy, depression of the blood sugar by D 860 is considerably delayed in the rabbit. In addition to this, there is a considerable initial increase in blood sugar (König).

β) **Diabetes after total pancreatectomy.** It is generally agreed that sulphonylureas do not lower the blood sugar in depancreatised mammals not insulinised. This is true for the pancreatectomised rat (Cox, Henley, and Williams), for the dog (Houssay and Penhos, Houssay and Migliorini, Fritz, Morton, Weinstein, and Levine also Fritz, Weinstein, Morton, and Levine, Schambye 1957, Caren and Corbo, M. A. Root 1957a, Tiszai and Szücs) and for the cat, (Gordon, Buse, and Lukens). BZ 55 did not produce a significant lowering of blood sugar in depancreatised dogs—hypophysectomised or adrenalectomised and therefore being highly sensitive to drugs affecting blood sugar (Houssay, Penhos, Teodosio, Bowkett, and Apelbaum). The same is observed in hypophysectomised and pancreatectomised cats (Gordon, Buse, and Lukens). The finding reported by Becker, Buddeke, and Müller that BZ 55 causes lowering of the blood sugar in completely pancreatectomised dogs can be explained by a potentiation of insulin, for the animals had received long-acting insulin 24 hrs before the experiment (see below). Kurtz, Holtzmann, and Meilman found depression of the blood sugar by D 860 if the drug was injected in the acutely pancreatectomised dog. However, the blood-sugar effect was delayed by 4—5 hrs.

Besides mammals, amphibia and birds deprived of their pancreas have been examined. In the toad, depression of blood sugar did not appear following pancreatectomy (Houssay and Penhos). Chicken and ducks not displaying elevated blood sugar after pancreatectomy and enterectomy show however, a decrease in blood sugar through D 860 (Mirsky and Gitelson 1957). This finding could be confirmed in the depancreatised hen (Hazelwood). In depancreatised geese with intact liver and enterectomised, there was no blood-sugar decrease through D 860. This is in so far remarkable since geese in contrast to ducks respond to pancreatectomy with diabetes (Mirsky and Gitelson 1958).

It can therefore be stated that in most species the removal of the pancreas, which is the source of the endogenous insulin, simultaneously diminishes the effectiveness of the sulphonylureas. It was therefore important to find out whether the effect of insulin injections was enhanced by sulphonylureas. This question was denied by FRITZ, WEINSTEIN, MORTON, and LEVINE for the accutely pancreatectomised dog still possessing some circulating insulin and for the chronically pancreatectomised dog constantly infused with insulin. In contrast to this, numerous other workers found potentiation of insulin through sulphonylureas in the pancreatectomised animal. HOUSSAY and MIGLIORINI also HOUSSAY, PENHOS, URGOITI, TEODOSIO, APELBAUM and BOWKETT; RODRIGUEZ-MIÑÓN and DE OYA; CAREN and CORBO also SCHAMBYE 1957a, either found a significant depression of the blood sugar in the pancreatectomised dog infused constantly with insulin or an increase and prolongation of the insulin effect after previous or simultaneous application of a sulphonylurea. The following observations of BECKER, BUDDECKE and MÜLLER and M. A. ROOT (1957a) also prove a potentiation of the insulin effect by sulphonylureas: BZ 55 causes blood-sugar decrease in the depancreatised dog if insulin had been given 16 or 24 hrs previously; D 860 showed a significant effect in the acutely pancreatectomised dog where insulin was still circulating in the organism (KURTZ, HOLTZMAN, and MEILMAN).

Particularly impressive is the insulin potentiating effect of sulphonylureas in the depancreatised dog continuously receiving insulin. This fact has been shown for BZ 55 and D 860 in the under-insulinised pancreatectomised dog by CAMPBELL and LAZIDINS, KIRTLEY et al. (1957), SIREK and SIREK; SIREK, SIREK, and BEST, SCHAMBYE, furthermore, RICKETTS, WILDBERGER and SCHMID also ROOT (1957a). The favourable effect is only found in the condition of hyperglycaemia and glucosuria while the general condition of the animals deteriorates after several weeks and finally distinct liver damage appears (s. p. 15). WILDBERGER and RICKETTS found that sulphonylureas normalise only the blood sugar and glucose excretion in the depancreatised dog given insulin not however nitrogen excretion as is characteristic when extra insulin is given. The authors conclude that sulphonylureas do not really potentiate insulin, but only have an effect on the liver which is present when exogenous insulin is applied. These findings exclude that the action of sulphonylureas on blood sugar in dogs deprived of pancreas and treated with insulin is caused by an inhibition of insulinase. The same effect has so far not been described for other species. It is therefore an open question whether the above behaviour is peculiar to the dog and is related to the special degradation of sulphonylureas occurring in this species (s. p. 13). The technical difficulties of total pancreatectomy and the different reactions of the various species explain why relevant experiments are still missing. It is only in the cat where the problem of insulin potentiation by sulphonylureas has been examined (GORDON, BUSE, and LUKENS). The negative results gained here have been explained by these authors to be owing to the severe diabetic state resulting from pancreatectomy in this species; due to this, a small side-effect could be overlooked.

For this reason the reaction of alloxan diabetic animals is of special interest, as this type of diabetes can be caused comparatively simply in various species.

γ) Alloxan diabetes. There is apparent discrepancy about the action of sulphonylureas in animals suffering from alloxan diabetes to be found in the literature. These contradictions can, however, be resolved on studying the papers carefully and relating the effect of sulphonylureas to the severity of the diabetes. The following must be emphasised: The severity of alloxan diabetes is solely dependent on the extent of β-cell destruction, i.e. the possibility of insulin production (WRENSHALL, COLLINS, WILLIAMS, and HARTROFT), while the number of intact α-cells is irrelevant.

Numerous investigators state that a single dose of a sulphonylurea, or its continuous application in the dog suffering from alloxan diabetes, is without effect (BÄNDER and SCHOLZ 1956, MOHNIKE, BIBERGEIL and CZYZYK, RODRIGUEZ-MIÑÓN and DE OYA); the same is true for the rabbit (MOHNIKE 1956, CZYZYK, KRACHT, and RAUSCH-STROOMANN; M. A. ROOT 1957; STEWART 1957b) and for the rat (v. HOLT, KRACHT, KRÖNER, and v. HOLT; MIRSKY, PERISUTTI, and JINKS; LANG and SHERRY, CHRISTOPHE, BELLENS and GEPTS; GORDON, BUSE, and LUKENS; DULIN and JOHNSTON; ROOT 1957).

This statement is, however, only valid for a severe and long-lasting alloxan diabetes. If one sub-divides a great number of alloxan-diabetic rabbits according to the severity of their diabetes, and treats them by continuously administering D 860 (1 g/kg), CREUTZFELDT and BÖTTCHER found the following: in mild diabetes tending to spontaneous remission, glucosuria and hyperglycaemia disappear even if the drug is withheld; in a moderately severe diabetes without acetonuria, hyperglycaemia and glucosuria diminish significantly for the duration of treatment and reappear after cessation. However, an increase in weight of these animals cannot be observed. In five animals of this group hypoglycaemic reactions with blood sugar values of 30 mg-% could be established (0.5—2 gr/kg D 860 orally) (BÖTTCHER). In rabbits suffering from severe alloxan diabetes and acidosis, D 860 was completely ineffective. Authors who have taken the severity of alloxan diabetes into consideration in their experiments agree with our results; thus, they also proved that sulphonylureas influence the blood sugar in mild and moderately severe alloxan diabetes of the dog (MAGYAR et al.; DE FRANCISCIS et al.) and of the rabbit (ACHELIS and HARDEBECK; BERINGER and KEIBL; MIRSKY, PERISUTTI and GITELSON) and in the rat (HULTQUIST et al.; DULIN and JOHNSTON, GONNARD and DALLION). v. HOLT, v. HOLT, and KRÖNER (1956) achieved a depression of the blood sugar with BZ 55 in the rat suffering from alloxan diabetes after removal of the supra-renals.

It is quite clear from these experiments that the sulphonylureas have a positive effect on alloxan diabetes if the organism produces some insulin which in itself is not sufficient for preventing diabetes. It is however questionable whether this is a true insulin potentiation. CREUTZFELDT and BÖTTCHER found no weight increase in spite of a lowering of the blood sugar and a decrease in glucosuria. This fact reminds one of the failure of sulphonylureas to normalise nitrogen excretion in the pancreatectomised dog treated with sub-optimal doses of insulin (WILDBERGER and RICKETTS), and excludes the explanation of this phenomenon by an implication of the insulinase system.

The same is true for the evidence that the effect of additional insulin on the blood sugar is increased by sulphonylureas in severe alloxan diabetes uninfluenced by sulphonylureas alone. AIMAN and CHAUDHARY found, with BZ 55 in rabbits severely affected by alloxan diabetes, a decrease in the blood sugar if the sulphonylurea was administered 24 hrs after the last insulin dose. Forty-eight hours later this effect could not be observed. An increased reduction in blood sugar by combining insulin with sulphonylureas has been described for the severe alloxan diabetes in the dog (MOHNIKE, BIBERGEIL, and CZYZYK; RODRIGUEZ-MIÑÓN and DE OYA) and rabbits (MOHNIKE 1956). This, however, could not be proved for severe alloxan-diabetic rats in the acute experiment (LANG and SHERRY). In contrast to this, prolonged treatment with sulphonylureas in severe alloxan-diabetic rats (v. HOLT, KRACHT, KRÖNER, and v. HOLT) and dogs treated with sub-optimal insulin doses (ROOT 1957) had a distinct effect on glucosuria and hyperglycaemia. Again, this effect cannot be explained by simple insulin potentiation, for CERLETTI and GREGOLIN found that simultaneous application of D 860 depresses the typical insulin effect; namely, the increasing of the respiratory quotient in alloxan-diabetic rats.

On the whole the observations on alloxan-diabetic animals correspond to those for the pancreatectomised animal. They emphasise the decisive role of a sufficient insulin production for the development of the blood-sugar-decreasing effect of sulphonylureas. On the other hand, it can be shown that in the presence of small amounts of exogenous or endogenous insulin, clear metabolic effects of the sulphonylureas are still demonstrable.

δ) **Pituitary and steroid diabetes.** Both the hormones of the adenohypophysis and the glucocorticoids act diabeticogenically in certain species on account of extra-pancreatic mechanisms. However, diabetes becomes apparent only if the *β*-cells can compensate no longer for the increased insulin requirement. Indirectly exhaustion of *β*-cells occurs, whereby they are stimulated by hyperglycaemia and not directly by hormones (for literature see CREUTZFELDT 1959). In the phase of idiohypophyseal and idiosteroid diabetes, the *β*-cell function is partially intact; the conditions are similar to mild alloxan diabetes. Insulin production has practically ceased in the phase of metahypophyseal and metasteroid diabetes, therefore comparable to conditions found in severe alloxan diabetes.

On considering this fact relevant publications may be understood. Thus, D 860 has an effect on the idiohypophyseal diabetes in the dog; that is to say, the appearance of diabetes is prevented or is less severe on simultaneous dosing with STH and D 860 (MIRSKY, GITELSON, and PERISUTTI 1959). The rapid decrease in the blood sugar characteristic for the normal dog receiving D 860 is here significantly weaker (MIRSKY, PERISUTTI, and GITELSON 1957). In rats where STH alone is not diabetogenic but only stimulates islet growth, STH premedication even increased the blood-sugar-decreasing action of D 860 (PASCHKIS, RUPP, and JASOVKSY). Also, in the idiosteroid diabetes in rats sulphonylureas had a small effect, e.g. simultaneous application of BZ 55 and cortisone resulted in lower blood-sugar values than with cortisone alone (v. HOLT, KRACHT, KRÖNER, and v. HOLT 1956).

The canine metahypophyseal diabetes showed no response to sulphonylureas (CAMPBELL and LAZIDINS, LAZARUS and VOLK 1958). Furthermore, the blood-sugar-decreasing effect of the same drug failed, or was strongly reduced in the metasteroid diabetes of the dog (LAZARUS and VOLK 1958), of the rabbit (RAUSCH-STROOMANN and KRACHT, LAZARUS and VOLK 1958) and the rat (PASCHKIS, RUPP, and JASOVSKY). The effectiveness of sulphonylureas in these types of diabetes is again dependent on some endogenous insulin production. If this is lacking owing to *β*-cell exhaustion, there is no blood-sugar-lowering effect. Weakening or delay in the acute blood-sugar lowering following sulphonylurea medication can already be proved if the insulin content in the pancreas is momentarily reduced; thus, already before degenerative changes of the *β*-cells occur. Therefore a blood-sugar decrease is missing, while hyperglycaemia produced by parenterally administered glucose in the rat leads to a *β*-cell degranulation (BRAUN, MOSINGER and KUJALOVA).

ε) **Starvation diabetes (,,Hungerdiabetes").** Prolonged fasting leads to a condition described as hunger diabetes in rats (CHERNICK, CHAIKOFF and ABRAHAM); here there is no hyperglycaemia or glucosuria; however, ketonaemia and decreased glucose tolerance occurs. Also inhibition of glycolysis in the liver (so called triosephosphate block of LAMPRECHT and TRAUTSCHOLD) is present. Simultaneously there is a degranulation of *β*-cells (NERENBERG) and a reduced insulin content of the pancreas (BEST, HAIST and RIDOUT, HAIST 1944).

MIRSKY, PERISUTTI, and GITELSON found that in fasting rats the blood-sugar-lowering effect of D 860 was reduced compared to normal rats, while the insulin effect was increased. Here too, the degree of the blood-sugar increase is closely related to the functional capacity of the β-cells. Other mechanisms also play a part in the influencing of hunger diabetes by sulphonylureas as described on p. 21; namely that inhibition of the triose-phosphate oxidation in the fasting rat premedicated with BZ 55 can be already minimised by 1/20 of the usual insulin doses (LAMPRECHT and TRAUTSCHOLD 1958 b).

ζ) Spontaneous canine diabetes and hereditary adiposity hyperglycaemia syndrome in the mouse. Spontaneous diabetes in the dog is according to the investigations of RICKETTS, WRENSHALL, HARTROFT and BEST (1954) a genuine insulin diabetes characterised by considerable reduction in β-cells and no insulin in the pancreas. Large doses of BZ 55 spread over several days are ineffective (GARBERS, APEL). APEL achieved control using D 860 in only one out of fourteen dogs receiving D 860 for three months.

Assuming that obese hyperglycaemia syndrome in the mouse is more like human maturiy-onset diabetes than any other form of animal diabetes, attention was called to the therapeutic value of sulphonylureas in this condition. WRENSHALL, ANDRUS and MAYER state that the insulin content of the pancreas is markedly increased in the obese hyperglycaemia syndrome in the mouse, although the β-cells in contrast to normal mice, are degranulated. This discrepancy can be explained by GEPTS, CHRISTOPHE and MAYER (1960) who found that the volume of islet tissue in these animals was six times as great as in their lean litter mates, but that individual β-cells had reduced insulin content in proportion to their diminished granules. This factor could not be conveyed if the total amount of pancreatic insulin was determined. Provided that this is considered, no difficulties exist in relating these results to those found in other forms of diabetes. CHRISTOPHE and MAYER (1959a and b) did not find either in the acute experiment, or during chronic application of BZ 55, an effect on blood sugar; while the lean litter mates showed the usual blood-sugar decrease. BZ 55 had also no effect on weight increase and synthesis of fatty acids and cholesterol.

3. Influencing of α-cells and the glucagon effect

The results gained from eviscerated and decerebrated animals discussed above show that the pancreas must play a decisive role in the action of sulphonylureas. The experiments by COLWELL et al. (1956, 1957, 1959) point in the same direction although their results have not been confirmed by other authors (HOUSSAY, PENHOS, URGOTTI et al. 1957, FOA et al. 1959). COLWELL found after infusing D 860 and BZ 55 in the pancreatic artery of the dog a more distinct lowering of the blood sugar than when infusing the same dose into the femoral vein. Respectively achieving significant effects by injecting sulphonylureas into the pancreatic artery in doses that were peripherally ineffective.

As the islets of Langerhans are composed in all species of two different cell types, the β-cells producing insulin and the α-cells glucagon, we will now discuss the role of glucagon. In the first reports on BZ 55 (ACHELIS and HARDEBECK, FRANKE and FUCHS; BERTRAM, BENDTFELDT and OTTO 1955), it was suggested that the sulphonylureas act by damaging or at least, functionally affecting the α-cells. This view arose under the impressions gained from the α-cell changes observed after synthalin (DAVIS 1952, s. p. 118), and also partially described for IPTD (v. HOLT, v. HOLT, KRÖNER and KÜHNAU 1954, s. p. 3) on the one side, and the recent results of glucagon research, on the other side. These views appear to have been supported by the morphological findings of FERNER and RUNGE

(1956a). Numerous other investigations in this field remain negative and the glucagon theory of sulphonylureas must now be refuted. For this reason, these studies will be discussed briefly; as the evidence for a diabetogenic effect of glucagon and the pathogenetic role of increased glucagon secretion in diabetes is controversial.

The degenerative changes in α-cells following short or prolonged application of BZ 55 and D 860 could not be observed for the following species: the normal and alloxan-diabetic rabbit (CREUTZFELDT and FINTER; CREUTZFELDT and BÖTTCHER, VOLK, WEISENFELD, LAZARUS and GOLDNER, BENCOSME, MARIZ and FREI), rat (GEPTS, CHRISTOPHE and BELLENS 1956b, GEPTS 1957, KRACHT and RAUSCH-STROOMANN, v. HOLT, KRACHT, KRÖNER and v. HOLT, HEINIVAARA also LUND-BAEK and NIELSEN, CREUTZFELDT, DETERING and WELTE, SCHÖLER and GAAREN-STRÖM also MOSCA), guinea-pigs (VAN CAMPENHOUT; BENCOSME, MARIZ and FREI), and for the dog (STRAHL and DORNER; BENCOSME, MARIZ and FREI) and calve (PFEIFFER, STEIGERWALD, SANDRITTER et al. 1957). The observed decrease in number and size of α-cells in rabbits treated over long periods with D 860 (CREUTZFELDT and FINTER 1956) was later found by the same authors also in rabbits treated with insulin and missed in rats chronically medicated with D 860 (CREUTZFELDT, DETERING and WELTE). Furthermore, the positive alkaline-phosphatase reaction of α-cells remained unchanged after D 860 medication in rats (CREUTZFELDT and LEHMANN; HEINIVAARA).

These morphological results correspond to the findings that the glucagon activity in pancreas extracts of rabbits (BERTHET, SUTHERLAND and MAKMAN) of dogs (CZYZYK also STRAHL and DORNER) and of calves (PFEIFFER, STEIGER-WALD, SANDRITTER et al. 1957) is not reduced on premedication with sulphonyl-ureas; according to STRAHL and DORNER, even increased. Even in the plasma, the glucagon concentration was normal in rabbits premedicated with sulphonyl-ureas (TYBERGHEIN and WILLIAMS). Therefore these results show that the possibility of functional inhibition of the α-cells by the sulphonylureas no longer exists. This possibility was discussed by FERNER and RUNGE and was first supported by the findings of SCHMID and BLOBEL who saw significantly smaller α-cell nuclei after eight-day D 860 treatment in rats. These could not be confirmed as KRACHT, v. HOLT and v. HOLT described unchanged α-cell nuclei after BZ 55 medication for 14—21 days; after four months, a significant increase in volume of the α-cell nuclei and after 7 months, normal values were again observed. PFEIFFER, STEIGER-WALD, SANDRITTER et al. (1957) saw six hours following D 860 medication in the calve, a temporary enlargement in the volume of α-cell nuclei and in the glucagon content of the pancreas. Both groups explained their findings as reactive stimulation of the α-cell system due to sulphonylurea hypoglycaemia.

Research was then done on the influence of sulphonylureas on the effect of injected glucagon. CREUTZFELDT and FINTER (1956) found a slight decrease in glucagon hyperglycaemia after high doses of D 860 in rabbits but it was not abolished. VOLK, GOLDNER, WEISENFELD and LAZARUS found the same in rabbits after BZ 55 and D 860; the difference could not be statistically ascertained. BERTHET, SUTHERLAND, and MAKMAN saw normal glucagon hyperglycaemia after low sulphonylurea doses. Also, man treated with therapeutic sulphonylurea doses, showed a normal glucagon reaction (STÖTTER et al. 1956, FAJANS et al. 1956, KIRTLEY et al. 1956, COX, HENLEY, FERGUS and WILLIAMS, MILLER and CRAIG, RECKNAGEL also CONSTAM et al., BUTTERFIELD et al.). GOLDNER, WEISEN-FELD and HUGHES found only mitigated hyperglycaemia. Thus is also proved that the in vitro findings of VAUGHAN mentioned above (s. p. 19) of phosphorylase inhibition by D 860 have no significance for therapeutic doses as was shown already by the results of MILLER, SOKAL and SARCIONE using the isolated perfused rat liver (s. p. 24). It is also unlikely that the glucagon degradation through sulphonylureas is greatly influenced. This possibility has been finally debarred by directly estimating the degradation of ^{131}I-labelled glucagon in vivo and vitro (BERSON, YALOW, WEISENFELD, GOLDNER and VOLK).

The effect of sulphonylureas on alloxan-diabetic animals mentioned in the detailed experiments discussed above (s. p. 24) will here be recalled. These showed that sulphonylureas and IPTD (s. p. 4) have no effect whatever in animals with severe alloxan diabetes. These animals have only lost the greater portion of their β-cells, while the α-cells are intact. This fact alone is enough to refute the hypothesis stating that α-cells play a part in sulphonylurea hypoglycaemia.

4. β-cells and insulin secretion

α) **Morphological findings in the β-cell system.** In contrast to the fact that no morphological change was found in the α-cells after sulphonylurea medication, the change in the β-cells was significant and contributed to illuminating the sulphonylurea mode of action.

Only few authors saw unaltered β-cells after sulphonylurea doses in rats (HEINIVAARA also LUNDBAEK and NIELSEN), and dogs (BERINGER 1957). However, there is strong proof that the sulphonylureas have indeed a specific effect on the β-cells system; they are "betacytotropic". The cells show degranulation, enlargement of nucleus and cell body, and accelerated mitosis; finally islet tissue volume expands which is known to be due to increased functional activity; but it is not yet known how these changes occur.

Degranulation. The phenomenon of β-cell degranulation was found in numerous species. In the rat, degranulation occurs several hours following a single sulphonylurea dose and can be seen during chronic medication (KRACHT and RAUSCH-STROOMANN; KRACHT, V. HOLT and V. HOLT; GEPTS, CHRISTOPHE and BELLENS 1956b; CREUTZFELDT, DETERING and WELTE; BÄNDER, HÄUSSLER and SCHOLZ, SCHÖLER and GAARENSTROOM; MOSCA also SANDRITTER et a.). Maximal degranulation is reached after 3—5 days of medication, later incomplete regranulation takes place; a sign of adaptation. This condition remains static for several months. Complete normality in the granular content is reached several days after discontinuing the drug (CREUTZFELDT, DETERING and WELTE). The degree of degranulation and the time needed for regranulation depends largely on the sulphonylurea doses given (BÄNDER, HÄUSSLER and SCHOLZ). Hypophysectomised rats react with stronger β-cell degranulation to single and chronic D 860 doses than do normal animals (CREUTZFELDT, DETERING, and WELTE). As these findings are due to a specific effect of the blood-sugar-decreasing sulphonylureas, those sulphonylureas not having a blood-sugar effect (1—2 C-atoms as R_2) do not cause β-cell degranulation in the rats (CREUTZFELDT, DETERING and WELTE). According to electron microscopical observations of GUSEK and KRACHT (1959a) on β-cells in rats medicated for several weeks with BZ 55 and D 860, there is a submicroscopical morphological substrate of an increased cell activity consisting of an increase of Golgi apparatus, and augmentation in the size of mitochondria and of RNA.

In other species, principally the same findings were made. Discrepancies in the temporal occurrence of degranulation, and in adaptation to duration of medication and regranulation are remarkable. Thus in rabbits after a single D 860 dose, there is no significant β-cell degranulation despite a blood-sugar decrease within the first two days of continual treatment (CREUTZFELDT and FINTER; FERNER and RUNGE 1956b; VOLK, GOLDNER, WEISENFELD and LAZARUS). Later degranulation is definite, and after 8 days, almost complete. This excessive degranulation is maintained for weeks; there is no adaptation as found in the rat. However, blood-sugar lowering can also be found during this time (CREUTZFELDT, DETERING and WELTE). Calves show a similar reaction as rats after a single D 860 dose. After rapid degranulation, regranulation occurs within 24 hrs (PFEIFFER, STEIGERWALD, SANDRITTER et al., 1957). This rhythm is repeated even on permanent daily medication despite no decrease in the blood sugar. Degranulation of β-cells has also been described in the dog (STAHL and DORNER); electron microscopical findings show a characteristic decrease of β-granules after a single sulphonylurea dose (LAZY and HARTROFT). For the guinea-pig, however, VAN CAMPENHOUT claims that sulphonylureas do not cause β-cell degranulation.

Enlargement of cell nuclei. Only those investigations will be mentioned that have quantitatively determined the size of β-cell nuclei revealing certain differences in the various species. In the rat, BZ 55 application for several days causes a significant increase in the volume of β-cell nuclei which can be demonstrated for several months (KRACHT and RAUSCH-STROOMANN; KRACHT V. HOLT and v. HOLT), and for D 860 (CREUTZFELDT, DETERING and WELTE). Only SCHMIDT and BLOBEL could not confirm this finding. Three hours after a single dose of D 860, CREUTZFELDT, DETERING and WELTE found that the nuclear volume of the β-cells was still normal, while SANDRITTER et al. could already demonstrate a nuclear swelling. In hypophysectomised rats even in the chronic experiment, the β-cell nuclei have the same size as in normal untreated rats despite the usual β-cell degranulation (KRACHT, v. HOLT and v. HOLT; CREUTZFELDT, DETERING and WELTE). (Untreated hypophysectomised rats are said to have a nuclear atrophy of the β-cells, according to KRACHT, v. HOLT, and v. HOLT while CREUTZFELDT, DETERING and WELTE found the nuclei to be of normal size.)

In the calf, PFEIFFER, STEIGERWALD, SANDRITTER et al. (1957) also SANDRITTER et al. found a significant increase of β-cell nuclei three hours after D 860 application which normalised after 24 hrs, although the plasma level of D 860 was not significantly diminished during this time. These nuclear enlargements can be repeated daily if sulphonylurea administration is continued. This phenomenon is said not to be caused by H_2O uptake (functional nuclear oedema), but by an "influx of protein in the nucleus" according to SANDRITTER et al. In the rabbit, no change in β-cell nuclear volume can be demonstrated after D 860 application for several weeks, despite considerable β-cell degranulation; although this animal reacts to cortisone with an increase in nuclear size (CREUTZFELDT, DETERING and WELTE).

Besides an enlargement in nuclei, an increase in cytoplasm of the β-cells was found following BZ 55 (v. HOLT, KRACHT, KRÖNER and v. HOLT) also D 860 (MOSCA).

Increase in β-cell mitosis. Augmentation of β-cell mitosis has been reported for BZ 55 and D 860 within the first week of application (GEPTS; CREUTZFELDT, DETERING and WELTE), but missed after prolonged application. Pre-mortal medication of the experimental animals with colchizin to arrest the course of mitosis still enabled proof of manifoldly increased mitosis after treatment with 500 mg/kg BZ 55 and D 860 for three weeks (KRACHT, KRÖNER, v. HOLT and v. HOLT; v. HOLT, v. HOLT, KRACHT, KRÖNER and KÜHNAU). The frequency of mitosis is twice to four times greater after BZ 55, while it is 10 times greater after D 860 than that of the normal animal according to JORES and KRACHT. These findings were not confirmed by MOSCA who also used the cholchizin method. He even found a decrease in the β-cell mitosis in rats after 25—70 days of treatment with 1 mg/kg D 860. Possibly this discrepancy is due to the double dose he used.

However, his findings are significant with regard to the mode of action of the sulphonylureas on the β-cell function (s. p. 41).

Islet volume. In normal rats receiving BZ 55 for several weeks, islet hypertrophy is found (KRACHT and RAUSCH-STROOMANN). This was confirmed by quantitatively measuring the islet volume by ASHWORTH and HAIST also GEPTS for BZ 55. No increase in islet volume was found in normal rats after D 860. Only in very young ones an increase was seen; however, not statistically significant (CREUTZFELDT, DETERING and WELTE). Similar reactions were observed in mice by GEPTS, CHRISTOFHE and MAYER such as significant enlargement of islet volume in young animals and not in older ones. Thus there appeared to be quantitative differences with regard to age, species and also between BZ 55 and D 860. CREUTZFELDT and GEGINAT were only able to find an increased islet regeneration with D 860 in partially pancreatectomised rats. The morphological substrate of this augmented islet volume consists of islet enlargement and neo-formation of islets from the epithelia of the small ductules (GEPTS; KRACHT, V. HOLT and V. HOLT; BÄNDER, HÄUSSLER and SCHOLZ; CREUTZFELDT and GEGINAT). Also the possibility of acinar-insular transformation is discussed (GEPTS; KRACHT, 1959, GUSEK and KRACHT; BÄNDER 1958 b). There are said to be acinar cells containing single β-granules in the marginal zone of rat islets following sulphonylurea medication, according to the electron microscopical investigations of GUSEK and KRACHT (1959 b). Here were also seen, similar as during embryonic development, undifferentiated cells. However, mitotic divisions play the main role in the increase of islet tissue; the α-β-cell relationship does not change even on prolonged sulphonylurea dosage in adult rats (GEPTS; CREUTZFELDT, DETERING and WELTE). MOSCA observed however, after D 860 in young rats, persistence in the high α-β-cell relationship characteristic for these young animals. He discusses whether this phenomenon is due to increased glucagon demand resulting from the sulphonylurea promoted blood-sugar decrease, or to an insufficient increase in the number of β-cells.

Histochemical results. The histochemically demonstrable zinc of the islets of Langerhans in the rabbit decreases rapidly after glucose injection and is thus a sensitive indication of insulin secretion (MASKE 1953, WOLFF, and RINGLER). MASKE (1956) found, however, despite a blood-sugar decrease after administration of a single D 860 dose, an increase of islet zinc; after 5—8 days of continual treatment a normal zinc content of the β-cell. This is remarkable: even if the rabbit is no ideal experimental animal owing to delay in the appearance of β-cell degranulation following sulphonylurea doses, it is possible that the results of MASKE indicate a different influence of the β-cells by glucose as physiological stimulant on one hand and the sulphonylureas on the other. SANDRITTER et al. did detailed histochemical research on calves and rats after D 860 medication. They found a significant decrease in staining intensity using Bahrsche's method for —SS- and —SH groups with which it is possible to estimate half quantitatively the insulin content. Here was already found a normal reaction in calves while the granular content of the β-cells was still greatly reduced. Rats showed parallelity of both reactions. The tyrosine and arginine reaction remained unaltered. Also there was no difference in the activity of acid and alkaline phosphatase in treated and untreated animals. LAZARUS (1959) histochemically compared glucose-6-phosphatase and acid phosphatase activity in degranulated β-cells in the rabbit, first after cortisone therapy, then after sulphonylurea treatment. Animals treated with cortisone showed no certain changes in enzyme activity in the β-cells; but after producing degranulation to the same degree by sulphonylureas (chlorpropamide), there was a decrease in glucose-6-phosphatase activity, while acid phosphatase was unchanged. LAZARUS discusses whether the decrease in glucose-6-phosphatase activity in the β-cell is adaptive or is the mechanism of sulphonylurea action on the β-cells.

Degenerative islet changes. The morphological β-cell changes show the sulphonylureas to be "β-cytotropic". If these are caused by a genuine β-cell stimulation, then theoretically the danger of a secondary β-cell degeneration through exhaustion exists, because some species react hypertrophically to increased demand, others degeneratively (comp. CREUTZFELDT 1959). Much research was done on this question. Most workers came to the conclusion that β-cell exhaustion does not occur; degranulation is reversible in dogs and rats even after therapy of several months duration (GEPTS; CREUZTFELDT, DETERING, and WELTE; BÄNDER, HÄUSSLER and SCHOLZ; CREUTZFELDT and GEGINAT; MOSCA). GEPTS (1957b) was not able to discover diabetes or islet degeneration when chronically administering combined doses of BZ 55 and cortisone in rats. Only KRACHT, v. HOLT and v. HOLT saw some hydropically changed β-cells in rats and dogs after BZ 55. GEPTS described for normal rats, after BZ 55 treatment lasting several months, the appearance of network consisting of reticulum fibres similar to an islet sclerosis. Corresponding observations were not made for normal rats after D 860, but extensively seen in partially pancreatectomised rats treated with D 860 (CREUTZFELDT and GEGINAT). However, these types of islet changes occur normally in partially pancreatectomised rats (FRIEDMANN and MARBLE; CREUTZFELDT and GEGINAT). They are only increased after D 860 doses; the same is true for islet regeneration. GEPTS also CREUTZFELDT and GEGINAT interpret this sclerotic picture as being rest-stroma of atrophied acinar tissue through islet proliferation. Islet hylanosis was never described.

To summarise. The morphological findings show increased activity of the β-cell system under the influence of sulphonylureas. Some contradictions are explained by species variance and different experimental set-ups. However, the question must remain open whether the increased β-cell activity is the result of simple β-cell stimulation as occurs physiologically through glucose, or if the effect of sulphonylureas on the β-cells follows a new principle. The following findings described above indicated the latter possibility; in the rabbit β-cell zinc is not reduced by D 860 and similar to β-granulation shows no decrease parallel to the blood-sugar depression until some days later; enlargement of the β-cell nuclei can only be proved in the normal, not however, in the hypophysectomised rat and not at all in the rabbit. During sulphonylurea degranulation, there is a decrease in glucose-6-phosphatase activity in the β-cells; this does not occur during cortisone degranulation. Also, the β-granulation is not normalised during prolonged sulphonylurea therapy. Thus the β-cells do not adapt themselves to treatment as is the case in rats under prolonged glucose or diabetogenic hormone therapy; if at all, islet hyperplasia occurs, and not degeneration caused by exhaustion with the diabetes. It is necessary to observe further physiological results before jumping to conclusions as to the mechanism of the β-cell effect.

β) **Pancreatic insulin content.** The insulin content of the pancreas was investigated after sulphonylurea doses in dogs (ROOT 1957), calves (PFEIFFER, STEIGERWALD, SANDRITTER et al. 1957), rats (DULIN and MILLER 1959) and in mice (GRODSKY and PENG).

ROOT found, after applying 250 mg/kg BZ 55 in dogs, after 24 hrs only a slight, after treatment for 2 days however, an excessive decrease in the pancreatic insulin content (determined by convulsion tests in the mouse). After 14 days of high BZ 55 doses (300 mg/kg/day) the insulin content of the pancreas was also greatly diminished. If non-toxic doses were given effecting therapeutic blood levels for BZ 55, a normal pancreatic insulin content was found even after 8 weeks. STAHL and DORNER also found no difference in the insulin activity of pancreas extracts in normal dogs and those treated with BZ 55 for a length of time.

Extensive investigations were carried out on calves by PFEIFFER, STEIGER-WALD, SANDRITTER et al. (1957) who found that 100 mg/kg D 860 causes a marked decrease in pancreatic insulin after $1^1/_2$ hrs; this returned to normal after 3 hrs (determined by the blood sugar level of rabbits). This behaviour is parallel to the reactions of −SS- and −SH-groups in the β-cell (SANDRITTER et al.). It has been suggested that the diminished insulin content may still be evident after continuous application lasting from 8 days to 4 weeks. However, the insulin content of animals treated for 8 days remained low for 72 hrs. If one takes this into account, it is not justifiable to speak in these chronic experiments of a repetitive decrease in the insulin content. The values obtained should not be correlated to untreated controls, but to animals subjected to premedication. If one uses a standard 24 or 48 hr value, one sees as in the dog experiments of ROOT that the pancreatic insulin content of animals (calves) treated with D 860 for 7 or 14 days is permanently lower than that of untreated animals. The renewed sulphonylurea application in this stage cannot lead anymore to a marked insulin liberation which is also apparent by the absence of the blood sugar decrease (PFEIFFER et al. 1957) in this experimental phase. Therefore the experiments of ROOT on dogs correlate with those of PFEIFFER et al. (1957) on calves. It can therefore be concluded that too high a dosage of sulphonylureas considerably reduces the insulin reserve of the pancreas present at the time of application. It is however, not clear whether the insulin turnover is also diminished as this is not apparent on only measuring the content of the pancreas.

The insulin content of the pancreas in normal and hypophysectomised rats has been determined by DULIN and MILLER who tested the pancreatic extract in adrenalectomised rats. They found that the insulin content was still unchanged 1−2 hrs after D 860 application; however, after 4 hrs, they found both in the normal and in the hypophysectomised animal a significant decrease in pancreatic insulin. If one compares these results with the −SS- and −SH-reactions of the β-cells measured by SANDRITTER et al., a temporal discrepancy is apparent as the histochemical reactions are diminished after $1^1/_2$ hrs and normal again after 3 hrs. A blood sugar depression preceeded the decrease found in the pancreatic insulin content in the experiments of DULIN and MILLER. This may be related to an increased synthesis of insulin.

Finally the experiments of GRODSKY and PENG on mice are to be mentioned. The authors found using a considerable number of animals, 2 hrs after a single dose of D 860, that no decrease in pancreatic insulin occurred despite an obvious depression in the blood sugar. The content of pancreatic insulin was determined with a method developed by BERSON and YALOW (1959) with the highly specific immuno-bio-assay for insulin. The negative findings of GRODSKY and PENG do not however mean that no insulin is liberated in the pancreas, because a decrease in the insulin content of 10−20% in the mouse is perhaps too slight to be estimated by their method. A similar quantity of insulin would be sufficient for lowering the blood sugar 30−40% in the normal animal, a depression comparable to the effect of sulphonylureas. Also in the rat, the decrease in pancreatic insulin was only 25% after 4 hrs (DULIN and MILLER). [The data on the insulin content in the rat pancreas vary between 6 and 16 U/kg body weight (HAIST 1944)]. A decrease in the insulin content of over 75% was only found in the calf and this corresponds to about 200 U of insulin (PFEIFFER, STEIGERWALD, SANDRITTER et al. 1957). In chronic experiments on dogs and calves, a considerable reduction in insulin (80%)

was obtained after high doses of sulphonylureas. Therapeutic doses did not influence the pancreatic insulin content in dogs (ROOT). It is therefore interesting to correlate the above findings with the behaviour of plasma insulin activity.

γ) Activity of the plasma insulin and cross-circulation experiments. In the investigations on plasma insulin level it must be emphasised that the results were achieved by indirect methods which only refer to an insulin-like activity of the plasma. It is furthermore important to discriminate between the values obtained from peripheral and portal blood as the endogenously liberated insulin (from β-cells) could possibly be bound in the liver and metabolised there (MORTIMORE and TIETZE; KAPLAN and MADISON; MADISON et al. 1959). If this is true, a significant increase in the periphery would remained unnoticed. However, the objection could be raised that following intravenous or intraportal application of [113]I labelled insulin in dogs the same ^{131}I activity in the plasma could be found (MARTIN, LEONARDS and MILLER).

An increase in insulin activity in the portal blood of dogs can be found regularly after D 860. This was measured using the convulsion test in mice (GOETZ and EGDHAL); the glucose uptake of the rat diaphram in vitro (BARROS BARRETO and RECANT) and the oxidation of ^{14}C-glucose by the epididymal adipose tissue of the rat in vitro (PFEIFFER et al. 1959b). The same finding was made by PFEIFFER et al. (1959b) using the epididymal adipose tissue test in portal blood in rats 30 mins following i.v. injection of D 860. HASSELBLATT and HARN found no increased insulin activity either in the portal or peripheral blood after infusion of D 860 in a peripheral vein (insulin activity was measured by the glucose uptake of the epididymal adipose tissue in the rat). However, slow insulin infusion in the portal vein leading to an equally strong blood sugar decrease caused a significant increase in the insulin-like activity in the portal vein. HASSELBLATT and HARN conclude from their experiments that at least in the rabbit, sulphonylurea hypoglycaemia is not instigated by augmented endogenous insulin secretion.

PFEIFFER et al. (1959a—c) examined for the first time simultaneously the insulin activity of peripheral and portal blood and demonstrated that in the dog (at least with a D 860 dose of 50 mg/kg) and in rats (100 mg/kg) the insulin activity in the portal blood increases to 3 times that of normal, while it is normal in the peripheral blood. Their results and those of other authors correlated with the view that pancreatic insulin decreases after sulphonylureas thus throwing some light on the controversies over insulin and sulphonylurea hypoglycaemia; the latter being difficult to connect with a marked increase in peripheral insulin activity. However, it must be admitted that some authors have described considerably increased plasma insulin activity in rats following D 860 (KRACHT, KRÖNER, v. HOLT and v. HOLT 1957) and following BZ 55 (v. HOLT, v. HOLT, KRACHT, KRÖNER and KÜHNAU) also in dogs after BZ 55 (R.-CANDELA and R.-CANDELA) when using the diaphragmatic test. There was no increase in plasma insulin had the rats been treated for 3 months with daily BZ 55 doses (v. HOLT, v. HOLT, KRACHT, KRÖNER and KÜHNAU). STUHLFAUTH et al. found on perfusing the isolated dog's pancreas with periston, increased insulin in the perfusate provided that BZ 55 had been added.

Indirect evidence for increased insulin activity in the portal blood has been advanced by the cross-circulation experiments of POZZA, GALANSINO, and FOA. When anastomosis of the pancreatico-duodenal vein of a donor dog medicated with BZ 55 is connected with an untreated recipient dog, a lowering of blood sugar could be found in both dogs although the recipient dog had a blood sulphonylurea level of only 2 mg-%. Connection of the mesenteric vein of the two dogs caused no blood sugar depression in the recipient dog. Therefore can be concluded that the factor instigating blood sugar decrease originated from the pancreatic vein.

δ) The action on various metabolic parameters influenced by insulin. Numerous experiments have been performed to find out whether the lowering of blood sugar following sulphonylurea administration in the normal organism is accompanied by the same metabolic changes as in the condition of hypoglycaemia. Agreements, also differences of opinion, were stated and either view expressed has been used for or against the concept of the stimulation of insulin secretion by sulphonylureas. It must however be stressed that peripheral (subcutaneous or intravenous) application of insulin cannot be compared directly with an intra-portal insulin injection or infusion. The problem of the stimulation of insulin secretion by sulphonylureas bringing the insulin to the portal vein in a physiological manner has attracted many research workers interested in metabolic problems. It has given impetus to work attempting to clear the role of insulin in liver metabolism which is still an open question. Special attention has been directed towards the speed of insulin application as one must assume that insulin secretion by the β-cells following drug stimulation does not occur abruptly, but will last for some time. For this reason, all metabolic changes occurring after rapid intravenous or intra-portal insulin injection should be compared with the effect of slow insulin infusion. If this point is considered, then some contradictory evidence found in the literature can be solved.

An increase in the arterio-venous blood sugar difference characteristic for peripheral insulin action was observed in the intact dog by MADISON and UNGER (1958) following D 860 application. FRAWLEY et al. (1959) however, found within the phase of acute blood sugar decrease, 30 mins after i.v. injection of D 860, no sign of peripheral glucose utilization, but a reversal of the arterio-venous difference although the used dogs had a porto-caval shunt. Only hepatectomised animals showed a significant increase in the arterio-venous blood sugar difference, e.g. an increased peripheral glucose utilisation after D 860 administration. It must therefore be concluded that the liver has a decisive, or at least modifying role in the mechanism of sulphonylurea action.

Blood sugar behaviour after a single glucose load the so-called glucose tolerance does not only reflect the peripheral glucose utilization, but is a resultant of glucose uptake by the periphery and the liver plus the ability of the liver to decrease glucose output. The influence that single or chronic sulphonylurea doses have on the glucose tolerance cannot clearly answer the question as to the site of sulphonylurea action. It will therefore not be discussed here (comp. p. 37 f.).

However, peripheral glucose assimilation can be determined by the gradient of the specific activity of plasma glucose after labelling the glucose pool with a small (not increasing the blood sugar) ^{14}C-glucose dose (DUNN et al. 1957, BERSON and YALOW 1957, ASHMORE et al. 1958, TARDING and SCHAMBYE 1958). Using basis conditions one sees an exponential gradient of the specific activity of plasma glucose due to continuous dilution of labelled blood glucose by the inflow of non-labelled glucose from the liver. If insulin is injected under these conditions, by which peripheral glucose assimilation is increased, then there is an increased inflow of non-labelled liver glucose. Therefore, specific plasma glucose activity momentarily rapidly decreases; a clear downwards slope is seen in the curve. If the inflow of non-labelled liver glucose is impaired, then the decrease in specific activity is slowed down and plateauing in the curve is apparent. From the behaviour of specific blood glucose following an insulin dose, or any other blood sugar depressing substance, it is said to be decisive whether the decrease in blood sugar is caused either by increased peripheral assimilation, or by inhibition of the

3*

hepatic glucose output. The limitations of these methods are discussed on p. 48.

When using this method, however, neither in the dog (TARDING and SCHAMBYE, SCHAMBYE and TARDING), nor in the rabbit (BERSON and YALOW 1957), nor in the rat (ASHMORE et al. 1958) could an increased peripheral glucose assimilation be demonstrated during D 860 hypoglycaemia. For this reason the decrease in blood sugar must be explained by glucose absorption or by inhibition of liver glucose output (s. p. 48). An increased glucose absorption in the periphery has only been seen by v. HOLT and v. HOLT (1958b) in rats. Despite this finding, these authors emphasise that after insulin application by a slow peripheral or intra-portal route, no increased peripheral glucose utilization can be found (v. HOLT, NOLTE and v. HOLT). This view is shared by REICHARD et al. based on their studies with isotopes. On the other hand, MADISON and UNGER (1958a) also DE BODO et al. reached the conclusion that under these conditions insulin causes a peripheral sugar utilization.

Further evidence for an increased peripheral glucose utilization originates from the investigations on the glycogen content of muscles in vivo. The numerous reports on the lack of glycogen uptake by the skeletal muscles after sulphonyl-ureas will not be mentioned here for glycogen uptake is of a variable magnitude also after insulin. However, while subcutaneous or intra-splenic (i.e. intra-portal) insulin injections regularly cause a significant increase of glycogen in the rat *diaphragm* (DULIN and JOHNSTON, CREUTZFELDT and SÜTTERLE), this effect cannot be demonstrated after sulphonylurea medication (v. HOLT, v. HOLT and KRÖNER 1956, CREUTZFELDT and SÜTTERLE; DULIN and JOHNSTON). More specific results could have been expected from ^{14}C-labelled glucose, but these results are not uniform which may be due to the experimental set-up or to the quantity of drugs given. ASHMORE et al. (1958) thus found no increase in ^{14}C activity in the skeletal muscle of the rat receiving D 860. According to MILLER, KRAKE and VANDER-BROOK an uptake of ^{14}C into muscle glycogen can only be expected if a sufficiently active ^{14}C-glucose dose has been given. In their experiments, MILLER et al. found an increase of $^{14}CO_2$ in the respiratory air demonstrating increased glucose oxidation. v. HOLT and v. HOLT (1958a—c) demonstrated in the same way with BZ 55 an increase in ^{14}C activity in muscle glycogen which was still present 10 hrs after medication. It was not demonstrable after 12 months of continuous treatment even if the animals had been untreated for 4 days previously.

BRESSLER and ENGEL examined the behaviour of the glycogen content in the dorsal adipose tissue of the fasting rat. This increases considerably after insulin, but they found no such change after D 860. Only if the rats were fed, the glycogen content was increased in the adipose tissue. Also KNITSCH and MOHNIKE (1958) found, after application of BZ 55 in not too high doses to starving rats, a charac-teristic glycogen increase in the peri-renal and peri-epididymal adipose tissue in the rat, in the re-feeding period similar to that found for insulin. An augmented incorporation of ^{14}C from labelled glucose in the fatty acids of peripheral adipose tissue, could not be demonstrated for the rat when D 860 was applied (ASHMORE et al.). Lipogenesis from ^{14}C glucose was even found to be inhibited in mice receiving BZ 55 (PROD'HOM and PLATTNER 1958, 1959). BÖCK, LINDNER, and OBENAUS have compared the insulin effect and that of BZ 55 on the glucose level of the intra-ocular fluid of the rabbit and found despite equal action on the blood sugar, a decrease in the sugar content in the intra-ocular fluid only after insulin, not however, after BZ 55.

A typical concommitant symptom of insulin hypoglycaemia is the decrease in anorganic *phosphorus* in the plasma as the result of the increased peripheral glucose utilization (SOSKIN, LEVINE, and HECHTER; NICHOLS); while the fall of plasma potassium is at least partly of hepatic origin. Also the decrease in *amino nitrogen* is mainly due to the peripheral insulin effect. MOHNIKE and BIBERGEIL found on intravenously applying sulphonylurea doses to dogs an extensive decrease in serum potassium, but only a brief depression in serum phosphorus that subsequently steeply rose. On oral sulphonylurea doses, dogs showed only a decrease in amino nitrogen while the serum potassium remained unchanged, and serum phosphorus was increased (MOHNIKE, CZYZYK, and BIBERGEIL). The poor effect on phosphorus and potassium is probably caused by insufficient action in the periphery of insulin liberated from the β-cells; additional phosphorus liberation from the liver is possible. The decrease in amino nitrogen could be explained by direct influence on amino acid metabolism, as after D 860 in pancreatectomised and alloxanised dogs without simultaneous blood sugar lowering, a decrease in amino nitrogen also occurs (MOHNIKE, BIBERGEIL, and CZYZYK).

GALANSINO et al. (1958) examined the behaviour of lactic and pyruvic acid in the blood of dogs receiving sulphonylurea and insulin, and found a significant difference. While insulin applied peripherally or by portal infusion increases lactate and pyruvate, i.v. injection of sulphonylureas caused a decrease in the latter despite an equal decrease in blood sugar. The decrease in the potassium level is very marked following insulin, but occurs after sulphonylureas only spuriously or not at all. The same is true for injection of chlorpropamide (FOA et al., 1959) and metahexamide (GALANSINO et al., 1959). This research team concludes from their investigations that the sulphonylureas have a specific liver effect which is not typical for insulin even after slow, intra-portal infusion. This effect is, however, only present if the β-cells are functionally intact.

In guinea-pigs, no significant difference in the blood concentration of lactate, pyruvate and α-keto glutarate behaviour could be shown between subcutaneous injection of insulin or of D 860 after 1, 2 and 3 hrs (ANDREU-KERN, SÖLING, and CREUTZFELDT).

As mentioned in the beginning of this section, the small or even absent peripheral effects during the sulphonylurea hypoglycaemia should not be used indiscriminately against the insulin secretion theory. The quantity of insulin reaching the periphery can be very small. MADISON and UNGER (1958a) demonstrated that the intra-portal insulin injection measured by the peripheral arterio-venous difference is far less effective than the i.v. injection. v. HOLT, NOLTE, and v. HOLT (1959) failed to find ^{14}C glucose incorporation into muscle glycogen when insulin was slowly infused by a portal or peripheral route, although the blood sugar fell in a similar way as during rapid injection, and these rapid portal, as the peripheral injections, caused an increase of ^{14}C activity in muscle glycogen.

If this reasoning is followed, it is only logical to doubt those findings that claim a high insulin activity in the venous blood after sulphonylurea medication (comp. p. 34).

It is of significance for our further discussion that peripheral metabolic effects, even in normal animals, are not wholly capable of explaining the sulphonylurea hypoglycaemia. It is highly probable that the seat of origin is essentially in the liver. Also, it is very probable that under some circumstances a pure insulin effect occurs in the liver (s. p. 48).

ε) **Glucose tolerance.** As has already been mentioned (s. p. 35), the behaviour glucose tolerance can only partly explain the mechanism of action, but is of interest in view of the possible exhaustion of the β-cell system through sulphonylureas. BELLENS et al. (1956,1958) found in rats and dogs increased assimilation of glucose i.v. injected following BZ 55. It was, however, only a temporary effect, as after two hours following BZ 55 application, glucose assimilation was already diminished in the dog (CHRISTOPHE and CONARD). Also repeated doses of BZ 55 reduced glucose assimilation in rats (DE MEUTTER et al. 1956, CONARD et al., 1957). The authors conclude from this finding that the pancreatic insulin reserve is reduced after one or several doses of sulphonylurea, as the co-efficient of glucose assimilation should be a measurement for insulin activity (CONARD 1955). The findings of BRAUN et al. (1959) favour the same view, for they failed to find a blood sugar effect of D 860 during an acute over-loading with sugar in rats. The decrease in oral glucose tolerance in normal rats and dogs treated for months with BZ 55 (V. HOLT, KRACHT, KRÖNER, and V. HOLT 1956, LEDERER and DE MEYER) and the decrease in intra-peritoneal glucose tolerance in partially pancreatectomised rats receiving D 860 for months (CREUTZFELDT and GEGINAT), and finally the decrease in the intra-venous glucose tolerance of normal and alloxan damaged (though not manifestly diabetic) rats given D 860 for months (LAZAROW and TREIBERGS) has similar significance. These results say nothing about the exhaustion of the islet system after prolonged sulphonylurea medication; this has always been feared for a β-cytotropic substance. The reduction in glucose tolerance is not progredient, but stays on the same niveau on continuing the therapy. The extent of the decrease depends only on the amount of sulphonylureas given daily (LAZAROW and TREIBERGS). Partially pancreatectomised rats that are (to begin with) latently diabetic, did not become manifestly diabetic (CREUTZFELDT and GEGINAT). Also in rats treated with alloxan without manifest diabetes, no diabetes occurred and in already diabetic animals spontaneous remission of alloxan diabetes occurred with and without D 860 treatment with equal frequency (LAZAROW and TREIBERGS). DULIN (1960) treated partially depancreatised rats for $8^{1}/_{2}$ and 12 months respectively with D 860. The severity of the diabetes increases and decreases with approximately equal frequency in these groups, as in the untreated and insulin treated controls. Contrary to these observations made on numerous rats is a finding of MOHNIKE (1957). He could produce diabetes in a dog premedicated with alloxan by administering BZ 55. Connected with this are the observations of v. HOLT and v. HOLT (1958). When normal rats treated for months with BZ 55 are force fed while continuing BZ 55 medication, severe glucosuria develops. This is not found in force fed control rats.

A further reason why one cannot conclude a β-cell exhaustion from the above mentioned findings of decreased glucose tolerance, is the fact that despite reduced glucose tolerance in partially pancreatectomised rats chronically treated with D 860, the blood sugar lowering effect of the drug was still obvious; it had only decreased slightly (CREUTZFELDT and GEGINAT).

It may well be possible that it is of great significance that the β-cell system shows a different sensitivity towards drugs according to species. This would explain many of the contradictions found in the literature: e.g. STEWART also BÄNDER, HÄUSSLER, and SCHOLZ; CREUTZFELDT, DETERING, and WELTE found an unchanged oral glucose tolerance in normal rabbits, rats, and dogs even after sulphonylurea medication for several months. SCHÖLER and GAARENSTROOM observed in one of their rat strains only a slight increase in blood sugar values after chronic BZ 55 application in contrast to another highly sensitive strain which displayed under the same conditions, after the 8th week diabetic blood sugar values with glucosuria. For this reason the observations of SCHÖLER and GAARENSTROOM will be discussed below (s. p. 41).

ζ) **The mechanism of β-cell influencing.** After the findings discussed above, there can be no doubt about an influence of the sulphonylureas on the β-cell system with consecutive insulin release. How can this be imagined? The usual view expressed assumes that sulphonylureas "stimulate" β-cells without defining the nature of this stimulation. Apparently, similar mechanism as in the physiological stimulus for insulin secretion is assumed. It must be emphasised that the precise nature of physiological insulin secretion is still not known (comp. reviews of LAZAROW 1957 and MASKE 1957). It is however known that the level of blood glucose controls the insulin secretion (GRAFE and MEYTHALER; ANDERSON and LONG; FOA et al. 1949). Thereby the insulin reserve, probably stored in the granula as a zinc complex is mobilised.

Several hypotheses have been proposed to explain the sulphonylurea effect on the β-cells. PFEIFFER, STEIGERWALD, SANDRITTER et al. (1957) take the view that sulphonylureas effect the liberation of a certain amount of soluble insulin present in the β-cells and only secondarily mobilisation of the insulin stored in the granules occurs. This procedure is activated by an increase in the sulphonylurea concentration in the blood and can be repeated rhythmically on each further dose. Against this explanation, it must be emphasised that there is no support for the view that soluble insulin in the β-cells could not penetrate freely anyway through the β-cell membrane.

MOHNIKE (1957) believes insulin release to be augmented by the sulphonylureas, but without the β-cells showing improved adaptability for physiological demand, e.g. blood sugar rise. MOHNIKE believes that an influence of the enzymes on the β-cells, respectively an appearance of metabolites causes the increased insulin release. WALLENFELS, SUMM, and CREUTZFELDT reached similar conclusions after research on numerous enzyme reactions in vivo and vitro. They believe that within the limits of their specific enzymatic equipment all metabolically active tissues are affected in the same way by sulphonylureas. The β-cells respond by increased insulin release. Other possibilities were discussed by WALLENFELS, SUMM, and CREUTZFELDT; namely, that under the influence of sulphonylureas metabolites are produced in the liver or in β-cells themselves which dissolve the insulin complex in the β-cell. This conclusion was drawn after the new investigations of SUMM, CREUTZFELDT, and WALLENFELS (1960), where under D 860 augmented incorporation of ^{14}C from ^{14}C-NaHCO$_3$ was found in the liver glycogen (s. p. 47). This finding suggests an increased turnover of metabolites and is not achieved by insulin. As sulphonylureas can inhibit ketogenesis in liver slices in vitro (RENOLD et al. 1959) one may conclude that there is an increased production of oxaloacetic acid, a substance that according to MASKE (1957) reacts more strongly with the zinc than with insulin. Thus it could liberate insulin from the zinc insulin complex. The activation of the malic enzyme found in the liver of man and rat by WALLENFELS, SUMM, and CREUTZFELDT also WALLENFELS, CREUTZFELDT, and SUMM could play a part in this process, especially if the activation also occurs in the β-cells which according to LACY (1960) is the case. However, it must remain open whether a mechanism analogous to the physiological insulin release is produced in this way, as the morphological findings are controversial as mentioned above.

A recent observation of WALLENFELS, BURCHARD, and SUND that BZ 55 in vitro in high concentrations can split the insulin-zinc complexes is of interest (s. p. 22). Thus one could theoretically explain very simply the sulphonylurea effect on the β-cells. At present the concentration required for splitting the insulin-zinc complex seems very high.

CREUTZFELDT and SÜTTERLE (1957) also considered a direct inter-action of the sulphonylureas with insulin; thus a combination occurs which can no longer be stored in the islets and which attaches itself particularly firmly in certain sites of action (liver). This hypothesis was formulated under the impression that special liver metabolic effects take place and also by the weak peripheral effects. We can explain this today, however, partly alone by the different effect of portally infused and peripherally applied insulin. STRAUZENBERG and HALLER (1959) believe in a similar theory and assume that there is a complex compound formed between insulin and the sulphonylureas which produces a change in insulin action. In favour of this, is the fact that it has been impossible to prove that the insulin release of the β-cells is followed by an increased production which would mean a continuously increased insulin turnover. The experiments by BÄNDER and SCHOLZ did not indicate an increase insulin turnover; they used labelled cystein together with D 860 and did not find an increased amount of this tagged substance in endogenous insulin. Furthermore, no increase in insulin activity could be found in plasma if the rats were treated for a considerable time with sulphonylureas although β-cells showed morphological signs of increased activity (v. HOLT, v. HOLT, KRACHT, KRÖNER, and KÜHNAU).

BÄNDER (1957, 1959 b) also HASSELBLATT and BLUDAU have discussed the mechanism of insulin release as being possibly a sensibilisation of the glucose sensitive receptors in the β-cells caused by sulphonylureas. This hypothesis explains why insulin secretion could start at normal blood sugar values and the level of the blood sugar could only be reduced to a certain level although the β-cells still contain sufficient amounts of insulin in order to compensate the blood sugar rise following glucose loading with normal speed. However, this concept neglects the fact that there is still sufficient circulating insulin at the time of glucose loading owing to the previous insulin mobilisation for assimilation of injected glucose. Apart from this, it must be noted that the blood sugar level rises already several hours following sulphonylurea application in the normal animal. In normal long-term treated animals, despite high sulphonylurea plasma levels, there is not always a permanently lowered fasting blood sugar level. On the contrary, they show a temporary blood sugar decrease daily, after each dose. PFEIFFER, STEIGERWALD, SANDRITTER et al. (1957) concluded from these experiments that the decisive effective factor of the sulphonylureas when acting on the β-cells is an increase in plasma concentration and not the absolute plasma level. In how far this view is applicable to human diabetes mellitus, particularly for those patients responding to sulphonylurea therapy, will be discussed on p. 82.

In this connection, it is interesting to record the observation of HASSELBLATT and SCHUSTER who found that a blood sugar decrease through sulphonylureas is significantly weakened by chlorpromazine and di-ethyl-barbituric acid (veronal), while insulin action remains unimpaired. To explain this phenomenon the authors assumed that veronal and chlorpromazine reduce the reaction of the β-cells. Besides this, disturbed phosphorylation of glucose in extra-pancreatic tissues, particularly the liver, may be important because chlorpromazine alone causes hyperglycaemia and interferes with the glucose tolerance. HASSELBLATT and HAUN (1960 b) recently relinquished this hypothesis. The authors were namely able to abolish the inhibitory action of chlorpromazine by cutting the right splanchnic nerve below the right supra-renal in the rabbit. The same effect could be achieved by administering the ganglioplegic acting pendiomid. However the inhibitory action of chlorpromazine and veronal was not changed through adrenalectomy. HASSELBLATT and HAUN postulated a local liberation of epinephrine through chlorpromazine and veronal in the liver, this led to glycogenolysis locally, thus abrogating the hepatic effect of D 860 that is said to be more important, especially in the rabbit, than a β-cytotropic effect (comp. also the peculiarity of the rabbit regarding cell changes s. p. 29 and 30). Chloralose anaesthetic which causes hyperglycaemia in the rabbit prevents the blood sugar depressing effect of D 860, while insulin is still capable of lowering the blood sugar (KÖNIG). It is likely that direct action on the pancreas leading to "anaesthesia" of the β-cells is possible and might be related to the fact that premedication with veronal (MARTINEZ) also with chlorpromazine (SIMOES and OSSWALD) protects the β-cells to some extent from the damaging effect of alloxan (premedicated animals therefore rarely show alloxan diabetes).

It is important to know whether this action on the β-cells is physiological or non-physiological, as this would answer the question whether permanent damage of the β-cell following sulphonylurea medication is possible. In this connection the observation of LAZARUS (1959) should be recalled (s. p. 31) who found that glucose-6-phosphatase activity found in the degranulation of β-cells after sulphonylurea decreases, but remains unchanged when cortisone is given. This finding favours the view that the action of hyperglycaemia and sulphonylurea is different on the β-cells, but not necessarily pathological. Completely unphysiological, however, would be the mechanism that has been discussed by FREINKEL and INGBAR based on their in vitro experiments on kidney slices. They assume that a localised histotoxic anoxia of the β-cell is causal for insulin liberation (s. p. 22). Actual findings on the islet tissue that would favour this concept are missing. However, it is known that certain β-cell poisons e.g., alloxan or dithizon are substances which are similarly "β-cytotropic" as the sulphonylureas. It is therefore theoretically possible that derivatives of the sulphonylureas exist which not only mobilise insulin from the β-cell (similar to the initial action of alloxan), but subsequently impair their function and eventually cause their destruction. This behaviour appears to be valid for D 860 and BZ 55 only under extreme conditions and is therefore of no practical importance (s. section on glucose tolerance on p. 37 f.). Few vacuolised β-cells have been found in the rat after 9 months of BZ 55 medication by v. HOLT, KRACHT, KRÖNER, and v. HOLT. MOSCA found a decrease in β-cell mitosis after high D 860 doses. Chronic application of more potent compounds such as chlorpropamide and metahexamide in low doses in rats and dogs regularly cause a diabetic blood sugar curve after glucose loading (BÄNDER 1959 a).

Low daily alloxan medication causes changes in the islets in rats which cannot be discriminated from those produced by sulphonylureas and consist of a β-cell degranulation without pycnotic nuclei or cytoplasmatic degeneration (SCHÖLER and GAARENSTROOM). According to this finding, no qualitative, but only quantitative difference appear to exist between β-cytotoxic substances of the alloxan type and the β-cytotropic substances of the sulphonylurea type. This view is supported by the experiments on animals given diabetogenic alloxan doses and premedicated with D 860. At first the animals do not exhibit a typical triphasic blood sugar curve in relation to the β-cell degranulation and diminished insulin content, because insulin release cannot follow the initial hyperglycaemia and therefore no transitory hypoglycaemia can result. Instead the blood sugar rises continuously and leads to severe permanent hyperglyaemia in all animals (KLIMAS and SEARLE). DE BASTIANI and GRANATA found the same with IPTD in the rabbit. This behaviour is all the more remarkable as it is known that the premedication with glucose in the rabbit (MASKE, WOLFF, and STAMPFL) and with epinephrine (MASKE, STAMPFL, and GAHN) are proceedings which physiologically lead to insulin secretion and to β-cell degranulation and which considerably reduce the frequency of diabetes caused by alloxan. MASKE had concluded from this that alloxan was not capable of damaging the β-cells if the zinc in the cell, due to premedication, was missing and alloxan was therefore incapable of inter-acting. In contrast to this, the β-cell degranulation caused by sulphonylureas is in no way protective for the β-cells. On the contrary, MOSINGER and BRAUN showed in a large series of experiments that a single dose of BZ 55 2—6 hrs before alloxan application considerably increased the number and severity of diabetic animals thus showing augmentation of the diabetogenic effect of alloxan. MEADE and KLITGAARD compared the toxicity of alloxan (measured by the mortality and the diabetogenity) in rats premedicated with glucose and insulin, also glucose plus D 860. In the animals treated with D 860 a significantly higher alloxan toxicity was found, corresponding to the increased alloxan sensitivity found in starving animals. It can therefore be concluded that the sulphonylurea action on the β-cells differs from that of glucose and that there is even an addition of their β-cytotropic characteristic with the β-cytotoxic action of alloxan. The reports of FISTER et al. of the weakening of the alloxan effect in rats through D 860, was contradicted by the fact that 3 groups of workers found the contrary (KLIMAS and SEARLE, MOSINGER and BRAUN, MEADE and KLITGAARD).

One may conclude from the data reviewed here to the question of the influence of sulphonylureas on the β-cells the following: firstly, it is more likely to have an effect on the metabolism of the β-cells and secondly, that those more effective sulphonylurea drugs e.g., chlorpropamide and metahexamide have to be viewed with restraint as they are automatically more closely related to β-cyto toxins.

5. The role of other endocrine organs

Extirpation of the supra-renals and the pituitary, or the addition of anterior pituitary lobe hormone and adrenal and thyroid hormones lead to interesting modifications in the action of sulphonylureas.

α) Thyroid. As mentioned on p. 15, thyroid changes are produced by high doses of sulphonylureas, more so by BZ 55 than D 860. These changes are similar to those after application of mild thyreostatica. These partially slight changes appear very slowly; therefore, thyroid inhibition cannot be the cause of the rapid blood sugar decrease following sulphonylurea application. An interesting connection between the thyroid and sulphonylurea effect was found by HASSELBLATT and BASTIAN; namely, that when premedicating mice with thyroxine, the sensitivity towards D 860 (measured by hypoglycaemic shock) was increased 20 times, while the sensitivity to insulin was increased only 1.67 times. These observations were confirmed for the normal rat by CREUTZFELDT and FINTER 1959: the same D 860 doses had a significantly stronger blood sugar effect after premedication with TSH or thyroxine for 5 days; D 860 doses that scarcely lowered the blood sugar in non-premedicated animals were highly effective after thyroxine application while the insulin effect was not increased. It was remarkable that there was no sensibilisation towards D 860 by thyroxine and TSH treatment found in hypophysectomised rats.

There is no satisfactory explanation for these findings. If the glycogen depletion of the liver, or the varied responsiveness of peripheral tissues should play an important part, then we do not understand that the insulin hypoglycaemia is not increased. A noticeably increased pancreatic insulin content after thyroxine doses discussed by HASSELBLATT and BASTIAN is scarcely credible; in fact, exactly the opposite is to be expected. One must either accept that thyroxine premedication alters the functional condition of the β-cells so that they react more strongly to sulphonylureas by insulin secretion, or that thyroxine influences the hepatic metabolism to such an extent that the hypothetical sulphonylurea action can be more effective. As alloxan diabetic rats did not react to D 860 doses either with a blood sugar lowering or recession of glucosuria, also after thyroxine premedication, they showed no blood sugar decrease on D 860 application and finally displayed unaltered glucosuria with prolonged combined doses of thyroxine and D 860; an influence on the β-cell function is more probable (Creutzfeldt and Finter 1959). Similarly the therapeutic value of sulphonylureas is less in a patient suffering simultaneously from diabetes and hyperthyroidism than in an euthyreotic patient (comp. p. 58). We can register at present that the thyroid hormone, contrary to the insulin effect modifies the action of sulphonylureas in the normal animals.

β) **Supra-renals.** Adrenalectomised animals show as after insulin, when compared to normal animals, a much stronger blood sugar decrease after sulphonylureas. This is true for rats (v. Holt, v. Holt, and Kröner 1956; Bänder and Scholz; Dulin, Morley, and Nezamis; Houssay and Penhos; Cox, Henley, and Williams; Houssay et al. 1957a), dogs (Houssay and Penhos; Houssay et al. 1957a), cats (Gordon, Buse, and Lukens) and toads (Houssay et al. 1957a). The blood sugar level decreases continuously until death, already on very small doses because the adrenergic counter-regulation caused by sulphonylureas is absent (s. p. 13). The crucial point is, therefore, the absence of the adrenal medulla. This is indirectly true for the behaviour of hypophysectomised rats suffering from extensive atrophy of the adrenal cortex and who do not react more strongly to sulphonylureas than do normal animals (s. p. 43 f.). The hypoglycaemic reaction of the adrenalectomised rat after sulphonylurea doses can be completely abolished by epinephrine injection and only partially by hydrocortisone (Dulin et al. 1956). As animals without adrenal medulla are 3—6 times more sensitive to sulphonylureas, totally adrenalectomised rats are 10 times more sensitive, one must assume that there is a reactive cortisone release compensating hypoglycaemia or a direct stimulation of the cortex through the sulphonylureas (Dulin et al. 1956). The increased sensitivity of adrenalectomised animals is also shown by alloxan diabetic rats previously not reacting to BZ 55 and after adrenal extirpation reacting to the drug with recession of glucosuria (v. Holt, v. Holt, and Kröner 1956). From these experiments, we see that the blood sugar lowering effect of the sulphonylureas is not achieved by an influence on the supra-renals. The supra-renals are only necessary for the prevention of severe hypoglycaemic conditions. Conversely, doses of glucocorticoids decrease the sulphonylurea hypoglycaemia (s. p. 26). As mentioned previously, the epinephrine effect is mainly peripheral because there is no decrease in the liver glycogen during sulphonylurea hypoglycaemia and epinephrine abolishes the blood sugar decrease in adrenalectomised animals receiving sulphonylureas despite the liver being practically without glycogen after suprarenal extirpation. Possibly the reason why the peripheral insulin effect after sulphonylurea doses in vivo is so difficult to prove is due to the powerful peripheral epinephrine effect.

γ) **Pituitary.** Sulphonylureas also have a blood sugar decreasing effect in hypophysectomised animals. While adrenalectomised animals, compared to their insulin sensitivity, are high susceptible to sulphonylureas, the hypophysectomised animal does not react, despite its well known insulin sensitivity, to sulphonylurea medication with a stronger blood sugar decrease than does the normal animal. These corresponding observations for rats (Bänder and Scholz; Cox, Henley, and Williams; Houssay and Penhos; Houssay et al. 1957b, Creutzfeldt, Detering and Welte; Dulin and Miller 1959), cats (Gordon, Buse, and Lukens), and toads (Houssay et al. 1957b) speak against a stronger insulin release from the β-cells of hypophysectomised animals after sulphonylurea doses, or at least against peripherally active larger amounts of insulin. Owing to the fundamental significance of this phenomenon, various experiments were made trying to explain it. First was found that there was even slightly more β-cell degranulation after D 860 doses in hypophysectomised rats than in the normal animal. However, there was no enlargement of the β-cell nuclei (Creutzfeldt,

DETERING and WELTE). One can conclude there to be a functional decrease in the β-cell activity. It must be assumed on account of the severe degranulation that the insulin reserve in the β-cells, which is the same in the hypophysectomised rat as in the normal animal, is released (HAIST 1942, also FRAENKEL-CONRAT et al.). Later, however, insulin could be slowly resynthesised resulting in a lower insulin turnover. For this speaks an atrophy of the Golgi apparatus of the β-cells, while β-granulation is normal following hypophysectomy (BATTS). Also there is no increase in islet volume in hypophysectomised rats constantly infused with glucose (HAIST 1959). Finally the relative resistance to sulphonylureas found in the hypophysectomised animal also cannot be explained by this, as hypophysectomised rats constantly treated for weeks with STH (which guarantees normal growth and according to BATTS normalises the Golgi apparatus of the β-cells within four days) also display no increased sensitivity to sulphonylureas (CREUTZFELDT, DETERING and WELTE). Admittedly, we know very little about hypophyseal influence on the β-cell function, but it is possible that a β-cytotropic factor exists not identical with the known anterior pituitary lobe hormones.

DULIN and MILLER (1959) found the pancreatic insulin content to be reduced to half that of normal after four weeks following hypophysectomy; this they regarded, contrary to other research workers, as being a sufficient explanation for the relative sulphonylurea resistence in hypophysectomised rats. They found the remarkably slight sulphonylurea sensitivity discussed here only in animals hypophysectomised several weeks previously; however, animals three days after hypophysectomy showed a stronger blood sugar decrease than normal rats. According to the insulin determinations by DULIN and MILLER, there is a decrease in the pancreatic insulin in the hypophysectomised rat receiving D 860 of about 0.35 U/kg in comparison to 1 U/kg in the normal animal. It must be stated that 0.35 U/kg are hardly tolerated by a hypophysectomised animal. According to our experience, already 0.1 U/kg of old insulin s.c. causes severe hypoglycaemic shocks in 80% of the animals, while 0.05 U/kg still produces a shock in 20%. An important part is certainly played by the direct sulphonylurea action on the adrenal medulla because also, hypophysectomised rats operated on some time previously, become highly sensitive to D 860 after adrenalectomy or removal of the medulla; while the same procedures do not influence insulin sensitivity (DULIN and MILLER). The observation that the expected increase in sulphonylurea sensitivity is still present 3 days after hypophysectomy, despite intact adrenal medulla, could also mean that extirpation of the pituitary causes a change in the liver metabolism decreasing the sulphonylurea action in this organ. It is however, unknown which hypophyseal factor could be responsible. It could not be due to ACTH as the sulphonylurea sensitivity shown by the adrenalectomised animal without local corticoid production is greatly enhanced. Likewise, medication of STH (CREUTZFELDT, DETERING and WELTE) and TSH and thyroxine (CREUTZFELDT and FINTER 1959) do not increase the sensitivity of hypophysectomised animals to sulphonylureas.

The pituitary, therefore, is unnecessary for producing the blood sugar decreasing effect of sulphonylureas, but it is capable of modifying the strength of the sulphonylurea effect in an unknown way. The findings in the hypophysectomised animal are arguments against the concept that the sulphonylureas act only by stimulating insulin secretion and are difficult to refute. It is therefore necessary to conduct further experiments in this direction. These observations again raise the question whether the β-cytotropic hormone of the pituitary really exists.

6. The role played by the liver

Our discussion on the site of action of the sulphonylureas gave rise to the opinion that the decisive site of action of these substances must be found in the β-cells of the pancreas. It was necessary to mention those findings which seem to contradict the view that simple stimulation of insulin secretion is the only mode of action. At first an account had been given of the various direct actions on the enzyme systems in vitro which however, presupposed high intracellular sulphonylurea concentrations. It had already been mentioned that little is known of the sulphonylurea concentrations attained at the site of action in vivo. Furthermore, sulphonylurea effects could be found in animals without pancreas or suffering from alloxan diabetes as long as small quantities of exogenous or endogenous insulin was present. It was also emphasised that only a few typical insulin effects occur in the periphery under sulphonylurea medication. This fact was not, however, sufficient evidence against the stimulation of insulin secretion because portal insulin secretion may have had different metabolic effects than the peripheral application, particularly as the speed of injection may have special significance. These differences may well have been caused by an influence on liver metabolism and it had to remain an open question whether this effect (doubted to date) on the liver was an indirect one of insulin on this organ. Modifications in the sulphonylurea action have also been found after thyroxine injection and following hypophysectomy; these are not found when insulin is released and may have been localised in the liver.

The part played by the liver in the sulphonylurea action deserves special considerations as the liver is the only source of blood glucose and occupies a special position in the carbohydrate metabolism. The result of the diminished glucose production in the liver would have the same consequence for the blood sugar as a peripheral increase in sugar assimilation. All these unsolved problems necessitate our attention on the insulin action on the liver.

α) Depression of the blood sugar in the hepatectomised animal. It must be emphasised to begin with that also the hepatectomised animal with intact pancreas produces a decrease in the blood sugar after sulphonylurea application. DULIN and JOHNSTON found in hepatectomised rats that were infused continuously with glucose, a blood sugar lowering, after 400 mg/kg D 860 s.c. of 40 mg-% lower than hepatectomised animals without D 860. They found in addition a decrease in the blood sugar in the hepatectomised dog which was infused with glucose after i.p. injection of 50—100 mg/kg D 860 (this reaction is however delayed when compared with that of normal dogs). SOBEL et al. even found in their hepatectomised dogs constantly infused with glucose after 125 mg/kg D 860 i.v., a blood sugar decrease which did not differ in time or extent from that of the normal dog. RICHTER reached the same conclusion using BZ 55 and D 860 in the rabbit after functionally isolating the liver. FRAWLEY et al. (1959) found in hepatectomised dogs infused with glucose after D 860, simultaneously with a blood sugar decrease, a rise in the peripheral arterio-venous blood sugar difference and a decrease of the serum potassium and phosphorus.

The results from these corresponding investigations clearly show that the sulphonylurea hypoglycaemia is independent of the presence of the liver in the organism. There is no blood sugar decrease found in eviscerated animals (liver and pancreas are missing) as shown by the results of the pancreotropic effect of the sulphonylureas and (at least when there is no liver) a peripheral insulin effect. This does not exclude that if the liver is present this organ is the main site of metabolic change, especially because a peripheral effect in the intact animal is unlikely.

Interesting in this connection is that rabbits poisoned with carbon tetrachloride show an increased blood sugar lowering after an oral D 860 dose (CREUTZFELDT and SÜTTERLE 1957a, SÜTTERLE; SÜDHOF et al. 1958b). As the insulin effect in the same animals is noticeably decreased (CREUTZFELDT and SÜTTERLE 1957a, SÜTTERLE), this observation cannot be explained by a weak counter-regulation following glycogen depletion of the liver (SÜDHOF et al. 1958b). These experiments show that the liver is involved, not only indirectly by insulin, in the development of hypoglycaemia following sulphonylurea application. Changes in the liver metabolism of the intact animal will be discussed in the following chapters.

β) **Liver glycogen.** BERINGER first stated that there was regularly an increase in liver glycogen during sulphonylurea hypoglycaemia in the fasting rabbit (BERINGER and LINDNER, BERINGER and KEIBL). This finding was confirmed in the guinea-pig (BÄNDER and SCHOLZ) and in the rat (v. HOLT, v HOLT and KRÖNER 1956, MILLER and DULIN; TYBERGHEIN, HALSEY and WILLIAMS; CREUTZFELDT and SÜTTERLE 1957a and b, FRY and WRIGHT; DULIN and JOHNSTON). This is remarkable, as at least in the rat (CORI and CORI; CREUTZFELDT and SÜTTERLE; BERINGER 1959) and in the mouse (SWENSSON), there is a decrease in liver glycogen when in fasting condition and under insulin, even if insulin is injected intra-portally (BÜRGER and KOHL, CREUTZFELDT and SÜTTERLE). However, various species react differently, and in the guinea-pig the liver glycogen remains unchanged, while in the rabbit there is an increase on insulin injection (BERINGER 1959). The increase in liver glycogen is no explanation for the hypoglycaemia instigated by the sulphonylureas. The evidence for this is as follows: animals having been fed, or given glucose and sulphonylureas, showed no increase in liver glycogen when compared to controls (BERINGER and KEIBL; TYBERGHEIN, HALSEY and WILLIAMS; CREUTZFELDT and SÜTTERLE). In adrenalectomised rats (v. HOLT, v. HOLT and KRÖNER 1956, DULIN and JOHNSTON; HENRY, KIM and HALL) and in hypophysectomised rats (CREUTZFELDT and SÜTTERLE), there is no increase in liver glycogen despite a blood sugar decrease. In contrast to this, it is possible to achieve an increase in the liver glycogen with sulphonylureas if adrenalectomised rats are treated with cortisone and epinephrine (HENRY et al.), while the decrease in the blood sugar is considerably less than in the untreated animal. Finally a simple calculation shows that the relatively small increase in liver glycogen cannot account for the considerable blood sugar decrease regularly observed. These findings only allow the conclusion that sulphonylureas have a specific effect on the liver metabolism not found with insulin. It is not linked to the presence of a functioning β-cell system. This is so as HENRY, KIM and HALL observed in alloxan diabetic rats previously showing no increase in liver glycogen with D 860, that after insulin premedication these animals reacted to D 860 with a significant increase in liver glycogen without concomitant blood sugar decrease. BERINGER and KEIBL found in severe alloxan diabetic rabbits no change in the blood sugar or liver glycogen after BZ 55. However, in moderate alloxan diabetes liver glycogen increase is parallel to the blood sugar decrease as in normal rabbits.

The explanation of increase in the liver glycogen by inhibition of glycogenolysis is unsatisfactory. This is because the evidence is contradictory in vitro and glycogen augmentation occurs only after high sulphonylurea concentrations (s. p. 19). The glucagon hyperglycaemia is not significantly reduced by sulphonylureas (s. p. 28). Glucose-6-phosphatase inhibition is also an unlikely causal factor, it can only be proved after 5 hrs in vivo, i.e. a long time after the decrease in blood sugar and the increase in liver glycogen (s. p. 20). Furthermore, inhibition of glycogenolysis should lead to a pathological increase in glycogen as this is the case in v. Gierke's disease. However, this is not so. Animals treated for a considerable time with sulphonylureas show only a normal or a slightly increased amount of liver glycogen (BÄNDER and SCHOLZ, CREUTZFELDT and SÜTTERLE; ROOT 1957b, CLARKE and SENMAN). However, there are some findings which support the view of increased fixation of liver glycogen. BÄNDER and SCHOLZ described a prolonged sustenance of liver glycogen in guinea-pigs in fasting conditions (this finding could not be confirmed in the rat by LANG and SHERRY); the thyroxine glycogenolysis is decreased by sulphonylureas (PERRINI and RIZZI; KÁLDOR and POGÁTSA 1959a). The post mortal glycogenolysis in the liver of rats treated with D 860 is delayed when compared to controls (KALDOR and POGÁTSA 1959b).

BERINGER and KEIBL explained the increase in liver glycogen under sulphonylurea as a sign of enhanced glucose assimilation by the liver; according to their view, sulphonylureas "guide the blood sugar stream" into the liver while insulin promotes the peripheral sugar metabolism. The decisive factor is therefore not glycogen storage, but an overall increased glucose utilization in the liver. Findings with ^{14}C-labelled glucose also speak for this. If one gives a small dose of ^{14}C labelled glucose i.v., before administering sulphonylureas, one finds increased incorporation of labelled glucose in the liver glycogen in rats and rabbits (BERINGER and HOFMANN-CREDNER; MILLER, KRAKE and VANDERBROOK; ASHMORE et al. 1958; v. HOLT and v. HOLT 1958a and c). This rise in the specific activity of liver glycogen under sulphonylureas also occurs if there is not an *absolute* increase in liver glycogen when compared to the controls, as this is the rule when compared to simultaneous glucose application. This rise is not found in adrenalectomised rats (ASHMORE et al. 1958). The ^{14}C incorporation into the fatty acids of the liver is increased at the same time if D 860 has been given after a test application of ^{14}C glucose (ASHMORE et al. 1958). The increased incorporation of ^{14}C into the liver glycogen from labelled glucose can be considered as being a specific effect for the sulphonylureas; for it does not occur under insulin. The site of insulin application for this effect is unimportant as subcutaneous injection (MILLER, KRAKE and VANDERBROOK; ASHMORE et al. 1958) also i.v. and intra-portal injections, and finally slow intra-portal infusion (v. HOLT, NOLTE and v. HOLT 1959) of insulin do not affect the specific liver glycogen activity when compared with controls.

Apart from the increased uptake of blood glucose by the liver as discussed above in the experiments with ^{14}C labelled glucose, the liver also shows increased gluconeogenesis under the influence of sulphonylureas. This has been demonstrated by an increase of the specific activity in liver glycogen after the injection of ^{14}C glycine (MILLER, KRAKE and VANDERBROOK) and after ^{14}C—NaHCO$_3$ (SUMM, CREUTZFELDT and WALLENFELS). Insulin was incapable of promoting incorporation of labelled glycine or labelled bicarbonate into liver glycogen. The evidence of gluconeogenesis has not explained the mechanism of sulphonylurea hypoglycaemia. The findings only mean that the sulphonylureas have a specific liver action not found in the case of insulin and which one can generally characterise as an activitation of glucose metabolism with an increased turnover of metabolites and glycogen. As has already been mentioned on p. 39, it is possible that the ability of the liver to effect increased CO$_2$ fixation when sulphonylureas have been given is also important for the insulin liberation from β-cells provided that similar effects could also occur in this organ (SUMM, CREUTZFELDT and WALLENFELS).

It can be said in conclusion that the studies on liver glycogen behaviour do not directly explain the occurrence of sulphonylurea hypoglycaemia. They do, however, show that sulphonylureas influence the glucose metabolism of the liver in vivo and in a way in which it is not possible to demonstrate for insulin even on portal application. It is, however, necessary to assume that exogenous or endogenous insulin must be present to produce these effects.

γ) **Fat and protein metabolism in the liver.** Injection of ^{14}C labelled glucose followed by insulin injected s.c. leads to a considerable incorporation of ^{14}C in the fatty acids in peripheral adipose tissue, but only to a moderate incorporation by the fatty acids isolated from the liver. D 860 causes, however, a more marked increase in ^{14}C-activity in the fatty acids of the liver, but not in the fatty acids of the peripheral tissues (ASHMORE et al. 1958). Liver slices of rats which had been treated for several days with D 860 incorporate ^{14}C labelled glycine in vitro into their proteins in much greater quantities than the liver slices of untreated controls (RECANT and FISÁKER). A single dose of D 860 does not yet show this effect on protein synthesis.

δ) **The action on the glucose output by the liver.** It has been reported that sulphonylureas cause a decrease in the glucose concentration in the canine hepatic veins, i.e. a decreased glucose output from the liver (ANDERSON et al. 1956, PURNELL et al., also TARDING and SCHAMBYE). The possibility exists, however, that glucose was absorbed by the intestinal territory supplied by the splanchnic nerve and experiments determining the glucose content of portal blood are especially interesting. ASHMORE et al. have taken this precaution and concluded that glucose liberation from the liver was reduced under sulphonylurea medication.

It is also possible to conclude from the above mentioned isotope investigations (s. p. 35 f.) on the decrease of specific plasma glucose activity after sulphonylurea medication (there was no proof of increased peripheral glucose utilization) that the decisive factor for this effect is liver glucose output. This is clear from the experiments of TARDING and SCHAMBYE also SCHAMBYE and TARDING. Here a constant plateau was seen in the specific activity curve spontaneously after D 860 injection in the dog. REICHARD et al. observed the same. We can therefore very probably accept the view that the blood sugar decrease after sulphonylurea dose is brought about in the liver. The crucial question is in how far this effect is actually specific for sulphonylurea action, or whether it is an insulin effect.

We cannot discuss in detail the old controversy existing since the discovery of insulin about an hepatic insulin effect. Some research will however be mentioned. While LUNDSGAARD found no increased ^{14}C glucose *uptake* by the liver in cats receiving insulin, DE DUVE believes that the rabbit liver has an increased glucose *uptake* under insulin. During the previous 2 years the question of glucose *uptake* by the liver under insulin action has been less discussed than an insulin effect on the glucose *output*. There are completely diverging opinions on this point, each side having significant experimental results and thus making it difficult for the author to be certain. This question is however of the greatest importance for the mode of action of sulphonylureas; thus, we can only answer both together. Only if the insulin has an effect on the liver glucose production, then the sulphonylurea hypoglycaemia can be based on a simple effect of insulin liberated from the *β*-cells and reaching the liver via the portal blood.

The research group of WEINHOUSE (DUNN et al., REICHARD et al.) assume on grounds of their isotope studies in which they always found plateau formation in the specific activity curve of plasma glucose after slowly applying insulin, that insulin momentarily decreases liver glucose output. SCHAMBYE and TARDING saw in similar experiments in the dog (also using portal infusion) no plateau formation. DE BODO et al. found one only rarely, and then it was not very marked so they did not believe it to be of significance. STEELE also SHOEMAKER et al. (1959a see also MAHLER et al.) said it was an artefact. The following research workers also using isotopes, the group of DE BODO (STEELE also DE BODO et al.), the group of ASHMORE (MAHLER et al., SHOEMAKER et al., 1959a and b) also the group of SCHAMBYE (SCHAMBYE and TARDING; TARDING and SCHAMBYE) concluded that insulin was not able to inhibit the hepatic glucose production. These controversial findings of the isotope method are very critically viewed owing to the unclear conditions of the glucose pool (MAHLER et al., SHOEMAKER 1959a, WRENSHALL and HÉTENYI). Therefore other investigations shall be mentioned where hepatic glucose output is measured directly. Here the results were also different. ASHMORE et al. (1958), SCHAMBYE and TARDING also SHOEMAKER et al. (1959b) saw no inhibition of hepatic glucose production even after portal insulin dose. Similar and very clear are the negative results from the experiments of SHOEMAKER et al. (1959b) using liver perfusion in vivo. Compared to this MADISON et al. (1959) found, following porto-caval cross-circulation in dogs (where there is no error in glucose uptake through the region of the splanchnic nerve) a decrease of the hepatic glucose output after insulin doses.

In judging the contradictory results of those experiments previously discussed, one should keep in mind that a positive result counts more in such complicated problems than many negative ones (STETTEN). This is true for the problem of insulin action on the liver as well as the problem of sulphonylurea action on the same organ. Also the question whether slow peripheral or intra-portal insulin application, in contrast to i.v. insulin injection, does not cause increased peripheral glucose utilization has so far been answered in different ways (s. p. 36). In these experiments one must take into account that portal insulin application is less effective on the blood sugar when compared to other methods of injection because insulin is bound in the liver (GALANSINO et al. 1958; MADISON and UNGER, 1958a; TARDING and SCHAMBYE, 1958). The possibility even exists that endogenous insulin liberated by the sulphonylurea action is altered and therefore more strongly bound to the liver than under physiological conditions (CREUTZFELDT and SÜTTERLE).

The discussion on the sulphonylurea action on the liver should only be concluded if the hepatic insulin effect is completely cleared. Until this aim has been achieved, it is the task of research workers to collect evidence for either view.

7. The influence on glucose absorption from the intestine

Although it has been shown by numerous experiments that the sulphonylureas acutely depress the blood sugar, also in the fasting animal, the possibility must be considered that inhibition of intestinal glucose absorption might be of additional significance. This possibility was supported by the investigations of FRIEDRICH et al. who injected BZ 55 i.v. 3 hrs before an oral glucose loading, and systematically determined over 5 hrs the reducing substances in the intestinal tract including the stomach. Glucose absorption was markedly delayed in animals treated with BZ 55 when compared to control rats subjected to a glucose load alone. LEE et al. also found a slightly delayed blood sugar rise after oral glucose dose in dogs premedicated with BZ 55. However, no differences were found if glucose was given i.v. KLIMAS and SEARLE (1958a) examined the effect of D 860 on glucose absorption from the small intestine of the rat (instillation of glucose alone with D 860 in the functionally eliminated intestine in situ) and found no difference as far as glucose absorption is concerned. BIRO et al. found under identical experimental conditions a distinct inhibition of glucose absorption from the small intestine. This difference can be explained by the high sulphonylurea dosage used (1800 mg/kg BZ 55 in the small intestine or parenterally). The differences found by FRIEDRICH et al. can probably be explained by the delay in the emptying time of the stomach; for SÜTTERLE observed in rats which had orally received 30 min. after D 860, a large amount of glucose solution, a surprisingly large quantity of fluid in the stomach. The same was observed in the new experiments of Kujalowá and Fabry who found after enteral and parenteral BZ 55 application no influence on the absorption rate of glucose instilled in the small intestine. However, when the stomach was included, distinct inhibition occurred. When using phenol-red, the authors were able to prove that BZ 55 and D 860 (500 mg/kg i.v.) caused a considerable delay in the emptying of the stomach, while lower doses did not show this effect. Similarly Lee et al. were unable to find a distinct effect in the time BZ 55 needed for the emptying of the stomach, or the effect it had on the peristalsis of the intestine. In any case the sulphonylurea effect on the glucose absorption from the alimentary canal appears to have a negligible role in the sulphonylurea mode of action.

III. Clinical observations with BZ 55 and D 860

a) Plasma level, degradation and excretion in man

1. BZ 55

BZ 55 is easily absorbed from the intestine. It is present in the blood as a non-acetylised sulphonamide to 85—97% (Franke and Fuchs; Achelis and Hardebeck; Ridolfo and Kirtley; Klaus and Stripecke; Wolff, Stewart and Crowley). However, 50—60% are bound to plasma proteins (albumins) (Kleinsorge 1956a; Quattrin, Jacono and Brancaccio, 1957). The distribution space is 7—11 litres according to Klaus and Stripecke; and 23.8 litres according to Stowers et al. (1958). After a single BZ 55 dose of 2—3 g, a plasma level of 10—15 mg-% was attained (Ridolfo and Kirtley, Stowers et al.). The plasma half-life time is differently quoted because it fluctuates widely (6—89 hrs.). The average half-life time was worked out to be approximately 40 hrs (Klaus and Stripecke, Baird and Duncan, 1957b, Stowers et al.; Fuchs et al.). During long-term therapy plasma levels between 6 and 20 mg-% are found (Quattrin et al. 1956, 1957; Wolff, Stewart and Crowley) using 3 grams over 20 mg-% daily (Fuchs et al.). Doubling the dose only leads to a plasma level increase of 5—6 mg-% (Hanusch and Jorke). Tubular reabsorption is 90—95% (Kleinsorge, 1956a; Quattrin et al. 1957). BZ 55 is also acetylised in the human organism. One finds about 33% of the entirely excreted sulphonamide in acetylised form (Ridolfo and Kirtley; Quattrin et al., 1957); according to Hanusch and Jorke, 50%. In diabetics who responded to BZ 55, a larger amount of conjugated sulphonamides were found in the urine than in those who did not (Wolff, Stewart and Crowley). Excretion in the faeces was only 5—8%; in the bile however, much higher BZ 55 concentrations were found than in the serum, so that enterohepatic circulation must be assumed (Quattrin et al. 1957).

BZ 55 is present in the urine and blood several days after the cessation of therapy. Cases suffering from renal sclerosis needed 11 days for complete elimination (Hanusch and Jorke). In a patient with anuria the blood level after i.v. injection of BZ 55 remained constant for 50 hrs (Stowers et al.). The clearance of BZ 55 decreases only if the glomerular filtration rate is strongly reduced (Klaus and Stripecke). The failure of the sulphonylurea therapy in the insulin deficiency diabetes (s. below) cannot be traced back to an insufficient blood-sulphonamide level as many authors have proved a sufficient BZ 55 level in juvenile diabetics.

Moeller and Hümmer also Moeller found that with a glomerular filtration rate of over 130 cm³/min (measured by endogenous creatinine clearance) a satisfactory control was never reached. If, however, the glomerular filtration rate values were less than 110 cm³/min. control was possible. Thus diabetics that responded to the therapy had a low BZ 55 clearance (under 2 cm³/min). Diabetics who responded poorly to the therapy had a higher BZ 55 clearance than those who responded well. MOELLER found contrary to WOLFF, STEWART and CROWLEY no correlation between response and degree of acetylisation.

2. D 860

D 860 is also easily absorbed. According to PFEIFFER, SCHÖFFLING, STEIGERWALD, DITSCHUNEIT and HEUBEL (1957), there are great individual differences in the rate of absorption. This can act on the rate of blood sugar decrease. D 860 is bound to serum albumin to 40—50% (WITTENHAGEN, MOHNIKE and LANGENBECK). Almost only unaltered D 860 is found in the serum; besides this, small amounts of carbonic acid can also be proved and occasionally also hydroxymethyl compounds (STOWERS et al. 1958; WITTENHAGEN et al. 1959). Degradation to carbonic acid in man is as in most other species (comp. p. 12). The distribution space for D 860 is 13 litres (STOWERS et al.) and is thus much smaller than that for BZ 55 found by the same authors. After a single dose of 3—4 g D 860, blood sugar levels of 20—30 mg-% are found within 3—4 hrs (PFEIFFER, SCHÖFFLING, STEIGERWALD, DITSCHUNEIT and HEUBEL, 1957; MOHNIKE and WITTENHAGEN, 1957; STOWERS et al., 1958). In patients suffering from liver disease, lower plasma levels are found than normally (SÜDHOF, ALTENBURG and SANDER). The plasma half-life time of D 860 is much shorter than that of BZ 55 and is only 3—8 hrs (BAIRD and DUNCAN, 1957b, STOWERS et al., SÜDHOF et al., 1958a). SÜDHOF, ALTENBURG and SANDER found, following long-term treatment for several months, that the rate of elimination of D 860 had increased by 20% compared to that at the commencement of treatment. Thus adaptation to medication occurred. Corresponding to the short half-life time, remarkably low D 860 fasting blood levels averaging 7 mg-% were found during prolonged therapy (BAIRD and DUNCAN; MOHNIKE and WITTENHAGEN). As the level is below that therapeutically effective, treatment using two daily doses is recommended where there is poor response (BAIRD and DUNCAN, 1957b). These authors had the best therapeutic results with possibly constant blood level values of 8—18 mg-%.

About 80% of the administered D 860 was found in the urine in oxidised form as carbonic acid (WITTENHAGEN and MOHNIKE, 1956; DORFMÜLLER 1956a; FAJANS et al., 1956). This degradation product can give a large flaky precipitate with sulphosalicylic acid or picric acid (Esbach's method). This can simulate protein excretion in diabetics receiving D 860. A method was produced by which it is possible to prove protein in the urine also in the presence of carbonic acid (DORFMÜLLER, 1956b; WITTENHAGEN, 1957).

Hardly any D 860 is found in faeces. WITTENHAGEN et al. (1959) found also here slight traces of the carbonic acid. An enterohepatic D 860 circulation can be assumed, as after i.v. D 860 dose the concentration in the duodenal content (containing diluted bile) is equal to that found in the blood and therefore, should be much higher in undiluted bile (SÜDHOF et al., 1958b). No exact research has been done on D 860 clearance. STOWERS et al. measured the plasma half-life time in various cases with renal disease and found a decrease in the elimination rate and a reduction in the glomerular filtration rate.

b) Results of the sulphonylurea therapy in diabetes mellitus

Since the first publication on BZ 55 therapy in diabetes (FRANKE and FUCHS; BERTRAM, BENDTFELDT and OTTO, 1955), and D 860 (MOHNIKE and STOETTER, 1956), countless reports have appeared in all parts of the world confirming these observations. New discoveries were however not included in later publications so

4*

that there is a unified picture today of the clinical oral diabetes therapy with sulphonylureas based on careful control of ten thousands of diabetics. It is difficult to estimate to what extent the sulphonylurea therapy has been applied throughout the world, as the indications vary greatly and also the conceptions in the different countries of the ideal diabetic control. In many clinics in the USA being influenced by the Joslin School, good diabetes control means fasting blood sugar values of under 110 mg-%, and postprandial values of under 150 mg-% after one hour, under 130 mg-% after 2 hrs, and under 110 mg-% after 3 hrs. Also glucose excretion must not exceed 2 g/24 hrs. A fair control is present when the fasting blood sugar values are under 130 mg-% and the postprandial blood sugar values do not exceed after 1 hr 180 mg-%, after 2 hrs 150 mg-%, after 3 hrs again 130 mg-% and the total glucose excretion in 24 hrs 5 grams. All values exceeding these are considered poorly-controlled (CAMERINI-DAVALOS, ROOT and MARBLE). Due to these very high standards of judging a good diabetes control, there are more diabetics requiring treatment than if the standards were lower. Added to this is that the relatively high fat and poor carbohydrate diet prescribed by many American diabetologists makes it difficult to control mild diabetes with diet alone and increases the daily insulin requirement. Only by this reasoning can the large number of patients treated with D 860 in the USA (according to O'DONOVAN, the Upjohn-Company in the USA sold D 860 in 1959 to over 500,000 diabetics) and the relatively high insulin dosage which could be replaced by sulphonylureas be understood (s. p. 53).

Great Britain goes to the opposite extreme. Here there is severe dietary control of over-weight diabetics and an additional insulin or sulphonylurea dosage is only justified if there is no improvement in metabolism after decrease in weight. The British believe that 40—50% of all diabetics can be treated by diet alone, 35—40% need insulin and only the remaining 10—25% require sulphonylurea treatment (BAIRD also DUNLOP et al.).

In Germany SCHÖFFLING, PFEIFFER et al. (1957a) compared the material of the Frankfurter diabetic out-patients in the time before and after introduction of the sulphonylurea therapy. They found that the per-cent of the patients treated by diet had only decreased slightly from 15.7 to 12.9%. These very low figures cannot be regarded as representative for those patients treated by diet alone in the whole diabetic population, as the mildest cases are not under the control of the diabetic out-patients clinic. Before the introduction of sulphonylurea therapy, 84.3% of patients were treated with insulin, 2 years later only 42.8%. 43% of the diabetics received D 860.

These figures of approximately 40% of all diabetics as aspirants for sulphonylurea therapy correlate to most continental European results. Increased positive results up to 90% are due to the investigator having chosen his patients from the beginning; therefore, nothing can be deduced (HEINSEN and HAGEN). Against the figural results of SCHÖFFLING et al. (1957a), the main contingent of diabetics treated with sulphonylureas today, are from the "diet group"; shown by the fact insulin production in all countries was first increased after the introduction of sulphonylureas, and only now is the production static or reduced. It cannot be said by this that most sulphonylurea treated diabetics take superfluous tablets. As many moderately severe diabetics used to protest against the daily insulin dosage, indicative insulin therapy was dispensed with. Here diabetics were satisfactorily stabilised in the clinic on diet alone, but at home did not restrict themselves to it and are now well compensated with diet plus sulphonylureas also at home. This group should not be treated with sulphonylureas according to many British authors. One must not overlook the fact that dietary restrictions require severe self-discipline in many people. However, it is remarkable that on performing the so-called double blind experiment, an astonishingly large number of patients responded to placebos (HURWITZ and McCUISTION). These observations show the importance of stern measures in the indication of sulphonylurea therapy in mild cases of diabetes.

The following data have been compiled from the whole world. As it generally corresponds, we will not mention each author separately. Some work has been done on BZ 55 some on D 860 and some on both substances as shown by the titles. The same basic conclusions were reached. The main difference between both preparations were the more frequent side-effects found with BZ 55 probably owing to its sulphonamide character and slight differences in effectiveness. As BZ 55, owing to its longer plasma half-life time, retains a higher blood level than does D 860 (s. p. 50); it is slightly more effective for long-term treatment than D 860 (BERTRAM 1958, HOFSTETTER and RAMEL, ILLIG 1958, MARK 1958). The stronger effectiveness was, however, only true for a small group of diabetics in whom a long-term sulphonylurea therapy was problematic in any case owing to an insufficient metabolic compensation (s. under secondary failures p. 59 f.). As a rule one can change from one preparation to the other using the same dose and control does not deteriorate (MOHNIKE and STÖTTER; HEINSEN and HAGEN, WEHLING 1956, MELZER and SACHSSE).

The following authors report of therapeutical results with BZ 55 and D 860 in a larger number of patients (compiled data does not claim to be complete, nomination is ordered according to publication date): BERTRAM, BENDTFELDT and OTTO 1955, 1956, 1957, JACOBI and KAMMRATH, SCHNEEWEISS et al., RAMEL and HOFSTETTER, BOULIN 1956, MOHNIKE and STÖTTER 1956, CONSTAM et al. 1956, MOREAU et al., HEINSEN and HAGEN, ROBBERS and SPECK, MELLINGHOFF 1956, DUNCAN et al. 1956, WOLFF et al., HUNT et al., McKENZIE et al., WALKER et al., COX et al. 1956a, CAMERINI-DAVALOS et al. 1956, 1957, McGAVACK et al. 1956, FULMER et al. 1956, 1957, DOLGER 1956, 1957, WEHLING 1956, MELZER and SACHSSE, FUCHS et al. 1957, HALLER 1957, STEIGERWALDT 1957, BOLLER and KÖCK, McKENDRY et al. 1957, MOHNIKE, ULRICH and JUTZI, SCHÖFFLING, STEIGERWALD et al. 1957a, SEIDLER et al. (STÖTTER), SUGAR 1957, GOLD 1957, CONSTAM 1957, ILLIG 1958, SCHRICKER 1958, BERTRAM 1958, HOFSTETTER and RAMEL, MEHNERT and CAMERINI-DAVALOS, v. UEXKÜLL 1958, STÖTTER 1958, O'DONOVAN.

1. Investigations on the controllability of diabetics using oral therapy

α) **Statistical results.** Already during the first clinical examination, it was seen that only certain diabetics responded to sulphonylurea therapy (BERTRAM et al. 1955, 1956, JACOBI and KAMRATH; MOHNIKE and STÖTTER 1956). Since then correlation has been proved between the control possibility with sulphonylureas and constitution (simply stated as body weight), age, age of manifestation of diabetes, duration of diabetes, length of previous insulin treatment, necessary insulin dose, also diabetic complications. As the observations are uniform they will be collectively dealt with. Recently O'DONOVAN (1959) confirmed them by statistics on more than 9146 diabetics treated with D 860. MOHNIKE, ULRICH and JUTZI (1957a and b) produced a conscientious statistical analysis of the conditions of controllability from the material of 1000 diabetics treated with D 860 as in-patients; of these, 600 could be well controlled. The results of these authors, which agreed with those of countless others, were based on the following data.

Body weight. First it was found that diabetics suffering from over-weight responded better to sulphonylureas than normal or under-weight diabetics. This difference cannot be ascertained in patients requiring under 10 U of insulin, but is very definite in those requiring 10—20 U. Normal or under-weight diabetics having an insulin demand of over 30 U cannot be controlled by sulphonylureas. Over-weight is a typical characteristic of the lipoplethoric diabetes with only a relative insulin deficiency (s. introduction). From these observations can already be seen that the type of diabetes plays a significant role. Numerically expressed, control of the adipose diabetic was possible in 72%, of thin diabetics only in 27.5% (MOHNIKE, ULRICH and JUTZI 1957 b). According to BERTRAM et al. (1957) the constitution is not important in mild cases but is of significance in patients requiring insulin.

Insulin dose. The greater the insulin demand the smaller is the chance of a beneficial sulphonylurea therapy. The best chance of success is with insulin requirements up to 20 U. An insulin demand between 20—30 U lowers the chances to 50%; over 40 U, there are only 20%. These reports of MOHNIKE, ULRICH and JUTZI principally correspond with those of most other authors. Differences are only present regarding the critical insulin dose which is minimal in a successful sulphonylurea therapy. While HÖPKER found this limit at 20 U, North American authors at 40 U (O'DONOVAN), Austrian authors (BOLLER and KÖCK) even at 60 U. Probably these high doses are due to the variable management of insulin therapy. Also many diabetologists were able to see, owing to the change-over to oral therapy, that many diabetics were over-insulinised. On slowly reducing the insulin, sometimes the amount of insulin could be largely diminished before glucosuria or severe hyperglycaemia appeared.

Length of diabetes and of insulin therapy. The length of diabetes and previous insulin treatment has only a slight effect on the controllability. However, a certain negative correlation is present based on the fact that in diabetes of longer duration with and without insulin therapy the severity, respectively the insulin demand, increases slightly. According to BERTRAM et al. (1957) the length of the previous insulin therapy is significant in an insulin demand of over 20 U.

Age of manifestation. There is a strong positive correlation between the age in which diabetes becomes apparent and the controllability. The chances of success are good if the age of manifestation is over 40—45 years. The *chronological age* should not alone be taken into consideration, as it is the sum of age of manifestation plus the length of diabetes. Therefore, control is determined by both criteria.

Sex. These criteria are of equal importance in both sexes. A sexual factor influencing the possibilities of control is not apparent.

Hereditary. BOLLER and KÖCK investigated besides the above mentioned criteria, the influence of genetic liability to diabetes as affecting diabetic control. Generally success was unimpaired if genetic liability to diabetes was present. It is, however, remarkable that the diabetic therapeutic failures in the group were those genetically liable to diabetes on the maternal side.

The most important factors determining diabetic control are, therefore, diabetic type (roughly proportional to body weight), insulin demand and age of manifestation. Simply expressed, the chances of therapeutic success are the greater the fatter the diabetic is, the higher the manifestation age, and the lower the insulin requirement. The influence of these three factors is well expressed in Fig. 1a and b from the paper of MOHNIKE, ULRICH and JUTZI (1957a) (s. p. 55).

MOHNIKE and STÖTTER (1956) also MOHNIKE, ULRICH and JUTZI (1957b) investigated the correlation between controllability and diabetic complications. Their results depend on some of the above analysed criteria so that the controllability of diabetes is essentially determined by these factors. There was only a 50% success in diabetics without complications (the groups consisted of mild diabetics and also of juveniles with a high insulin demand). If retinopathy was present, only 30% could be controlled as here there were hardly any mild cases. 77% of the hypertensive diabetics could be controlled. This can be explained by the combination of over-weight and hypertension. When hypertension and retinopathy were both apparent 64% were successfully controlled. Only 44% of the diabetics suffering from nephropathy (with or without retinopathy or hypertension) could be controlled. This is again explained by the afore mentioned factors (early age of manifestation, high insulin demand). Considering these figures and the above mentioned criteria, certain prognosis on the controllability can be made. This prognosis is still of questionable value for the individual as not one of the criteria is 100% certain, and even on considering the most important criteria, unknown incalcuable factors play a part.

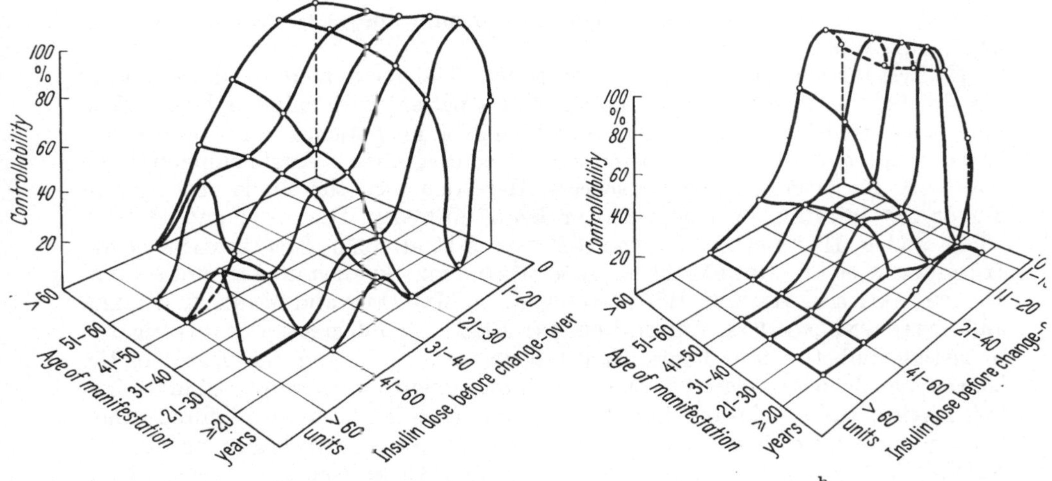

Fig. 1a and b. Controllability of diabetics with D 860 (in %) in relation to the age of manifestation of the diabetes (in years) and the insulin requirement (in units) for over-weight (a) and normal and under-weight (b) patients. After MOHNIKE, ULRICH and JUTZI (1957a)

This still does not mean that for the *practice of diabetic treatment* every non-sulphonylurea treated diabetic should be subjected to a therapeutic trial. In fact, one can exclude at the start the following from sulphonylurea treatment: juvenile diabetics (age of manifestation under 40 years) with an insulin demand of over 20 U or (in the case of recently manifested diabetes) with glucosuria of over 50 g/day under standard diet and definite acetonuria.

It stands to reason that this is also the case if acidosis is present. Also those diabetics with a manifestation age of over 40 are not suitable for sulphonylurea treatment under the following conditions: 1. history of coma diabeticum, 2. glucosuria of over 50 g/day on a standard diet, 3. definite acetonuria respectively heavy acetonuria and glucosuria after insulin is withheld. Thus, acetonuria is an important criterium for the controllability of diabetes in practice. Finally acetonuria and tendency to ketoacidosis are typical for insulin deficiency diabetics who do not respond to sulphonylurea therapy. Most diabetics belong to this type with manifestation before the age of 40, also 20—30% of those that fall ill later. As exception to those general rules previously described that are only meant to fill statistical gaps, are some observations on juvenile diabetics. Only single observations have been published on sulphonylurea treatment in the recently manifest child and juvenile diabetic. FERRET and IZARD were able to compensate metabolism satisfactorily with D 860 alone in a ten-year old child with blood sugar values of over 500 mg-% and acetonuria, for an eight month period of observation. A similar case of a child being successfully treated with D 860 is described by LARSON. Besides countless unsuccessfully treated children and juveniles, many research workers found single cases where at least temporarily a control was reached with D 860, or combined with small insulin doses response to sulphonylurea therapy (OTTO 1956, MOHNIKE and STÖTTER 1956; CONSTAM et al.; HEINSEN and HAGEN 1956, BEASER 1956; WEHLING 1956, CAMERINI-DAVALOS et al. 1957, LESTRADET et al., 1957; BERTRAM 1958b). Owing to the rareness of these positive observations, change-over experiments with juvenile diabetics are no longer justifiable. An exception being, if the insulin demand is very low. Rarely, diabetics suffering from acidosis were successfully controlled (BROGLIE et al., HALLER) partially after introductory insulin doses. According to general experience, it is not adviseable.

β) **Test methods for judging controllability.** The above mentioned criteria are not sufficient to forsee the controllability of a patient with sulphonylureas. Also much time is needed for optimally controlling in or out-patients. For these reasons, it was soon tried to correlate blood sugar decrease after a single sulphonylurea dose with the later therapeutic success. Here one used the single oral dose of 3 g or i.v. injection of 1 g D 860 or BZ 55 (MIRSKY, DIENGOTT and DOLGER 1956a and b, HUNT et al., CAMERINI-DAVALOS et al. 1956, BRAVERMANN et al., HEINEMANN et al., DUNCAN et al. 1956, PFEIFFER, SCHÖFFLING, STEIGERWALD, DITSCHUNEIT and HEUBEL 1957, SACHSSE also MEHNERT and MARBLE, HALLER and STRAUZENBERG 1958, MEYER-LEDDIN). Blood sugar decrease was investigated in fasting diabetics four hours after tablets were given and the degree of the blood sugar decrease related to the success of a long-term therapy. All investigators reached the conclusion that this method of testing has only a limited value. It is only possible to separate a certain group of diabetics at the beginning who will certainly not respond to sulphonylurea therapy. These would be those patients who only show a slight blood sugar decrease (under 30% from the initial value). In agreement with this fact is that in diabetics in fasting conditions already without sulphonylurea doses there is a blood sugar decrease averaging 25% after 4 hrs (SACHSSE; HALLER and STRAUZENBERG).

If the diabetic has a chance of successful control with sulphonylureas, the blood sugar level must show a decrease of more than 30% according to PFEIFFER et al.; according to HALLER and STRAUZENBERG also MEYER-LEDDIN even more than 40—50%. However, even in these strong blood sugar reductions there are still many therapeutic failures. Thus the practical value of the test is low, especially as it gives no indication of a possible secondary failing of the sulphonylurea therapy. According to MEHNERT and MARBLE the fasting blood sugar during the test day must also be taken into consideration. The higher the fasting blood sugar is, the stronger must be the decrease in the blood sugar after 4 hrs if there is to be a chance of success (at 120 mg-% fasting values, 20% decrease is sufficient, at 250 mg-%, however, 60% are required; in other words, the blood sugar must practically fall to normal values). Also MEHNERT and MARBLE see the value of the test more as a possibility for excluding a certain diabetic group from sulphonylurea therapy at the beginning. Besides the time saved by this method, it has also the advantage of showing the cooperative patient why he is not suitable for sulphonylurea therapy. This is especially important in American patients. WILD-HACK also propagates normalisation of the blood sugar after 4 hrs if a beneficial prognosis can be made as to the result of oral therapy. He emphasises however, that about 50% of the patients who do not come under these criteria later respond to sulphonylurea therapy.

γ) Therapeutic successes in special cases of diabetes and effect in rare disturbances in the carbohydrate metabolism. Especially interesting is the reaction of rare types of diabetes and other unusual disturbances in carbohydrate metabolism to sulphonylurea treatment. Owing to the rarity of these conditions, the problems have no practical significance. However, observations on these conditions show interesting points on the mode of action of these drugs.

Diabetes following pancreatectomy. Patients suffering from mild diabetes following partial pancreatectomy respond well to sulphonylureas (MOHNIKE and STÖTTER 1956; MILLER and CRAIG 1956). In more severe diabetes following pancreas destruction through pancreatitis or partial pancreatectomy or carcinoma of the pancreas, no blood sugar decreasing effect with D 860 could be proved (MOORHOUSE and KARK; STEIGERWALD, PFEIFFER, SCHÖFFLING and DITSCHUNEIT; JACKSON et al.). Also after total pancreatectomy, no effect on the blood sugar or glucosuria could be achieved either by oral or intravenous sulphonylurea doses (OGRYZLO and HARRISON; COX et al. 1956a; FAJANS et al. 1956, MILLER and CRAIG 1956, PURNELL et al.; GOETZ et al. 1956, CREUTZFELDT, KÜMMERLE and KERN; McGULLACH and GOEBERT). In several patients permanent sulphonylurea doses were given in order to reduce insulin. In the case of OGRYZLO and HARRISON this was hardly successful, and in those of COX et al. (1956a) also PURNELL et al. completely unsuccessful. Also the blood sugar decrease following i.v. insulin dose in two totally pancreatectomised patients was not intensified by simultaneous i.v. injection of 2 grams D 860 (CREUTZFELDT, KÜMMERLE and KERN). Likewise, the blood sugar curve was not modified following combined infusion of insulin and glucose by D 860 (McGULLACH and GOEBERT). Here, observations in man correspond to those found in animal experiments. Contrary to the insulin potentiating effect of sulphonylureas (comp. p. 24) described for the dog however, this could not be proved in man.

Bronze diabetes. In 9 cases of diabetes in patients suffering from haemochromatosis, sulphonylureas alone or in combination with insulin were given. In all cases a certain effect on hyperglycaemia and glucosuria was not found; it was also not possible to reduce insulin (JACOBI and KAMMRATH; MILLER and CRAIG 1956; MOHNIKE, ULRICH and JUTZI 1957b; CREUTZFELDT and SCHLAGINTWEIT; STEIGERWALD, PFEIFFER, SCHÖFFLING and DITSCHUNEIT 1957; HOFSTETTER and RAMEL). If from the general view that bronze diabetes is a real pancreas diabetes following β-cell damage by haemosiderin deposits, then this uniform finding of various investigators correlates with the other observations, namely that the sulphonylureas are ineffective in insulin deficiency diabetes. It is possible that in mild cases of bronze diabetes a certain effect can be achieved comparable to the positive results in mild alloxan diabetes (comp. p. 24 f.).

Steroid diabetes. In a series of cases where diabetes appeared during steroid therapy, the sulphonylureas were practically without effect (STÖTTER and CREUTZFELDT; DOWNIE et al. 1956; BERGENSTAL et al.; CREUTZFELDT and SCHLAGINTWEIT). Only MOORHOUSE and KARK described one case where a slight blood sugar decrease occurred through D 860. CREUTZFELDT and SCHLAGINTWEIT found only on the first day of sulphonylurea therapy, in 3 of their 4 cases, a transient recession of glucosuria of 50%; also in the case of BERGENSTAL et al. a slight, but completely insufficient effect was present. Metabolic recompensation was achieved in no case. One can conclude from this that sulphonylureas have no strong effect on the complex metabolic disturbances produced by the glucorticoid therapy. As, however, steroid diabetes in man only appears if an increased insulin demand due to

β-cell inadequacy cannot be compensated, these observations clearly show that in man sulphonylureas require a functional β-cell remnant for their anti-diabetic effect.

Cushing syndrome with diabetes. Several authors attempted controlling patients suffering from morbus Cushing and diabetes with sulphonylureas. The results are contradictory. MOHNIKE and STÖTTER; MILLER and CRAIG; BREDNOW and JORKE; MOHNIKE, ULRICH and JUTZI 1957 b reported of good response in the Cushing diabetic. Other authors found sulphonylureas ineffective (BARTEL-HEIMER and MARING, FAJANS et al. 1956). Probably the possibility of a sulphonyl-urea effect depends on the degree of the functional reserves in the β-cells system. According to the nomenclature of experimental diabetology, there is a chance of therapeutic success in the so-called idiosteroid diabetes, while metasteroid diabetes is refractory to sulphonylurea therapy. This corresponds to the animal experimental findings (comp. p. 26).

Diabetes with acromegalia. Also in patients with diabetes and acromegalia caused by intra-sellar tumours, varying successes were seen. In some cases the trial was successful with sulphonylureas (MOHNIKE and STÖTTER; MOORHOUSE and KARK; BREDNOW and JORKE; FIELD and FEDERMAN; LACHNIT and TRETEN-HAHN; BERGENSTAL et al. 1957). Other authors saw no effect of the sulphonyl-ureas in diabetics with acromegalia (MOHNIKE and STÖTTER; BARTELHEIMER and MARING; FAJANS et al. 1956; FIELD and FEDERMAN, an own unpublished case). Again, the different results can be explained by the severity of the respective diabetes and also by the degree of the β-cell insufficiency. While patients re-sponding to therapy had as a rule only mild diabetes, failures had stronger glucosuria. Here there is also good parallelity to the experiences gained in the animal experiments (idio-and metahypophyseal diabetes s. p. 26).

Hyperthyroidism. According to MOHNIKE, ULRICH and JUTZI (1957) also STÖTTER (1958), diabetics suffering also from hyperthyroidism respond less well than do other diabetics, the remaining criteria being equal. VON UEXKÜLL (1958), however, found no difference in therapeutical response in diabetics with and with-out hyperthyroidism.

Abnormally high insulin requirements (insulin resistance). In a series of cases with abnormally high insulin requirements (over 200 U/day), and in which no antibodies against insulin could be proved, sulphonylurea therapy was commenced. MILLER and CRAIG (1956) achieved a moderate effect of D 860 in a case of lipo-atrophic-diabetes with 500 U insulin demand. CREUTZFELDT and SCHLAGINTWEIT were able to decrease the insulin requirement with combined treatment of insulin and D 860 from 600 to 60 U/day in a patient with a liver cirrhosis and hepatogenic insulin resistance not caused by antibodies. It was also possible in 2 other cases with cirrhosis of the liver and diabetes, having abnormally high insulin require-ments without demonstrable antibodies, to reduce the insulin doses by admin-istering D 860 (SCHÖFFLING 1957, BILHAN). In a fourth case with insulin resistance (320 U) following jaundice, the BZ 55 dose only led to a transitory reduction in the insulin requirement to 30 U (UHRY et al.).

The case of FRIEDLANDER (FRIEDLANDER also FRIEDLANDER and BRYANT) is slightly different, as here there was found no liver damage by biopsy. However, there was simultaneously an insulin allergy and increased plasma insulin binding. Doses of D 860 succeeded in reducing the insulin demand that was partly over several thousands units per day by 75%, and in a second attempt by 33%. ACTH also reduced abnormal insulin requirements. Therefore, FRIEDLANDER believes that D 860 acted as an inhibitor in his unusual case on the insulin binding factors. Besides these impressive cases, it was diversly possible, by combined doses of sulphonylureas and insulin, to improve a continuously bad metabolism with insulin requirements of 70—120 U and to even replace the insulin (KOTZ et al.; ANGELI 1957; SILVER and NAGEL; CONSTAM 1957). Many similar cases have probably not been published. The observations show that in cases of insulin resistance or abnormally high insulin requirements where often great therapeutical difficulties are present, sulphonylureas should be tried. Hereby, the effect is only apparent after several days and when using very high doses. The cases with so-called hepatic insulin resistance seemed to have the best chance of success. Nothing is known about the mode of action of the therapeutic successes, as the origin of the hepatic insulin resistance is still unclear.

Diabetes renalis. Renal glucosuria in a child (SAUERBREI) and in an adult (CREUTZFELDT and SCHLAGINTWEIT) remained unchanged during sulphonylurea dosage for several days. Therefore, the pathological disturbance of glucose reabsorption is as little influenced as the normal renal glucose threshold.

Diabetes with islet cell adenoma. The combination of diabetes with islet cell adenoma is very rare. GITTLER et al. described a case complicated by liver cirrhosis and a colon tumour where there was very little insulin in the pancreatic tumour. However, they found for diabetes an unusually strong blood sugar depression after D 860 doses and suggest a sulphonylurea loading as a diagnostic test for a suspected islet adenoma.

PFEIFFER et al. (1969 b and c) observed after i.v. doses of D 860 and meta-hexamide in a non-diabetic with a large islet cell adenoma a blood sugar decrease of unusual duration. This is contrary to the rapid re-increase in the blood sugar found in the metabolically normal patient after sulphonylurea injection (comp. p. 75). At the same time an increase of plasma insulin activity, which speaks for insulin release from the tumour, was found to be due to the sulphonylureas. After the extirpation of the tumour, the blood sugar lowering effect following sulphonyl-urea injection was normal. As the estimation of plasma insulin activity is only possible in few places, it is interesting to know whether the continuous blood sugar decrease and missing re-increase for many hours is proof of an islet adenoma. According to FAJANS and CONN (1959), it is only so with certain limitations. A clear hypoglycaemia of shorter duration is, however, seen in a case of morbus Addison (FAJANS and CONN), and in some cases of liver cirrhosis (KAUP comp. p. 75). As both diseases can show spontaneous hypoglycaemia, these must first be exempted. In any case, here is an interesting diagnostic possibility and its value must be further examined. In two own cases with islet cell adenoma in non-diabetic persons, the injection of one gram D 860 i.v. produced severe hypo-glycaemic shock, after 30 respectively 45 mins which made glucose injection necessary. Therefore, it was not possible to wait for the missing re-increase. After these experiences we believe that the appearance of real hypoglycaemic shock after injection of 1.0 g D 860 in the normal person is highly suspicious for hyper-insulinism because we have never seen such an event in healthy subjects before.

v. Gierke's glycogen storage disease. In a case having a glycogen storage disease which did not react to glucagon with a blood sugar rise, BULGARELLI found a clear blood sugar decrease following BZ 55. This observation is theoretically interesting as it shows that a blood sugar decrease following sulphonylurea doses also occurs if liver glycogenolysis is inhibited, shown not only by the pathological glycogen storage, but also in their special case by a negative glucagon test.

2. Lasting success, indication and contra-indication, treatment

α) The problem of the so-called secondary failures in diabetes therapy. Generally the metabolism remains compensated even for months and years in patients that respond well to sulphonylurea therapy. HEINSEN and HAGEN (1956) were the first to indicate the possibility that sulphonylureas lose their effect in a series of cases on longer medication, e.g. after some time there is a re-increase in the blood sugar and glucosuria. First it is often possible to compensate the metabolism for a while by increasing the sulphonylurea dosage or sometimes by a change-over to another drug. (CHRISTOFFEL was able to continue treatment successfully with BZ 55 in most D 860 secondary failures.) Finally, however, the cases were totally refractory. This phenomenon of mitigation of the sulphonylurea effect was greatly discussed and rechecked. It was one of the main topics of discussion in the colloquium in Hamburg in 1957 (comp. BERTRAM and KUNTZE). In special papers the following authors have stated their point of view: PFEIFFER, SCHÖFFLING, STEIGERWALD, TRESER and OTTO, 1957; EDLEN et al., 1957; HEINSEN, 1958; WELLER, 1958; OTTO-BENDTFELDT and OTTO; DOTEVALL, 1958; STRAUZENBERG, HALLER and MEYER; MEHNERT, CAMERINI-DAVALOS and MARBLE; MOSS et al., 1959.

The first alarming observation has lost its horror by these detailed analysis. As was rightly feared by several authors, this could be a general phenomenon appearing sooner or later in all patients treated with sulphonylureas thus rendering sulphonylurea therapy in diabetes only temporarily useful. The generally accepted reason for this being an exhausion of the β-cells through the continuous stimulation, thus a real insulin deficiency diabetes with absolute insulin deficiency developed from a stable maturity-onset diabetes with only a relative insulin deficit. The frequency of these findings varied (up to 14%).

In the meantime, it has been seen that completely different aspects were conglomerated. First those metabolic deteriorations already present in the first weeks after the beginning of treatment (termed secondary failures in the narrow sense by some authors contrary to those not controllable primary failures) can be neglected as they are rare. More important are the so-called late therapeutic failures first apparent after 6—8 weeks. Only this group is of interest and according to the general terms described as the secondary failure group. In the majority of cases secondary failure occurs between the fourth to sixth month of treatment (PFEIFFER et al., 1957). STRAUZENBERG et al. (1958) described coincidence in the time secondary failures became manifest and the quality of previous control, e.g. in badly controlled diabetics metabolic decompensation appeared after 3—4 months, while in well controlled diabetics only after 16 months.

Exogenous factors were found to be the most frequent cause of secondary failure. Primarily the adherence to *diet* was not strict. HEINSEN (1958) emphasises correctly that in the case of dietary mistakes one should refrain from speaking of the failure of tablet therapy as one must then also talk of an insulin therapeutic failure when the condition of an insulin controlled diabetic deteriorates owing to non-adherence to the prescribed diet. Here is only shown that a successful permanent therapy with sulphonylureas is only possible if the rules of diabetes diet are strictly abided by. Secondly, infections, traumas, and operations are important; they also increase insulin requirements as is well known. Increasing tablet dosage usually does not have the same effect as increasing the insulin dose of diabetics injecting it. Therefore, there is danger of decompensation, and is often the beginning of a permanent sulphonylurea resistence. It is, however, remarkable that the insulin requirements are later not more than before the sulphonylurea therapy.

Finally there remains a group of patients in which no cause for the mitigation of the sulphonylurea effect can be found. Analysing these cases, almost all authors concluded that the majority were not optimally controlled from the beginning, e.g. always elevated blood sugar values and glucosuria of 10—20/24 hrs were present (PFEIFFER et al. 1957; OTTO-BENDTFELDT and OTTO; STRAUZENBERG et al.). Thus, here are mainly concealed primary failures, patients that should never have been put on permanent sulphonylurea therapy. OTTO-BENDTFELDT and OTTO found no single case among their 24 secondary failures having previously responded optimally to sulphonylureas, while 60% had only shown just passable metabolic compensation from the beginning. STRAUZENBERG et al. had 4.2% failures among 1000 diabetics. On clearing the state of metabolism, only 0.6% of the well controlled patients showed secondary failure, 7% in the moderately controlled, 13% in the unsatisfactorily controlled. From this is clearly shown that stern criteria must be used when applying permanent sulphonylurea therapy if the numbers of secondary failures are to be kept low. If these conditions are observed, the whole problem loses its significance. However, the fact that secondary failures do exist shows how important a careful control of the diabetics treated by tablets is. General experience shows that it is senseless in the case of secondary failures to increase the sulphonylurea dose to over 2—3 g/day. It is even pointless in combined doses of insulin and tablets (STRATMAN). It is advisable in most cases to change-over to insulin. Recently it was reported that the addition of biguanides (often in very low doses which produce no side-effects) compensated the metabolism again; thus, the oral therapy could be maintained (comp. p. 136).

Of great theoretical interest is the question whether the insulin requirements are greater following secondary failure of the sulphonylurea therapy than before the beginning of tablet treatment. Single observations on increased insulin requirements were published. On analysing larger groups of patients, it was seen that these were exceptions. PFEIFFER et al. (1957) found in 41 of their secondary failures previously treated with insulin an average increased demand of only 0.7 U insulin; STRAUZENBERG et al. saw in 19 of their diabetics previously insulin treated an average increased demand of 1.7 U. There were also cases that required less insulin than before. Only in exceptional cases was the insulin requirement greatly increased. It is significant in this connection that diabetics permanently injected with insulin show a greater increase in their insulin demand. PFEIFFER, SCHÖFFLING, STEIGERWALD, TRESER and OTTO (1957) found an average increase in the insulin demand of 8.3 U, SCHNEEWEISS, of 8.6 U in a larger group of patients. The fact that insulin requirements do not increase in secondary failures speaks against β-cell exhaustion as being their common cause. In the process HEINSEN (1958) describes as metamorphosis of a secondary insulin deficiency diabetes, the insulin deficit must grow larger and thus also the insulin requirement. Only in the extremely rare cases where this is so, β-cell exhaustion is to blame for causing secondary failures; this would correspond to similar animal experimental observations (s. p. 37 f.). The animal experiments have shown that neither after partial pancreatectomy (CREUTZFELDT and GEGINAT) nor following doses of alloxan (LAZAROW and TREIBERGS), i.e. after reduction of the β-cells, is the latent diabetic metabolism changed to a manifest diabetes by sulphonylurea doses.

Why the secondary failures occur in the other cases where insulin requirements are not intensified—this group being much larger—cannot be said for certain.

β) **Indication and contra-indication.** *Indications* in using sulphonylurea treatment are given from the above mentioned criteria for controllability. Thus, primarily those whose diabetes becomes manifest after the age of 40 can be considered, showing an unsatisfactory metabolism on diet alone, e.g. still excreting glucose and showing postprandial blood sugar values of over 180 mg-%. Here the insulin requirements as a rule should not exceed 30 U. These are mostly elderly patients suffering from mild diabetes. In obese patients, sulphonylurea therapy has the advantage over insulin of causing no, or only slight increase in weight

(HALLER and STRAUZENBERG). Therapeutic attempts are furthermore justified in certain special forms of diabetes, and when abnormally high insulin requirements not based on antibodies are present. Under certain circumstances, one must accept in old, solitary patients having difficulties with the daily insulin injections, a sub-optimal control with sulphonylureas; as irregularly, or wrongly dosed insulin, has greater dangers (especially hypoglycaemia) than the sulphonylureas.

Not indicated are the sulphonylureas in juvenile diabetics and older patients with acidosis tendencies, e.g. in insulin deficiency diabetics further in acute diabetic complications due to infections and operations. This is primarily so where diabetes is found for the first time during an infection or necessary operation. To avoid risks one must reach a satisfactory insulin control and wait for the complications to subside.

However, it is not necessary to interrupt the sulphonylurea therapy in every diabetic controlled with sulphonylureas who undergoes an operation or infection. Conscientious control is much more necessary in these cases and to arrest impending decompensation with insulin. Namely it has been shown in many cases that sulphonylurea therapy can be continued without danger. This is particularly true for banal infections.

Also in *surgical complications* arising in diabetes (diabetic gangrene, boils, abscesses, abdominal surgery and urological intervention) PRÖSCHER could observe 92 patients showing excellent results on sulphonylureas and diet alone. PRÖSCHER saw good healing tendency in abscesses and gangrene after BZ 55 as after D 860. Thus this is not based on bacteriostatic action but must be connected with the metabolic effect. Other authors, however, saw poor healing tendency in diabetic gangrene after sulphonylureas and thought this complication to be a contraindication (MILLER and CRAIG, MELLINGHOFF 1956, DUMMER, 1957, BOLLER and KÖCK, STRAUZENBERG and HALLER 1959b). Finally one must decide in each case whether sulphonylurea treatment can be continued or not. In every case optimal control is essential. If this is so, even operations can be performed under sulphonylureas, as insulin therapy can be introduced at any time. Under circumstances, sulphonylurea therapy is much simpler to handle than insulin because the parenteral feeding necessary in the insulinised diabetic pre- and post-operational is often not necessary (CANARY et al., 1959).

Extensive research on the question of possible success in treating tubercular diabetics with sulphonylureas has been done (KÖNIGSTEIN and SUESS; MOHNIKE, ULRICH and JUTZI, 1957b; BLECHER, 1958; WELLS and BOCK; IRSKENS, 1958; SCHLIACK and SCHILLING; PFAFFENBERG). In general it may be said that control is possible under the same criteria as in non-tubercular diabetics. Only in feverish tuberculosis the therapeutic prognosis is unfavorable. IRSKENS, however, had the impression that with otherwise equal criteria, tubercular patients responded principally less well to sulphonylurea therapy than controls. MOHNIKE, ULRICH and JUTZI found this especially in cases with productive cirrhotic lung tuberculosis. On reaching an optimal metabolic state, permanent sulphonylurea therapy in tubercular diabetics is possible according to corresponding views. The course of tuberculosis is the same as under insulin therapy. However, regular metabolic control is indicated as PFAFFENBERG saw more secondary failures in tubercular diabetics than are known for the non-tubercular. Incompatibility with the usual tuberculostatic drugs is unusual. Only BRAUCH reported of the appearance of strong headaches and vertigo on simultaneous dosing with p-amino-salicylic acid and BZ 55 in one case.

Some authors considered sulphonylurea therapy in *arteriosclerotic changes* (cerebral and coronary sclerosis) to be more advantageous than insulin therapy provided that a satisfactory metabolic state had been attained through the sulphonylureas (STOETTER, 1958b; STRAUZENBERG and HALLER, 1959b). The danger of an insufficient blood supply to the organs arising by the additional glycopenia that can never be completely prevented under insulin is negligible with sulphonylurea therapy as here hypoglycaemic reactions are very rare. STOETTER (1958b) diversely saw about 2 weeks after commencing D 860 therapy, even recession of attacks of angina pectoris in diabetics. It is interesting that recession of angina pectoris in non-diabetics receiving D 860 was described (SINGH and BARDHAN). Improvements in the ECG are also cited; they are believed to be caused by a blood lactate decrease through D 860. Negative influence of the sulphonylureas has not been found.

The sulphonylureas apparently do not have a specific effect on *serum lipid changes* in diabetes. They might have been important in indicating sulphonylurea therapy in arteriosclerosis. BÖHLE et al., however, saw in a successfully D 860 treated diabetic displaying metabolic improvement a decrease in the total lipids and cholesterol. Other authors were not able to see a systematic decrease in the serum lipids (MUNRO and MURRAY; McGAVACK et al., 1956; MOHNIKE, ULRICH, BIBERGEIL and CZYZYK, 1957; ZEFFREN and SHERRY; LACHNIT and TRETENHAHN; HALLER, 1957; DUNCAN and BAIRD, BASTENIE et al.), even if in single cases clear depressions combined with metabolic improvement were observed. Also in patients suffering from essential hypercholesterolaemia no decrease in the serum cholesterol level with D 860 doses could be reached (WADDELL).

To date, it cannot be decided whether the sulphonylureas are contra-indicated in the other *diabetic complications*, for these run such a long course. Especially it cannot yet be said whether the sulphonylureas prevent the appearance of complications. Finally, it has not been decided whether the late development of complications are influenced in any way by insulin control, or whether they occur anyway. There is no reason to assume that diabetic *retinopathy* deteriorates under sulphonylureas (BERTRAM et al., 1956; MOHNIKE, ULRICH, BIBERGEIL and CZYZYK, 1957). Regarding those haemorrhages which suddenly start and suddenly stop, this particular question cannot be yet answered. On investigating capillary fragility in diabetics during D 860 therapy (STICH, MARX and EHRHARDT, 1957) and BZ 55 treatment (FREY) no increase in capillary fragility was found as was first feared in the case of BZ 55 by PHEMISTER.

Marked diabetic, or other *nephropathies*, are taken by many to be a clear contra-indication for sulphonylurea therapy. This point of view seems to us to be justified for two reasons. First, in the case of renal insufficiency, delayed excretion may occur and sulphonylureas accumulate in the organism; there is danger of protracted hypoglycaemia (BENDTFELDT and OTTO; HANUSCH and JORKE). Secondly, single cases have been described where deterioration of nephropathy occurred following sulphonylureas (MOHNIKE, ULRICH, BIBERGEIL, and CZYZYK, 1957; STRAUZENBERG and HALLER, 1959b).

Diabetic *neuritis* is no contra-indication. BOLLER and KÖCK have the impression that insulin treatment has a better effect on neuritis than the sulphonylurea therapy. This has not been generally published so that one must judge each case on its own merits. Especially as BRENEMAN saw a case of diabetic neuritis of three months standing which disappeared 8 days after D 860 therapy had been started.

General experience shows that acute and chronic *liver diseases* are no contra-indications against a sulphonylurea therapy. Meanwhile many diabetics with liver cirrhosis have been treated with sulphonylureas without negative effects on the liver function. The publication of BOLLER and KÖCK also KÜHNLEIN on the observations of their 2 patients whose liver cirrhosis deteriorated during this therapy, are the only ones of this kind. However owing to the variable course of liver cirrhosis the sulphonylureas are not necessarily to blame. Some authors have even reported of a beneficial effect on chronic hepatitis (s. p. 84). However it is advisable to change-over to insulin in the case of severe hepatitis or a decompensating liver cirrhosis. Sulphonylureas may be used in compensated liver cirrhosis as in many of these cases there is a marked hepatic insulin resistance partially responding well to sulphonylurea therapy.

Pregnancy is a clear cut contra-indication for sulphonylurea therapy. This view is based on following the practical reasoning, sulphonamides generally pass through the placenta. In the case of foetal death described by LASS, 2.9 mg-% BZ 55 were found in the placenta, 1.8 mg-% in the foetal liver. Then also abortions and anomalies were produced in rats using very high doses of BZ 55 (s. p. 16). Added to this, however, one is only seldom faced with this problem because as a rule pregnant diabetics are too young to show a response to sulphonylureas. There are some female diabetics around 40 having very mild diabetes who can be well controlled with sulphonylureas. Some such cases have been treated, meanwhile, with BZ 55 (GHANEM and MIKHALL) and D 860 (SUGAR, 1957; Moss et al., 1959b) and no complications arose during pregnancy. On the other hand, some cases of foetal death had been described when pregnant diabetics were treated with BZ 55 (GHANEM and MIKHALL; LASS), but no connection with the sulphonylurea therapy could be proved. Final conclusions cannot be drawn from these limited observations. As metabolism oscilates in pregnant diabetics and as diabetes is dangerous for the foetus, one should on the principle of nil nocere dispense with sulphonylureas during pregnancy.

γ) **Combination therapy with insulin.** At the beginning of sulphonylurea therapy numerous authors tried to combine insulin and sulphonylureas in young patients not responding to sulphonylureas alone. Only in a few cases was a second insulin injection avoided by this, or a more stable metabolism produced than by insulin alone. Thus, a combination therapy based on these experience is of doubtful value. Especially stabilisation of the labile metabolism of juvenile diabetics with tendency towards hypoglycaemia on one hand, and acetonuria on the other (brittle diabetes), was not possible on the addition of sulphonylurea doses—for exceptions see especially FABRYKANT 1959. Only in abnormally high insulin requirements do combination treatments seem indicated, as thus, large insulin doses can be dispensed with (s. p. 58). If the insulin requirements are only slightly increased and only slight insulin amounts on addition of sulphonylureas are reduced, combination therapy is still not justified.

Recent experiences show new indications. It is not surprising that *older* diabetics responding insufficiently to sulphonylureas alone can reduce insulin on combination treatment of insulin and sulphonylureas. According to this, MOHNIKE, ULRICH, BIBERGEIL and CZYZYK (1957) were able to reduce insulin doses on combination treatment, especially in older, over-weight patients. STRATMANN found in secondary failures (older diabetics) lower insulin requirements than before the commencement of sulphonylurea treatment if after resumption of insulin therapy sulphonylureas were given. However, as the patients inject themselves with insulin anyhow, combination therapy should only be used if *better* metabolism is attained than by insulin alone. In a series of cases this is actually the case. FABRYKANT (1957, 1958, 1959) treated on the whole 46 labile and 85 stable diabetics with combined insulin and D 860 doses for 12—14 months. He saw, especially in the older patients, a more balanced metabolism and an increased feeling of well-being. Also VOLK and LAZARUS (1959) reported shortly of a group of 12 maturity-onset diabetics, where not only was insulin reduced by D 860, but also metabolism was more balanced than by insulin alone even in relatively high doses. These observations indicated an effect of sulphonylureas in certain diabetes types that cannot to the same degree, be attained by insulin. The cases of improvement in labile juvenile diabetics, excepting the larger series of FABRYKANT, are rare and difficult to interpret, as they often appear only after weeks or months of combination therapy. Here one must consider the influence on the liver metabolism. On the other side, beneficial effects of combination treatment are more frequently found in maturity-onset diabetics that are not optimally controlled either with sulphonylureas or insulin alone, having, however, certain β-cell reserves of great interest for further research. Either it means that endogenous insulin mobilised from the β-cells has a different effect in certain diabetics than injected exogenous insulin, or that sulphonylureas favorably influence the metabolism in maturity-onset diabetics in a specific way. In any case, the findings support the view that some forms of human diabetes are caused by the disturbances that can be more favourably influenced by sulphonylureas than by exogenous insulin (comp. p. 81 f.).

Thus the report of SILVER and NAGEL (1957) is remarkable. The authors treated 20 maturity-onset diabetics (69—87 years) suffering from this disease for over 15 years without simultaneous reduction in the insulin dose (average demand 32 U) for several months with additional D 860 doses. After 4 months, the fasting blood sugar started to fall and after 8 months the insulin could be dispensed with in 17 cases (in one special case the insulin requirement was 120 U before commencing combination therapy). Also in the remaining 3 cases, a remarkable reduction in insulin was possible. It follows that this improvement seen after months is connected with a primarily slow activation of the β-cells atrophied by years of insulin therapy. Possibly thus real β-cell regeneration occurred (s. p. 81). It must be emphasised that these ideas are purely theoretical. The limited observations in this field demand the greatest interest.

Lately FAJANS and CONN (1959 b) proposed treating patients with latent diabetes (proved by a decreased glucose tolerance) prophylactically with sulphonylureas and thus by timely β-cell activation, preventing the manifestation of diabetes. The authors believe in the possibility of diabetes prophylaxis through sulphonylureas after investigating 12 young patients with "asymptomatic diabetes" where there was improvement in glucose tolerance after 2—17 months of D 860 therapy. However, restraint is necessary as glucose tolerance is subjected to spontaneous oscillations and thus gives uncertain indications as to therapeutic success. Also reduced glucose tolerance does not definitely indicate later manifestation of genuine diabetes mellitus.

The question of combined insulin-sulphonylurea therapy is surely of interest for the therapeutic diabetologist. However, this must be approached conscientiously and with utmost criticism so that problematic extention of sulphonylurea therapy to uncontrollable limits be avoided.

δ) **Treatment.** The effectiveness of the sulphonylureas is limited. As was described in the paragraph on the pharmacology (s. p. 13 f.), there is only a limited positive dose-effect relationship in the healthy animal. From a certain dose upwards (in long-term therapy about 4 tablets = 2 grams BZ 55 or D 860), no increase in effect, even in the diabetic, is possible. Besides this, it is not possible to improve glucose tolerance in the diabetic through sulphonylureas, but only to reduce the fasting blood sugar values and thus achieve on the whole a low blood sugar niveau; consequent dietary adherence is also the basis of sulphonylurea therapy. In normal and over-weight patients, no increase in weight is desirable. A *first control* of untreated, or previously only insulin treated diabetics can be attempted if the above mentioned criteria (comp. p. 55) are fulfilled by the patients, and if during the trial period with consequent diet, no glucosuria nor blood sugar values of over 180 mg-% appear throughout the day. Keeping to the standard diet following dosages, are indicated; dosage on the first day 3×2 tablets to 0.5 g. BZ 55 or D 860. This dose is kept to if no effect on the blood sugar or glucosuria appears. After 4—5 days (exceptions 7 days), the therapeutic experiment must be stopped as then usually no satisfactory control can still be reached. If decrease in glucosuria and fasting blood sugar is apparent, the dose is reduced to 2×2 tablets and decreased to the maintenance dose of 3, 2 or even 1 tablet. Owing to the short half-life time of D 860, it is sometimes expedient to divide the daily dose. Often metabolic balance is achieved also with D 860 with a single morning tablet. More than 3—4 tablets should not be given as permanent treatment as these are usually sub-optimally controlled patients where no metabolic balance is achieved even with high doses. In such laboriously controlled patients, the danger of secondary failure is relatively great (comp. p. 59 f.).

On observing that in some cases metabolism remains compensated for days and even weeks after discontinuing sulphonylureas, the so-called *intermittent therapy* was advised in special cases (BERTRAM, BENDTFELDT and OTTO, 1955, 1956; BROGLIE et al., 1956; MURRAY and WANG). MURRAY and WANG looked for the duration of remission after an initial course of 2 weeks treatment with sulphonylureas and found in the case of D 860 an average remission of 2 weeks (1—58 days) and in the case of BZ 55, 3 weeks (4—56 days). Apart from the fact that one also found prolonged improvement in mild diabetes following adherence to a severe diet after discontinuing insulin, today there is no reason for this form of treatment. The reason was based on the possible toxicity of the substances, thus the least possible amount was given. Now experience has shown us that toxicity is only slight, especially of D 860 and the intermittent therapy no longer seems advisable. Also it makes control difficult and has no clear advantages to permanent therapy. If a diabetic does not respond satisfactorily to a sufficiently dosed sulphonylurea therapy, one should change-over finally to insulin. All attempts at an improved initial position by introductory insulin doses or by strict dietary adherence, are problematic. By this an only just sufficient control is reached that can lead to later metabolic disturbances resulting in secondary failures.

When *changing over* in the previously insulinised patient, great care is necessary. The above mentioned criteria for control must be carefully observed (s. p. 55). Patients with acidosis tendencies, or coma history, also juvenile diabetics can be excluded from the beginning. These have only a slight hope of successful oral treatment and are in the danger of acute metabolic decompensation. The change-over can either be abrupt by discontinuing insulin, or gradual by a temporary combination of insulin and sulphonylureas.

1. The abrupt insulin discontinuation is adviseable if following the general criteria for controllability (s. p. 53 f.) success of sulphonylurea therapy is probable. Principally a 2—3 day insulin withheld trial should preceed this. Thus one has a picture of the individual insulin/glucose equivalent and sometimes one can exclude those cases that have superfluously been treated with insulin and in which, of course, oral tablet treatment is redundant. If acetonuria and rapid metabolic decompensation occur unexpectically during the withheld experiments control with sulphonylureas should not even be attempted. If this is not the case, sulphonylurea doses are commenced after 2—3 days according to the above cited dose scheme (3×2 tablets D 860 on the first day, then decrease of dosage according to the blood and urine sugar values).

2. If there is any doubt about the controllability of a patient, one should not abruptly depose insulin. However, if residual glucosuria persists, either one administers 3×2 tablets in addition to insulin and waits to see whether the residual glucosuria is influenced; or decreases insulin dosage by 30—40% and simultaneously administers sulphonylureas whereby in positively reacting cases glucosuria must not occur. During the following days, a gradual decrease in the insulin dosage is attempted while the sulphonylurea therapy is continued. Very responsive patients might react with hypoglycaemia, therefore very careful control and observation of the patient are necessary during this time. The rate of insulin reduction depends on the strength of tablet action on the blood and urine sugar.

The question whether the change-over to, or control with sulphonylureas can only be performed on, in- or also on out-patients is answered in various ways. Numerous authors believe this to be to risky in out-patients, other disagree with this. SCHÖFFLING, PFEIFFER, TRESER et al. (1957) state that change-over or control must be partially carried out in out-patients as not enough beds are available in the town hospitals. They treated 758 out-patients without complications and found their results equal to those seen in the in-patients. However, the patients were selected from the beginning by the criteria for their controllability. Their blood and urine sugar values were ambulatorily controlled every 2 days to foresee possible metabolic decompensation. Experienced diabetologists carried out the treatment having all the facilities of a large diabetics' out-patient clinic. Today after some diabetics have been finally changed over to the sulphonylurea therapy, the following rules can be made: diabetics who fulfill the criteria for controllability and excrete no acetone can commence being controlled by sulphonylureas as out-patients if the doctor is experienced in diabetology and if there is possibility of regular blood and urine sugar control. Optimal control should be reached to prevent the secondary failing of sulphonylurea therapy. However, in diabetics controlled by insulin, an ambulatory change-over attempt should not, if possible, be made. This is so because it is not possible to determine exactly the minimum insulin requirements in out-patients or the danger of metabolic decompensation following abrupt insulin withdrawal, or finally hypoglycaemic reactions when insulin is reduced by administering with sulphonylureas. These possibilities present no problem in the clinic, but are dangerous in out-patients (DUNCAN and BAIRD; MÜTING, 1957). This fact warns against a change-over in out-patients.

Control is optimal only when the lowest maintenance dose has been found as the danger of side-effects increases with the dosage; this is especially evident in the more toxic sulphonylureas (chlorpropamide and metahexamide s. p. 87 f. and 91 f.). Further control during permanent therapy is of course possible in out-patients, but must be carried out with at least the same care as for insulinised patients. Here special attention to allergy, blood picture changes and liver function must be paid. As there should be no sugar in the urine in optimally controlled diabetics, intelligent patients can regulate themselves with a simple qualitative urine sugar test more easily than during insulin therapy where residual glucosuria is according to many authors important as a shock buffer.

Generally the daily *maintenance dose* during permanent therapy is 0.5—1 gram (1—2 tablets) of D 860. Half a tablet is sufficient only for a very few patients; 10—20% require 3—4 tablets according to the various statistics (SCHÖFFLING, PFEIFFER, TRESER et al., 1957; SEIDLER et al. STÖTTER 1957). More patients can be compensated with half a tablet of BZ 55 daily. Most, however, require 1 to 2 tablets as with D 860. Higher BZ 55 doses are seldom necessary. Thus we see

5*

in the long-term therapy a slightly stronger effectiveness of BZ 55 (BERTRAM, 1958a) which is connected with its longer half-life time. The price of this is, however, more side-effects.

3. Side-effects, hypersensitivity reaction, cases of death

From most papers published on BZ 55 and D 860, especially, however, from the Anglo-American reports, is seen that side-effects, and more so hypersensitivity occur more frequently on a BZ 55 than a D 860 therapy. CAMERINI-DAVALOS, ROOT and MARBLE observed side-effects in 9.2% of their 279 cases treated with BZ 55. KIRTLEY (1957) published a collective statistical report of over 7193 cases in the USA treated with BZ 55 of which 5.4% developed side-effects. According to BERTRAM (1958) these figures are more optimal in Germany. Correlating observations throughout the world showed fewer side-effects for D 860. SCHÖFFLING, PFEIFFER, TRESER et al. (1957) found that in Frankfurt the number of side-effects which led to interruption of oral treatment was 1.6% of 758 patients; this correlates to O'DONOVAN's findings in the USA of 1.5% of 9168 patients. Owing to this, BZ 55 was not on the market in the UK and in the USA. In the following paragraph the different side-effects of BZ 55 and D 860 will be discussed separately.

α) Hypoglycaemia. Seen as a whole, hypoglycaemic reactions following BZ 55 and D 860 are rare. They were observed on changing over from insulin to sulphonylureas on simultaneous dosage of both. Low blood sugar values (under 60 mg-%) were also diversely seen when sulphonylureas alone were given without subjective shock symptoms. Later single shock conditions with unconsciousness and paralysis of a hemiplegic type were seen. These conditions can run a protracted course especially after BZ 55 administration owing to its slow elimination; they were similar to the shock following long-acting insulin. Even if this condition is rare (more so than during insulin therapy), one must know of its existence and introduce the therapy with large parenteral glucose doses.

Following BZ 55, severe hypoglycaemia with unconsciousness was described by BENDTFELDT and OTTO (1956), SEIDLER et al. (1957), CAMERINI-DAVALOS, ROOT and MARBLE (1957), MELLANDER (1957), PETERSEN (1957) MÜTING (1957) and LAMBERT (1957). A case of HOFFSTETTER and RAMEL (1957) ended fatally. This patient was, however, not a diabetic but suffered from Addison's disease and was receiving BZ 55 in order to stimulate the appetite. The great sensitivity of patients with renal insufficiency is not surprising when compared to animal experiments (s. p. 43).

LOUKOPULOS et al. also MCKENDRY saw one case of unconsciousness *after D 860*. MCKENDRY's patient (84 years old with cerebral sclerosis) died during hypoglycaemia. The lowest estimated blood sugar value was about 26 mg-%.

β) Skin reactions. Nearly all authors observed allergic skin reactions in some patients during sulphonylurea therapy. These consisted of pruritus, urticaria, toxic exanthema, erythema nodosum and dermatitis; these were more frequently seen following BZ 55 (3—5% of the cases) than after D 860 (0.4—0.6%). WOLFF et al. (1956) found the largest number of skin reactions with 11% in Great Britain. These differences are due to the sulphonamide character of BZ 55. Three cases of photo-allergic eczema were described after BZ 55 (BURCKHARDT and SCHWARZ, SPECK, SCHREUS and IPPEN). CAMPBELL (1960) who saw in Indians 5 cases of photo-allergy after BZ 55 insisted that these were never caused by D 860 (but seen after chlorpropamide application). Dangerous conditions only healed after long time e. g. a generalised epidermolytic reaction (STERZING) and a severe generalised dermatitis with facial, glottis and laryngeal oedema (FELLER and KÜPPER). While most of these skin changes usually appeared at the beginning of sulphonylurea therapy, KRESBACH saw an expansive resistant exanthema similar to erythema figuratum first appear after 2 years of treatment with D 860.

Patients showing skin changes after BZ 55 could often tolerate D 860. Sometimes patients were allergic to both sulphonylureas; this can not, of course, be due to the p-amino group. Such cases of "crossed allergy" have been described by BERTRAM, BENDTFELDT and OTTO (1957), WALKER et al. (1957) also SCHÖFFLING et al. (1957). Some advise anti-histamine doses on the appearance of skin reactions and continuation of the sulphonylurea therapy. In mild cases, one can try this. As a rule one should desist, as skin reactions are sometimes only the beginning of severe general toxic reactions. Thus following skin reactions after BZ 55 occurred: polyneuritis of the Landry's type (DOMANOWSKY et al. 1958), fatal encephalomyelitis (BARTELHEIMER 1957), and one lethal case with intensive perivascular cerebral oedema (MAIER 1957). Also in most of the reported cases of agranulocytosis following BZ 55, a skin reaction was the first symptom (AARSETH and WILLUMSEN; JACKSON and HERMAN; NEUDECK 1957, PAGE et al., VARELA FUENTES et al., WENDEROTH and BALZEREIT).

γ) **Haematopoetic system.** When judging haematological changes following sulphonylureas, two factors must be taken into consideration. First, blood damage caused by the sulphonamides (this has been known since their use as chemotherapeuticals). Secondly, owing to the complexity of its metabolic disturbances, diabetes itself can cause changes in the haematopoetic system and in blood coagulation (STICH, MARX and EHRHARDT). Slight changes in the number of leucocytes and thrombocytes also occur in diabetics treated with insulin or on diet. One cannot speak of a general damaging bone marrow effect of the sulphonylureas. Against this is the experience over years with hundred thousands of patients.

BZ 55. A series of severe cases of leucopenia and agranulocytosis have occurred in the form of a BZ 55 hypersensitivity reaction. Thus there are reports of severe leucopenia and agranulocytosis following BZ 55 (recovery after discontinuing treatment) by AARSETH and WILLUMSEN, BERTRAM et al. (1957); JACKSON and HERMAN; KAEDING (1959), PHEMISTER (1957); PRINZ and GUTSCHKER; TONIELLI et al., WENDEROTH and BALZEREIT. Also in the fatally ending case of FIELD and FEDERMANN (1957) due to BZ 55 hypersensitivity with interstitial myocarditis and focal milliary granuloma, leucopenia occurred. Fatal agranulocytosis following BZ 55 was observed 9 times to date (AARSETH and WILLUMSEN; KAEDING 1959; NEUDECK 1957; POSSNER 1959; WALDMANN 1957; WENDEROTH and BALZEREIT; PAGE et al., also VARELA FUENTES et al.). Anuria occurred simultaneously in the cases of PAGE et al., also VARELA FUENTES et al. Their evidence shows that BZ 55 can have dangerous side-effects. However, if the large number of patients treated meanwhile with BZ 55 in Europe are taken into consideration, these effects were relatively rare. The conditions in the USA during 1955—56 following BZ 55 were far more serious. In 7193 cases 59 of leucopenia and agranulocytosis were seen (KIRTLEY 1957). In Great Britain, the frequency of haematological damage, besides leucopenia, also thrombopenia (PHEMISTER 1957, RONDANINI 1958) led to a warning note against BZ 55 therapy (DUNCAN, NABARRO, OAKLEY and WOLFF 1956).

D 860. The conditions are more favorable for D 860 treatment. Some mild forms of leucopenia, always transitory, cannot be proved as bone marrow damage caused by D 860. The careful haematological studies of SEIDLER et al., (1957), STICH, MARX and EHRHARDT (1957) also SCHÖFFLING, PFEIFFER, STEIGERWALD et al. (1957) showed no difference in the white and red blood picture and in the number of thrombocytes in diabetics treated with D 860, respectively insulin or diet. Also disturbances in the porphyrin metabolism could not be proved. STICH, MARX and EHRHARDT also STEIGERWALD, PFEIFFER et al. (1957) could even treat patients suffering from porphyria cutanea tarda and diabetes with D 860 without deterioration of the former.

There are two cases described in the whole literature where at least in connection with D 860 therapy, severe fatal disease of the haematopoetic system occurred and must be discussed. In JOST's (1959) case, increasing aplastic anaemia developed after 4 weeks of D 860 therapy with a moderate decrease of leucocytes and thrombocytes. Despite the fact that D 860 was discontinued and blood transfusions were given, the anaemia could not be influenced. Death occurred 3 months later owing to myocardial infarction. In BROD's case (1959), bone marrow depression occurred after 3 months of D 860 therapy, changing to a fatal myeloblastic leucaemia following ACTH therapy. SAUER and LANDBECK then described two cases of allergic thrombocytopenia following a 9 and 12 months' D 860 therapy. It was cured after the drug was discontinued. Therefore blood pictures are also necessary during D 860 therapy.

δ) **Liver damage.** Most authors treating larger number of diabetics with BZ 55 and D 860 made liver function tests and watched the possible liver damage. One cannot suppose there to be any liver toxicity of both the sulphonylureas from all published investigations (MEHNERT and GEORGII 1959a).

BZ 55. BZ 55 has not been in the market in the USA owing to its bone marrow damaging effect and ostensible liver damage (2 fatal cases of jaundice were observed, KIRTLEY 1957). After 5 years' experience with this substance, no convincing evidence has been found for the occurrence of liver damage. Single cases of jaundice (e.g. WILD and LINDEN) can probably be explained as intercurrent hepatitis because they were limited in number (contrary to the observation made with chlorpropamide and metahexamide s. p. 90 f. and 93). PULLOCH's case of jaundice (1958) appeared with other severe allergic reactions (fever, thrombocytopenia, exfoliative dermatitis) and cannot be regarded as a liver toxicity of BZ 55. In the fatal case of jaundice described by CAMERINI-DAVALOS, ROOT and MARBLE, cholostatic hepatosis was present. Besides this case, only WILD and LINDEN saw one case of cholostatic hepatosis following BZ 55. This complication cannot be regarded as being typical for BZ 55, as even in WILD and LINDEN's patient an allergic skin exanthema and ascending polyneuritis was present. The slight increase in alkaline serum phosphatase and bromsulphonephthaleine retention after BZ 55 found by MARBLE and CAMERINI-DAVALOS (1957) showed no progredience on continuing therapy and was not confirmed by later investigations in patients treated with BZ 55 (QUITZOW et al., 1957, BERTRAM 1958, SACHSSE 1958). ILLIG, V. UEXKÜLL and WAGNER more often found, however, pathological liver function tests in diabetics receiving BZ 55 than those given insulin or D 860. The systematic decrease in serum albumin and total protein described by MÜTING (1957) was not found by other workers.

Bioptic and autoptic investigations in patients treated with BZ 55 for a length of time showed no histological liver changes that could have been caused by the therapy (GEPTS 1958b, CREUTZFELDT 1958, SACHSSE 1958, CABARROU et al., BERINGER and THALER 1959).

In already present liver diseases, BOLLER and KÖCK saw deterioration in the liver function tests through BZ 55. QUITZOW et al., however, saw no further changes. These observations must be judged with reservation as processes of the liver have an uncertain course (more to this question on p. 85).

D 860. No toxic liver damage has been described for D 860. However, single cases of jaundice were seen under D 860 medication and explained as intercurrent virus hepatitis (MOHNIKE, ULRICH and JUTZI 1957 c, SEIDLER et al., 1957, GREIF 1958) as the same number was also found in untreated diabetics. The case of acute liver dystrophy described by SEIDLER et al. could also have been caused by virus hepatitis. This conclusion seems justified on the grounds of universal experience. Only recently has the first case of cholostatic hepatosis, bioptically ascertained, following D 860 application been described (BAIRD and HULL). It seems redundant to count the many papers published on the liver function of treated diabetics and where no deterioration was found. FÜRTHMÜLLER et al. (1957) did detailed research on the behaviour of serum protein fractions under D 860.

Again we must mention here some reports describing that liver disease deteriorates under D 860 therapy (KÜHNLEIN 1957, MEHNERT and GEORGII 1959, LAWRENCE). From this, we only conclude that the possibility of liver therapy with sulphonylureas in non-diabetics (comp. p. 84) as described by some authors is questionable.

Bioptic and autoptic findings in diabetics that were treated with D 860 for a length of time also showed no reason for believing this substance to have a liver damaging effect (CREUTZFELDT 1958, SACHSSE 1958, CABARROU et al. 1958, BEBER and BEBER). The observed liver changes are related to the diabetes and are equally frequent in untreated or insulinised diabetics.

ε) **Kidney changes.** FRAENKEL and SCHULZ described slight changes in electrolyte excretion under BZ 55. They found a positive sodium balance when loading with sodium. MOHNIKE, ULRICH, BIBERGEIL and CZYZYK (1957) saw under D 860 a transitory increase of sodium excretion and an increased diuresis. According to OTTO (1957) there is increased citric acid excretion in the urine under D 860 when the doses exceed 1 g/day (not, however, under BZ 55). There is no explanation for this.

There are only a few reports of more severe kidney damage. Here there was hypersensitivity, localised in the kidney. FELLER and KÜPPER found oliguria and proteinuria during a severe allergic reaction to BZ 55. The patient recovered. The cases of agranulocytosis following BZ 55 administration described by VARELA FUENTES et al. also PAGE et al., died showing symptoms of anuria. KLEIBEL and FRANK saw 2 cases of acute glomerular nephritis under BZ 55, one died. Finally SCHNALL and WIENER described a case where an acute nephrotic syndrome developed under D 860; when the drug was discontinued, recovery was complete.

Experience shows us that neither D 860 nor BZ 55 has a direct toxic effect on the kidneys. However, the use of these drugs is not adviseable owing to the danger of their accumulation in the presence of renal insufficiency; especially because some cases have been described where diabetic nephropathy deteriorated (MOHNIKE, ULRICH, BIBERGEIL and CZYZYK 1957, STRAUZENBERG and HALLER 1959 b, comp. p. 63).

ζ) **Nervous system.** D 860 and BZ 55 generally have no central nervous effect. Whenever large doses were given there were occasional complaints of headache, drowsiness and of tinnitus, independent of the blood sugar value. These symptoms are similar to those often seen after chlorpropamide administration, though essentially slighter (s. p. 90).

BZ 55. There are single reports of severe central nervous damage on an allergic basis, rare however, when considering the total number of successfully treated cases. BARTELHEIMER (1957) described a fatal case of encephalomyelitis; MAIER (1957) described a fatal case with a severe cerebral perivascular oedema. Both cases first reacted to BZ 55 therapy with exanthema. The same case history was found in the case of severe polyneuritis of Landry's type described by DOMANOWSKY et al. and that of ascending neuritis seen by WILD and LINDEN (this case was complicated in addition by cholostatic hepatosis). PURTSCHER (1957) observed a patient who suffered from headache, paraesthesia and visual disturbances with papilloedema four months after commencing BZ 55 therapy. When discontinuing BZ 55 therapy, the side-effects disappeared. Mild polyneuritis following BZ 55 therapy was seen by WILD and LINDEN also GOOR and SCHREUDER. The correlation between these and BZ 55 is concluded by their rapid disappearance following withdrawal, while diabetic polyneuritis is usually of long duration and difficult to treat.

D 860. There are no reports of central or peripheral nervous damage caused by D 860. Only ELLENBERG saw typical diabetic neuropathies appear shortly after successful diabetic control. However, he states the fact that similar observations have been made also after successful insulin treatment. In both cases neuritis disappeared despite continuation of therapy.

η) **Thyroid gland.** As described on p. 15, the sulphonylureas have a mild thyreostatic effect on animals; BZ 55 a stronger one than D 860. Also in man, the thyroid ^{131}I uptake is decreased by BZ 55 and slightly less so by D 860 in high doses (3—4 g). There is no significant effect on the ^{131}I uptake during a permanent therapy using 1—2 gms/day (RENOLD et al. 1956, BROWN and SOLOMON 1956, McGAVACK et al. 1956). McGAVACK et al. (1957) showed in further research that a permanent BZ 55 therapy of 2 grams leads to a transitory lowering of the protein bound iodine and of the basal metabolic rate, also to a decreased ^{131}I uptake. When continuing the therapy, normal values are again obtained. D 860 produced no such effects even when 2 grams were given daily.

The thyreostatic effect of the sulphonylureas seemed to have no significance in practice. STRATMANN was the only one who reported of 3 diabetics treated with BZ 55 in whom the already present goitre increased so greatly in size that therapy had to be discontinued. One case has been described for BZ 55 (MAMOU) and one for D 860 (MONTENORO) where *myxoedema* appeared and subsided when discontinuing therapy.

The slight thyreostatic effect of sulphonylureas is not sufficient to be of therapeutic value in the case of hyperthyroidism; for as mentioned on p. 58, hyperthyreotic diabetics generally do not respond satisfactorily to sulphonylurea therapy.

ϑ) **Gastro-intestinal disturbances, intestinal flora.** Feeling of repletion, sickness and nausea are extremely rare during BZ 55 or D 860 therapy. If they do appear, then only under the high commencing doses; they disappear on reaching the maintenance dose of 1—2 g. Again, these side-effects are more frequent following BZ 55 (1.1% of over 7000 cases of KIRTLEY 1957) than after D 860. MOHNIKE, ULRICH, BIBERGEIL and CZYZYK (1957) were only forced to discontinue therapy in 3 out of 1000 cases treated with D 860 owing to gastric intolerance; SCHÖFFLING, PFEIFFER, TRESER et al. (1957) in 6 out of 758 patients. According to BOLLER and KÖCK, those patients having stomach history complained of this intolerance. Sometimes antacida are useful for removing these complaints. HENNING et al. proved that BZ 55 and D 860 stimulate ventricular peristalsis and acid secretion. This is similar to the effect found after insulin and differs only in that it is of longer duration and occurs intermittently.

GELFAND (1959) reported of 2 diabetics with ulcus history who suffered from ventricular haemmorhages after BZ 55 administration. Also BEASER (1957) found in a patient with an ulcus, deterioration of this condition; and in a 75 year old man, without any previous symptoms, the perforation of a duodenal ulcer after 135 days of D 860 treatment of 2.5 g/day! Luckily these complications seem to be rare.

After introducing BZ 55, it was often feared that this sulphonamide could damage the coli flora; this would mean that BZ 55 was inferior to the non-bacteriostatic D 860.

MEHNERT (1956), MEHNERT and MEHNERT (1956) also BENDTFELDT et al. (1957) did, in fact, find a slight decrease in coli flora under BZ 55 and an increase of entero-cocci. Only PRESSER and RITZERFELD found no significant changes. However, no practical significance results from this. No cases are known where BZ 55 has influenced the intestinal flora in a negative way for the organism, e.g. as intestinal disturbances or avitaminosis.

ι) **Intolerance to alcohol.** Despite the fact that animal experiments showed no certain antabuse effect (comp. p. 17), some authors observed a decrease in the alcohol tolerance in diabetics that were controlled by BZ 55 (BERTRAM et al. 1955, 1957) or D 860 (DOLGER 1956). BÜTTNER and PORTWICH even described certain antabuse symptoms following alcohol intake in diabetics under D 860; the symptoms could also be reproduced in normal control subjects. The enzymatically estimated blood acetaldehyde level was increased 3—4 times. However, CZYZYK and MOHNIKE (1957) found no difference in the acetaldehyde level after alcohol intake following BZ 55 or D 860 administration.

These findings have no great practical significance. The few patients showing this intolerance must either abstain from alcohol or sulphonylureas.

c) Clinical experimental research
on the mechanism of action of the sulphonylureas

In this paragraph we must differentiate between those investigations made in metabolically normal patients and in diabetics. This is so as the results found in the metabolically normal patients should not differ from those found in animal experiments. Compared to this the conditions found in maturity-onset diabetics who respond to sulphonylureas are of great interest, as this type of diabetes cannot be reproduced in animal experiments. Therefore, metabolic improvement in maturity-onset diabetes can only be investigated in human patients. It can be discussed whether the sulphonylureas intervene at a significant metabolic point for the pathogenesis of this form of diabetes; primarily inhibition of abnormal hepatic glucose reduction is assumed. Also the resolving of an insulin release disorder of the β-cells (not yet proved) must be discussed.

The first clinical investigations confirmed by countless papers already show juvenile diabetics with tendency to acidosis scarcely responding to sulphonylurea therapy; a large number of older diabetics without tendency towards acidosis respond with decreased blood sugar and glucosuria. We see from the papers of WRENSHALL, BOGOCH and RITCHIE mentioned in the introduction, on the pancreatic insulin content in juvenile and older diabetics, also on the plasma insulin content of the various types of diabetes (BORNSTEIN and LAWRENCE, SELTZER and SMITH 1959b) that there is a correlation between therapeutic success and endogenous insulin reserves (WRENSHALL and BEST etc.). There is also the possibility that the sulphonylureas are only able to correct a certain metabolic defect characteristic for the maturity-onset diabetes.

Our review will therefore be along the same lines as the animal experimental part. First we must look for proof of pancreatic insulin mobilisation in the normal and diabetic patient; then for the metabolic changes characteristic for the insulin effect accompanying hypoglycaemia; finally for the effect on hepatic metabolism.

1. Plasma insulin determination

The results of plasma insulin determinations in man are contradictory. On one hand, no increased insulin activity was found in peripheral blood when using the diaphragm method to 120 mins after D 860 administration orally and i.v., either in normal subjects (RENOLD et al., 1957, SELTZER and SMITH, CUGADDA et al.) or in diabetics of the maturity-onset type (SELTZER and SMITH, CUGADDA et al., WEAWER et al.). The same authors found the diaphragm method useful when a significant increase in plasma insulin activity was found on orally administering glucose in normal and diabetic subjects (CUGADDA et al., SELTZER and SMITH 1959a and b); or i.v. injection of 0.1 U/kg insulin (RENOLD et al. 1957). Even with the help of glucose uptake of the epididymal adipose tissue in the rat no increased plasma insulin activity could be found following i.v. BZ 55 doses, either in the peripheral or hepatic venous blood, in healthy human subjects. After glucose injection increased plasma insulin activity was seen (HUMBEL et al.). On the other hand positive results contradict these negative findings. VALLANCE-OWEN et al. also GAMBASSI and PIRELLI saw, when applying the diaphragm method, in healthy subjects and maturity-onset diabetics (not juvenile diabetics) a remarkable increase in plasma insulin activity parallel to the blood sugar decrease after oral and i.v. sulphonylurea administration. PFEIFFER et al. (1959b and c) found the same using the adipose tissue method.

The discrepancy that some found no increased plasma insulin activity after sulphonylureas but following glucose administration in the same diabetics (SELTZER and SMITH, CUGADDA et al.) or in metabolically normal subjects (HUMBEL et al.), while others found an increase after sulphonylureas and none following glucose in the same diabetic (PFEIFFER et al. 1959b and c) is striking. This discrepancy cannot, therefore, be based on the insensitivity of the used methods. Thus the question must remain open whether in normal subjects or diabetics responding to sulphonylureas, liberated pancreatic insulin reaches the peripheral circulation. YALOW et al. recently published a further paper on this question. They determined the concentration of insulin in the blood by the new immunobioassay method and found after i.v. and after oral dose of D 860 an elevation in healthy and diabetic subjects. However the plasma insulin concentration was increased to a significantly greater extent following glucose administration by the same routes to the same subjects. A further, to date unanswerable question is whether the insulin release in the diabetic is important only during the first application of the drug, or also during permanent therapy. In normal subjects, increased plasma insulin activity following BZ 55 given for several days was only found by AIMAN and KULKARNI using the diaphragm method.

2. Potentiating of the insulin effect and insulin degradation

First it must be cleared whether the effect of endogenous or exogenous insulin is increased by the sulphonylureas. Clinical observations show that the insulin dose in the juvenile insulin deficiency diabetic cannot be reduced in most cases by additional doses of sulphonylureas. This speaks against an insulin saving effect caused by delayed insulin degradation. Insulin sensitivity in metabolically normal subjects and diabetics is, according to numerous investigations, not increased after a sulphonylurea dose (KIRTLEY et al., FAJANS et al., 1956, HEINEMANN et al., CONSTAM et al., 1956, COX et al., 1956a, BASTENIE et al., BUTTERFIELD et al., 1957, MOHNIKE, CZYZYK and ULRICH 1957). Also in 2 totally pancreatectomised humans the blood sugar decrease was not steeper or stronger after i.v. insulin administration if 2 grams D 860 were injected i.v. simultaneously (CREUTZFELDT,

KÜMMERLE and KERN). Some workers however, describe an increased insulin sensitivity; this means a steeper and more rapid blood sugar decrease following sulphonylureas in diabetics who did not respond to sulphonylurea therapy (BARTELHEIMER and MARING; MIRSKY and DIENGOTT; HALLER 1957). In practice this effect should be meaningless; thus, the sulphonylureas should not influence the controversial insulinase. Research on changes in insulin degradation following sulphonylureas performed in man with the help of ^{131}I labelled insulin had negative results (COX et al. 1956a, BOLINGER and GRADY; WEAWER et al.). Therefore, there is no proof for the inhibition of insulin degradation as assumed by MIRSKY, PERISUTTI and GITELSON, and said by these authors to be the cause of the second phase of sulphonylurea hypoglycaemia (not, however, of the initial blood sugar decrease) that at least in the diabetic lasts longer than insulin hypoglycaemia (comp. also p. 21).

3. Acute blood sugar decrease and effect on various metabolic parameters influenced by insulin

The varying strength and speed of the blood sugar decrease in normal and diabetic patients following single oral, or better still i.v. sulphonylurea dose, shows how significant the functional capacity of the β-cell system is for the acute blood sugar decrease. In healthy subjects, dosed orally with D 860 the blood sugar decreases rapidly within the first hour and regains its normal value within 2 hrs (DIENGOTT and MIRSKY). The blood sugar curve reminds one of the effect of i.v. injected insulin; the only exception being that with high sulphonylurea doses contrary to insulin, there is a delayed rise of the blood sugar. In diabetics responding to sulphonylurea therapy, there was no initial blood sugar lowering; instead, the blood sugar decreased gradually, but continually, over 4—5 hrs (MIRSKY, DIENGOTT and UNGER). As the degree of blood sugar decrease depends largely on the severity of the diabetes, it was used as the so-called "quick tablet test" for judging the possible therapeutic success (s. p. 56). Most impressive was the varied blood sugar decrease in normal subjects and in diabetics after i.v. injection of 1—2 grams BZ 55 (PFEFFER et al. 1957) or D 860 (KAUP; DE MEUTTER et al. 1958, UNGER and MADISON 1958a and b, also WILLE). The corresponding experimental results clearly show that impairment of islet function characteristic for diabetes, minimises the blood sugar decrease after sulphonylureas. This observation is one of the strongest arguements for the stimulation of insulin secretion by sulphonylureas even in man. There is hardly any other explanation for the rapid blood sugar decrease in the metabolically sound. Difficulties arise in judging the situation in diabetics. This is because, also in diabetics responding to sulphonylureas, PFEIFFER et al. (1959a) also VALLANCE-OWEN et al. (1959) found the same increase in insulin activity in peripheral blood as in the normal subjects; the blood sugar did not, however, decrease correspondingly. Besides, the insulin plasma activity was already normal while the blood sugar was still decreasing. This discrepancy again causes us to think of a specific effect on the hepatic glucose output; this could play an important part in maturity-onset diabetes. KAUP investigated whether the blood sugar decrease following i.v. BZ 55 administration was influenced by cirrhosis of the liver. He concluded that in patients with cirrhosis of the liver, with and without diabetes, the initial blood sugar decrease did not differ significantly from patients with a normal liver with and without diabetes. However, patients with liver cirrhosis, with and without diabetes, had a lower insulin sensitivity (WAIFE et al., KAUP; CREUTZFELDT 1959d). Besides, in cases with cirrhosis of the liver, the interval until the blood sugar regained its normal level was greater following sulphonylureas than insulin (KAUP).

PFEFFER et al. (1957) and later UNGER and MADISON (1958b) also ZAROWITZ and EIS suggested that the sulphonylurea loading should be used for diagnosing mild diabetes. According to UNGER and MADISON, metabolically normal subjects should show a blood sugar decrease of 25% 20 mins after 1 gram D 860 given i.v. If the decrease is only 15—24%, the 30 mins value must at least show a blood sugar lowering of 25%. A slighter blood sugar decrease indicates the presence of diabetes. We do not yet know whether this test can show the extent of the meta-bolic disorder which is also of interest for the clinician and can be seen by the result of a usual glucose tolerance test. Our experiences show this not to be the case. In our normal control subjects we found a blood sugar decrease of 20% and more during the 20 or 30 mins values. Also in cases of mild diabetes these values were not attained, however it was not possible to differentiate between the varying severity of the diabetes (WILLE). According to BARROS BARRETO and RECANT, healthy subjects receiving steroids for several days already show a reduction, or at least a temporal shift of the maximal blood sugar decrease, after injection of sulphonylureas. Possibly one can define a real hepatic glucose tolerance disturbance in patients with a liver disease and in those with a real insulin deficiency using the i.v. sulphonylurea test. This seems so because KAUP found a normal initial blood sugar decrease and a delayed re-increase in patients with cirrhosis of the liver (frequently showing pathological glucose tolerance) after sulphonylurea injection. WILLE compared the absence of glucose assimilation and blood sugar reduction following D 860 injection in 19 cases with cirrhosis of the liver, and found that in most cases where glucose tolerance was already impaired, there was a normal D 860 test. Recently has been shown that an especially strong and extended blood sugar decrease after injecting D 860 is found with islet adenoma (GITTLER et al., PFEIFFER et al. 1959a and b, FAJANS and CONN, own observations). This observation has a practical significance in diagnosing per-nicious hyperinsulinism (comp. p. 59). According to own experiences in two cases with islet adenoma the appearance of real hypoglycaemic shocks after i.v. injection of D 860 indicated the presence of an islet adenoma.

Also in man, as previously in animals, countless experiments were made during sulphonylurea hypoglycaemia to prove an increased *peripheral glucose assimilation*. Only GOETZ et al. (1956) saw following an i.v. dose of D 860 in healthy subjects an increase in the arterio-venous blood sugar difference (simul-taneously there was a decrease in inorganic phosphorus in the serum). Other workers found this to be unchanged in healthy subjects and diabetics after sulphonylurea administration (with and without previous glucose dose) (BERINGER and LINDNER, MCKENZIE et al., PURNELL et al., VOLK et al. 1956, WEAVER et al., STOWERS et al. 1958, BUTTERFIELD et al. 1957, RECANT and FISCHER, MADISON et al. 1959, CRAIG et al., STRAUZENBERG and HALLER). They all agree that the estimation of the arterio-venous blood sugar difference varies greatly. Besides, MADISON et al. (1959) showed that after slow peripheral insulin infusion (0.0006 to 0.1 U/min) no increase in the arterio-venous difference was found in the healthy subject, although the blood sugar decreased. CRAIG et al. (1959) found the same following i.v. injections of very small insulin doses. BUTTERFIELD et al. (1958), therefore, investigated the peripheral glucose uptake using a special technique before and after several days of D 860 treatment in maturity-onset diabetics. They found the blood sugar threshold, above which glucose is assimilated, similar as after insulin, significantly lowered.

Also in healthy and diabetic subjects, investigations using ^{14}C-labelled glucose were carried out and the decline of the specific activity of plasma glucose followed after injection of insulin and D 860 (JACOBS et al.). After D 860 the sharp decline in the activity curve characteristic for insulin was absent. Only a marked plateau was seen, thought to be a sign of reduced hepatic glucose output. The curves were, however, identical with those found after a s.c. insulin dose; here also was the influence on hepatic glucose output more important than the peripheral assimilation. The experiments of SEARLE et al. (1959) principally the same, had different results. The plateau was not always found after insulin, but regularly after D 860. Healthy subjects showed even after D 860, increased peripheral assimilation. This was absent in diabetics despite an obvious blood sugar decrease. During further observations SEARLE et al. (1960) found the following: despite the missing peripheral effect (measured by the behaviour of the specific activity of plasma glucose) following D 860 in diabetics and controls, the same amounts of labelled glucose were oxidised to $^{14}CO_2$ and expired as after the same blood sugar effective insulin dose. They can argue from these experiments that insulin is liberated from the β-cells by sulphonylureas. RENOLD et al.(1957) also GOETZ (1957) tested the respiratory quotient and the nitrogen balance in diabetics receiving sulphonylureas. No change was found in either case.

The muscle glycogen content of diabetics receiving sulphonylureas does not increase (BERINGER and LIDNER). Diabetics treated with insulin show a higher muscle glycogen content than do diabetics treated with sulphonylureas (BERINGER and HELMER).

A slight improvement in *glucose tolerance* in diabetics was only seen at the beginning of the sulphonylurea therapy (BASTENIE et al. also JENSEN et al. 1958). It is generally agreed that the oral and i.v. glucose tolerance of diabetics treated for a longer duration with sulphonylureas is not improved though glucosuria and blood sugar values are decreased (STÖTTER et al. 1956, DUNCAN et al., KIRTLEY et al., FAJANS et al., MILLER and CRAIG 1956, MOORHOUSE and KARK 1956, RENOLD et al. 1956, VOLK et al. 1956, MOHNIKE, CZYZYK and ULRICH; BAIRD and DUNCAN; BASTENIE et al., BUTTERFIELD et al. 1957, HALLER; STOWERS et al. 1958; SPANÁR, BALÁZ and ADAMEC). The blood sugar curves were lower after treatment because the initial values were lower. However, the course remained unchanged—typically diabetic. From this we see that the effect of the sulphonylurea therapy was mainly on the lowering of the fasting blood sugar.

The results of the decrease of anorganic serum *phosphorus* do not correspond. A slight lowering in the healthy subject and in the diabetic was found by GOETZ et al., MOHNIKE, CZYZYK and ULRICH (1957) also FRAWLEY et al. (1957); and not found by the others (RENOLD et al. 1956, McKENZIE et al., CROWLEY et al., STRAUZENBERG and HALLER). LACHNIT and TRETENHAHN observed a stronger decrease in serum phosphorus after glucose dose in diabetics premedicated for some days with sulphonylureas. A single dose of sulphonylureas is not sufficient for this effect (JENSEN et al., SPANÁR et al.). The serum *potassium* falls slightly according to GOETZ et al., MONIKE, CZYZYK and ULRICH (1957), SZÜCS and TISZAI also STRAUZENBERG and HALLER. However, the changes are very slight in the diabetic. STOWERS et al. compared the decrease of serum phosphorus and potassium after a dose of glucose with and without previous D 860 dose. No significant difference was found.

The blood *amino acids* were reduced in normal subjects and in diabetics after sulphonylureas and also after insulin (MOHNIKE, CZYZYK and ULRICH, DE MEUTTER et al. 1958, FRAWLEY et al. 1959). CROWLEY et al., however, saw no changes in the amino acids. According to LOHMANN, different effects are found in individual diabetics; a decrease or increase of amino acids can only be proved if a blood sugar reaction occurred.

The behaviour of several *metabolites of carbohydrate metabolism* were investigated (pyruvic acid, α-keto-glutaric acid and lactic acid). After sulphonylurea injection the metabolically normal controls do not show the abrupt rise in pyruvic acid and lactic acid which is typical for insulin (RENOLD et al. 1956, MOORHOUSE and KARK 1956). HENNES et al. even found, as in the animal experimental results of GALANSINO et al. 1958 (s. p. 37), a decrease in pyruvate after D 860; the α-keto-glutarate was uncharacteristic. M. MILLER et al. (1957) found that normal controls showed no pyruvate or lactate increase found after insulin, following D 860 administration; but, that in the diabetic, neither insulin nor D 860 influences the blood concentration of lactate and pyruvate. Thus the difference found in normal controls is not significant STEIGERWALD et al. (1957) determined the metabolites enzymatically following oral D 860 dose and i.v. insulin dose. They were the first who found in the metabolically normal controls and in the diabetic an increase of pyruvate and believed this to confirm the insulin secretion theory. They believed difference in degree and time of this increase to be caused by the oral application of the sulphonylureas. The lactate changes were uncharacteristic. A very impressive decrease in the blood concentration of α-keto-glutarate was found in the metabolically normal and opposed by an increase displayed by the diabetic after D 860. This behaviour is explained by an additional hepatic action. GIALRONI-GRASSI et al. found in diabetics treated with D 860 and dosed with glucose and insulin a reduction of the blood pyruvate; an increase was found in non-treated diabetics following glucose and insulin. A strong argument against the assumption that large amounts of insulin become peripherally active after sulphonylurea administration was found in the investigations of SEGAL et al., also FRAWLEY et al. (1957) on the distribution of infused *pentoses* (xylose and arabinose). The authors found the following in the metabolically normal: contrary to the rapid disappearance of injected glucose from the blood stream after D 860 injection, they found no influence of the sulphonylureas on the decrease of the plasma pentose level. Insulin, however, led to a rapid lowering of the blood pentose level. These findings were less significant as an argument against a missing peripheral insulin effect under sulphonylurea action according to the recent investigations of FRAWLEY et al. (1959). These authors namely found, in the meantime, that in normal patients receiving insulin intra-portally during an operation, an effect on the decrease of infused pentoses was also not found; an effect was present on peripheral insulin application under the same conditions. Here alone the fact that the insulin, secreted on sulphonylurea stimulation, first reaches the liver is responsibile for the behaviour of pentoses after sulphonylurea administration.

From these investigations, we see again that it is nearly impossible to prove or refute a peripheral insulin effect following sulphonylurea doses. Therefore, to conclude this paragraph, the corresponding animal experiments should be referred to (s. p. 35 f.). The results that show the sulphonylureas to have a positive effect on hepatic metabolism also in man, and especially in the maturity-onset diabetic, are important. In how far this is also only transmitted by endogenous insulin, cannot be decided before we know more about the action of insulin on the liver.

4. Effect on hepatic metabolism in man

Possible inhibition of the *hepatic glucose output* after sulphonylureas can be assumed from the above mentioned investigations on normal and diabetic subjects; namely, a decrease in the specific plasma activity following a dose of ^{14}C-labelled glucose (JACOBS et al., also SEARLE et al. 1959) (s. p. 76 f.). Also when measuring the hepatic venous glucose level directly using a heart catheter, the following is found: the glucose production in the splanchnic area in the metabolically normal (KIBLER and GORDON, RECANT and FISCHER, CRAIG et al. 1959) and in the diabetic (KIBLER and GORDON) after sulphonylurea dose is strongly and permanently inhibited. Naturally not only the hepatic glucose output is measured, but also the glucose uptake from the whole area supplied by the portal vein. Thus it is not astonishing that CRAIG et al. (1959) also found a reduction of glucose production on dosing with small amounts of insulin. This observation corresponds with the older results of BEARN, BILLING and SHERLOCK. These authors underline, however, that only juvenile diabetics (hepatic sensitive diabetes) show a prompt inhibition of glucose production with insulin. In the older stenic, relatively insulin resistent diabetic, without ketosis tendency, glucose production of the splanchnic area is hardly influenced by insulin (hepatic insensitive diabetes). Just this diabetic type responds well to sulphonylurea therapy. Thus a relative specifity of the sulphonylureas to the hepatic glucose output can be assumed; this is significant for the mechanism of action in the diabetic. BASTENIE et al. (1957) mathematically analysing the behaviour of blood sugar after insulin dosage and intravenous glucose loading in diabetics before and during sulphonylurea therapy, concluded the following: hepatic glucose output is hardly influenced by insulin doses in the diabetic; sulphonylureas, however, are highly effective in this respect.

A further indication of the influencing of hepatic glucose production is given by experiments with *fructose*. This sugar does not stimulate insulin secretion (POZZA et al. 1958) and is practically only used in the liver for which no insulin is necessary (comp. PLETSCHER, FAHRLÄNDER and STAUB 1951). When loading with fructose, part of the fructose is changed to glucose which is compensated by the metabolically normal; thus, there is no blood sugar rise. In the diabetic, however, this leads to hyperglycaemia (PLETSCHER et al. 1951, PLETSCHER 1953). Different research workers came to the same conclusion; namely, that the blood glucose rise defaults after fructose loading in the diabetic previously treated with sulphonylureas. Hyperglycaemia after glucose loading remains unchanged (RENOLD et al. 1956, MOORHOUSE and KARK 1956, MILLER and CRAIG 1956, MOORHOUSE et al. 1957, BONHOTE 1957, BAIER 1959). M. MILLER et al. (1957) could, most impressively, prove the inhibition of glucose output following fructose infusion in the diabetic by catheterising an hepatic vein. The corresponding results state that sulphonylureas inhibit gluconeogenesis from fructose in the liver. BAIER suggests that possibly increased fructose degradation is the cause of the phenomenon as he simultaneously saw a rise of the α-keto-glutarate. The fact that sulphonylureas inhibit (RENOLD et al. 1956) not only the change of fructose to glucose, but also that of galactose to glucose, speaks for an influencing of gluconeogenesis.

We do not know of any quantitative investigations of the *liver glycogen* content in human diabetics receiving sulphonylureas. However, BERINGER and KEIBL described for fasting conditions after sulphonylurea administration an increase in the histochemically visible liver glycogen, found in the liver biopsy. Repeated biopsies in the diabetic showed the glycogen reaction in the liver cell to be clearly increased after several days of sulphonylurea therapy and it remained constant during further therapy (BERINGER and THALER).

Few investigations have been made on *enzyme activities* in liver biopsies in human diabetics treated with sulphonylureas. The greatly increased glucose-6-phosphatase activity found in human diabetics (PATRICK and TULLOCH, GELI and ALP, WALLENFELS, CREUTZFELDT and SUMM) analogous to conditions found in alloxan diabetes (LANGDON and WEAKLEY) is reduced after sulphonylurea treatment (PATRICK and TULLOCH, WALLENFELS et al., 1959). Insulin therapy has the same effect. However, in the cases of WALLENFELS et al. (1959 comp. also SUMM), D 860 was more effective than insulin. WALLENFELS, CREUTZFELDT and SUMM investigated in all, the activity of 22 enzymes in the precinct of glycolysis, of the hexose-mono-phosphate-shunt and the citric acid cycle. Many enzymes in untreated diabetics were adaptively increased. This change can be partially or totally reversed by insulin therapy. Sulphonylurea therapy has partly the same effect. However, D 860 therapy shows the additional effect of increasing the activity of those enzymes catalysing speed-limiting processes. Thus augmented activity was found for hexokinase, fructose-6-phosphate-kinase, phosphotriose-isomerase, and for the malic enzyme. These effects specific for sulphonylurea therapy work together with the normalising of many changes of the enzymatic pattern of the diabetic liver. The latter produced also by insulin causes an improvement of glucose liberation. Further investigations of this kind on human liver biopsies may reveal the sulphonylurea mode of action on the diabetic liver, and also more about the role of the liver in the diabetic metabolism as maturity-onset diabetes cannot be reproduced in animal experiments.

Thus, the investigations on the influence of sulphonylureas on *ketone synthesis* will be briefly mentioned. KINSSEL et al. described a reduction in ketonaemia through D 860 in non-acidotic diabetics receiving a ketogenic diet. Also CATTANEO also BOSHELL et al. found in maturity-onset diabetics who responded to sulphonylurea therapy, an impressive decrease in the blood ketone bodies following sulphonylurea dose. BOSHELL et al. were able to prove an inhibition of ketogenesis in the human liver, already seen by them in rat liver slices in vitro through sulphonylureas. The diminished effect is explained by the fact that the patients receive glucose during the operation while the rats were in a fasting condition.

5. Influence on the glucagon effect

Numerous authors examined whether the glucagon hyperglycaemia in the metabolically normal or diabetic is weakened or abolished by sulphonylureas. Many workers found a normal glucagon reaction following one, or long-term sulphonylurea treatment (STÖTTER et al. 1956; FAJANS et al., 1956; KIRTLEY et al., 1956; Cox et al., 1956a; MILLER and CRAIG, CONSTAM et al., RECKNAGEL 1956; BUTTERFIELD et al., GORMAN and WEAVER). A slight decrease in the glucagon effect was found by GOLDNER, WEISENFELD and HUGHES in a larger group of metabolically normal and mildly diabetic patients. Here they do not assume the influence of the sulphonylureas on the glucagon, but that it is the result of a stronger insulin effect. There is no such effect in severe diabetes. IZZO investigated the nitrogen balance in maturity-onset diabetics receiving daily glucagon injection and found an increased protein catabolism. BZ 55 doses did not influence the negative nitrogen balance under glucagon.

6. Influence on adreno-cortical function

Various research workers discussed whether one, or long-term sulphonylurea treatment had an effect on the excretion of 17-ketosteroids and corticoids in the urine in diabetics. No significant change in the increase or decrease of steroid excretion could be found (PFEIFFER, SCHÖFFLING and STEIGERWALD, 1956; RAUSCH-STROOMANN and SAUER, 1956; RENOLD et al., 1956; CONSTAM et al., DUNCAN et al., 1956; MORTIMORE et al., 1956; WENGER, 1957; GUTMAN et al., IZZO). Also the 17-hydroxycorticosterone plasma level was not elevated in diabetics receiving sulphonylurea doses (RAUSCH-STROOMANN and SAUER, 1957). Then the increase of plasma 17-hydroxycorticoids following ACTH infusion or long-acting ACTH injection was not significantly modified by sulphonylureas

(WENGER, 1957; GUTMAN et al.). Finally, SPANÁR et al. found a stronger increase in the plasma cortisol level. GUTMAN et al. described for diabetics receiving sulphonylureas a slight elevation of 17-ketosteroid excretion in the urine after ACTH dose.

We can conclude from the investigations that the adrenal cortex is not significantly influenced by therapeutic sulphonylurea doses.

7. Islet-cell system in diabetics receiving sulphonylurea therapy

Despite the fact that changes in the islets of Langerhans in diabetics receiving sulphonylureas belong to the field of pathological anatomy, they will be mentioned in this paragraph as they are of interest in connection with the sulphonylurea mode of action in man. Reports on islet morphology comprise 39 diabetics treated with BZ 55 and D 860 up to 29 months (FERNER and RUNGE, 1956b; CREUTZFELDT, 1956; GEPTS, 1958a and b). The results correspond entirely. Namely, no changes were found that could with certainty be attributed to the therapy. The α-cells were normal; the β-cells showed the usual morphological diabetic criteria. Besides normally granulated β-cells, all degrees of degranulation and vacuolation (so-called hydropical degeneration) were present. Islets totally and partially hyalinised were found irregularly. From the slight augmentation of islet hyalinosis, contrary to untreated diabetics found by GEPTS, no conclusion can be drawn from the few cases examined. The α-β-cell relation was not different from the untreated controls of the same age. The cases investigated by CREUTZFELDT and GEPTS, including also diabetics not responding to sulphonylureas, coincide with the findings in maturity-onset diabetics and the concept of insulin deficiency diabetes. This is namely that a strong reduction in β-cells renders successful sulphonylurea therapy impossible. From these investigations one can only assume that a certain initial amount of insulin producing tissue must be present; not, however, that the sulphonylureas can stimulate the existing β-cells in any way. This is because degranulation and hydropical degeneration were not increased in treated, compared to untreated diabetics. There is no reason for assuming an influence on the α-cells. Also stronger islet regeneration could not be positively proved in the treated diabetics. However, this question is difficult to answer as islet buds also occur frequently in untreated diabetics, and a quantitative judgement is not possible. GEPTS (1958b) sometimes found augmentation and swelling of the centro-acinar cells and of the small pancreatic ducts, and believes a regeneration of islet tissue to be possible in single cases. Further observations are necessary here. However, it can already be stated that such changes are rare and do not allow for the hope that sulphonylurea therapy significantly increases the insulin producing tissue in the human diabetic.

8. Conclusions about the mode of action in man and animal from the experiments

Roughly, the findings correspond in the metabolically normal and in the diabetic. The many opposing findings only show the complexity of the problem. Today, the glucagon theory (FRANKE and FUCHS) is obsolete, also the insulinase theory (MIRSKY) and the possibility of hypophyseal inhibition. In animal and man, the sulphonylurea effect on carbohydrate metabolism depends on the existence of intact β-cells; thus on a sufficient endogenous insulin production. It is, however, questionable whether the mechanism of action can be explained simply by insulin liberation or even by continuous stimulation of insulin secretion. The insulin release is possibly only important in the acute experiment in the healthy organism. In the diabetic its significance is doubted in the acute experiment and especially so during long-term treatment. A weighty arguement against the principle of action being a stronger insulin effect during long-term therapy is the fact, that diabetics successfully treated with sulphonylureas increase less in weight than those treated with insulin (STRAUZENBERG and HALLER). These differences in weight gain are apparent in normal and over-weight patients.

The liver, rather than the periphery, is the *site* of the metabolic effect of the sulphonylureas. Research is too young on the subject to be able to explain the influencing of hepatic glucose production by sulphonylureas (taken for granted) by a portal insulin effect alone (MADISON et al., 1959; PFEIFFER et al., 1959). It is possible, however, that the complex questions will be resolved in this sense. The hypotheses is not proved to date, that there is a complex formation between the sulphonylureas and endogenous insulin resulting in a liver effective factor, thus explaining the double effect on the β-cells and on hepatic metabolism (CREUTZ-FELDT et al., STRAUZENBERG and HALLER). However, there are numerous obser-vations pointing to a direct effect of the sulphonylureas on the liver (comp. p.19f., 45f., 78f.) modifying the effect of endogenous insulin in a characteristic way; however, they require a certain amount of endogenous insulin to become effective. In the diabetic responding to sulphonylurea therapy, the hepatic effect could predominate which is only secondary in a normal person, because this type of diabetes is characterised by a large hepatic glucose production. Here it is re-markable that the liver glucose output in the maturity-onset diabetic can hardly be inhibited by insulin (hepatic insensitive diabetic according to BEARN, BILLING and SHERLOCK). Also the blood sugar decrease after sulphonylureas, despite normal increase in plasma insulin activity (PFEIFFER et al., 1959; VALLANCE-OWEN et al.), is greatly delayed and relatively weak in the diabetic in contrast to the healthy controls.

On the grounds of the relatively high pancreatic insulin content and the normal or even increased plasma insulin activity in the maturity-onset diabetic, it has been discussed that in this type of diabetes, the β-cell response to the physio-logical secretion stimulus, e.g. blood sugar level, is reduced (LAZAROW 1957, et al.). The morphological substrate for this could be membrane changes (LACY and HARTROFT). Then the glucose would only penetrate the β-cells and stimulate insulin secretion if it had attained a pathological blood level. The sulphonylurea effect should consist in raising the sensitivity of the β-cell for the glucose stimulus (HASELBLATT and BLUDAU, BÄNDEG, 1959b) or in rendering the thickened mem-brane more permeable for glucose (LACY and HARTROFT). Against this hypotheses, speaks the simple observation that elevation of the blood sugar in the diabetic in the case of infection or a glucocorticoid therapy regularly causes a rapid metabolic disturbance as the absolute capacity of the β-cells is also reduced in the maturity-onset diabetic. As this is so, it is difficult to imagine the diabetic suddenly being able to produce permanently more insulin under the influence of sulphonyl-ureas.

Despite countless experimental data and more or less well founded, mostly one-sided theories, we must confess that to date the sulphonylurea mechanism of action has not been cleared satisfactorily. One can only say that the sulphonyl-ureas act on *various* tissues and metabolic processes. The basis of this is, perhaps, enzymatically similar processes, but it depends on respective conditions whether one certain effect is dominating. The conditions for a sufficient effect in vivo are in any case, a minimum number of functional β-cells. It is almost certain that in the acute experiment, and if the β-cell system is intact, insulin secretion is in the foreground. It is, however, probable that on chronic dosing, especially in the diabetic a specific effect on the liver gains in importance and plays a significant part in improving diabetic metabolism. This question cannot be fully answered until we know more of the effect of insulin in hepatic metabolism and also more about the pathogenesis of human diabetes, especially the so-called hyperfunctional diabetes of the older patient.

d) Sulphonylureas as therapeutics in non-diabetic diseases

1. Dermatological diseases

D 860 (KABELITZ and KAPPEL) and also BZ 55 (NEUMANN) have been successfully used in the treatment of psoriasis. Continual improvement occurred after 1—3 weeks; after discontinuation, deterioration frequently occurred. The daily dose was 1—3 tablets (0.5—1.5 grams). Hypoglycaemia was rarely seen and was never severe. In 19 patients treated with BZ 55, psoriasis disappeared completely in two cases, 14 showed significant, and two only slight, and one no improvement (NEUMANN). In 25 patients receiving D 860, 17 showed improvement or disappearance of the disease, while 8 did not respond to therapy. Nothing is known of the mechanism of action of the sulphonylureas in the influencing of psoriasis. NEUMANN discusses some metabolic effect.

HÄGGBLOM reported the healing of a dermatitis hepatiformis in a diabetic by BZ 55 which simultaneously had a beneficial effect on the diabetes of the patient.

COHEN and COHEN saw in 2 diabetics treated with D 860 a surprising improvement in the also existing acne. Thus they chose 23 non-diabetics suffering from pustular acne, chronic staphyloderma, recessive furunculosis, sycosis vulgaris, hidradenitis suppurativa and other suppurating skin infections; all were resistant to antibiotics and x-ray treatment. The treatment lasted months with 0.5—1 gram D 860 daily. From 26 patients, 8 showed excellent, 12 good and 5 a fair improvement. In one case, treatment was discontinued owing to gastro-intestinal side-effects. Blood sugar changes were not seen. Sometimes there was subjective complaints similar to those found with hypoglycaemia that disappeared after sufficient carbohydrate administration. As D 860 has hardly any bacteriostatic properties (s. p. 14), its beneficial effect on resistant acne and other suppurating skin diseases can therefore not be brought about bacteriostatically. The authors discussed the possibilities of a disturbance in the carbohydrate metabolism involving only the tissues of the skin (skin diabetes) as causing this resistant skin change. They argue of a specific effect of the sulphonylureas on these peripheral metabolic disturbances. From these experiences, there are interesting indications in dermatology for the sulphonylureas. This would justify a critical analysis on more material.

2. Diseases of the liver

At first it may seem strange that the sulphonylureas are at all discussed as possible therapy for liver diseases as one of the main problems in introducing these as oral anti-diabetic drugs was the possibility of liver damage. Therefore it must be recalled, that already 20 years ago the first papers on a protective sulphonamide effect on toxic liver damages were published. LEACH and FORBES described an effect of sulphanilamide, sulphathiazole and sulphapyridine on the time of survival and on necrosis of the liver following acute tetrachlorcarbon poisoning in the rat. Their findings were confirmed using sulphanilamide and sulphaguanidine by WILSON et al. (1952) in the acute CCl_4 poisoning of the mouse. Nothing is known of the mode of action of this protective effect. The bacteriostatic property plays no decisive role, for other strong bacteriostatic sulphonamide derivatives do not have this effect (WILSON, 1952). Increase in liver glycogen was not observed. Possibly here is either a direct reaction of the sulphonamides with the administered toxic substance, or competition with the poison at those cell structures or enzymes that are damaged by the poison (LEDUC and WILSON). Thus it is probable that the mechanism of this effect is only a competitive one and not a real sulphonamide liver protective effect.

Therefore it is not surprising, in the face of these older findings, that sulphonylureas also reduce liver necrosis in the acute poisoning with various hepatic toxins. This was shown for acute CCl_4 poisoning with BZ 55 (v. EICKSTEDT), for acute allyl alcohol poisoning with BZ 55 (v. EICKSTEDT; EGER and REINCKE) and D 860 (KIRNBERGER et al., EGER and REINCKE) and for the acute thioacetamide poisoning with D 860 (KNICK, RUCKES and EMRICH, GEORGII et al.).

KALDOR et al. (1960), however, found no influence of D 860 on the extent of necrosis of CCl_4 poisoned rats but an increased hepatic glycogen content. As, however, the effect achieved by sulphonylureas does not differ from that of the other sulphonamides it is naturally not connected with the blood sugar decrease or hepatic glycogen increase. The results are not so favourable in experimental cronic poisoning. Possibly the above discussed competitive effect of the sulphonylureas cannot assert itself after repeated daily poisonings. On the other hand, it must also be considered that the evaluation of the protective effect from the survival time or histological control of the liver changes, or from serum electrophoresis following chronic administration of such severe liver toxins, is of doubtful value. KNICK, RUCKES and EMRICH found no changes in the histological picture of liver damage following long-term thioacetamide poisoning with simultaneous D 860 doses, and even gained the impression of a slight liver protective effect from the results of the functional tests and estimations of enzymes (KNICK and RUCKES). However, GEORGII et al. saw more intense change in the liver after administering thioacetamide and D 860 for many months than after thioacetamide alone. RÖTTKER investigated the influence of D 860 on liver regeneration in the rat, incidental to 3 months of thioacetamide poisoning, and found no difference from the control group. HESSE found that D 860 had no effect on the development of CCl_4 cirrhosis in the rat. PETZOLD and STÖHR, however, described reduced connective tissue proliferation after BZ 55 in rabbits chronically treated with CCl_4. Their experimental results are questioned by the extraordinary fact that only pure BZ 55 has this effect and not the sodium salt (even more easily absorbed in rodents than the pure substance) (comp. p. 11).

Finally the effect of D 860 on the experimentally produced fatty liver degeneration in the rat was investigated. KIRNBERGER et al. found in the dietary fatty liver (protein deficiency) a significant weak lipotropic effect if D 860 was administered with the noxious food. PETZOLD also described a lipotropic effect of D 860 in the liver regeneration test in the rat where simultaneously some histochemical enzyme reactions were influenced.

A real liver protective effect of the sulphonylureas cannot be certain on the grounds of these experiments. This does not refute, however, the possibility of a therapeutic effect of these drugs in liver diseases in man. As is known, no animal experiment can reproduce the hepatitis and liver cirrhosis found in man. We can at least see from the above experiments that the sulphonylureas have no liver damaging effects; thus, the above mentioned clinical observations are confirmed (comp. p. 70f.).

Independently from the animal experiments, some authors also investigated sulphonylurea action on liver diseases in man. Here they started out on the assumption that hepatic glycogen augmentation through the sulphonylureas must have a beneficial effect on the damaged liver. KNICK and EMRICH first reported of the beneficial effect of D 860 (3 grams over 3—6 weeks) in 6 cases of chronic hepatitis and 6 cases of liver cirrhosis without diabetes. The effect was apparent by a decrease in serum bilirubin, improvement in the serum lability tests, in the serum electrophoresis and the bromsulphonephthalein retention test; hypoglycaemia did not occur. PFEFFER et al. (1958) treated 14 non-diabetics with acute, and 16 with chronic hepatitis and 13 non-diabetics with cirrhosis of the liver with BZ 55 (1 g daily for several weeks). They believed, on grounds of laboratory findings and some liver biopsies, to see definite improvement in the cases of acute and chronic hepatitis. A certain effect was not found in the cases with liver cirrhosis. In 7 patients, hypoglycaemia occurred at night. MAGYAR et al. (1957) treated 9 patients with chronic hepatitis (2 of which were diabetics) and 3 with liver cirrhosis (1 of which was diabetic) for 10 days with BZ 55 (commencing with 2.5 g then 1 g daily). They saw no distinct improvement and also no deterioration in the liver function tests. LÁSZLÓ et al. (1959) dosed 50 patients suffering from acute hepatitis with D 860 and saw a rapid decrease in serum bilirubin and quicker recovery time; however, this was only of 4 days when compared to a similar group of controls.

No final conclusion can be drawn from these results. The findings in acute and chronic hepatitis must be accepted with reserve as these cases show a tendency towards spontaneous improvement; thus, therapeutic effects are difficult to judge objectively. The beneficial effects seen by KNICK and EMRICH in cases with cirrhosis of the liver could not be confirmed by PFEFFER et al. (1958). We also saw no improvement in the liver function tests (also no deterioration) in 10 diabetics with liver cirrhosis receiving D 860 for several months because of their diabetes. Also other workers saw no negative effect of the sulphonylureas on the course of liver disease in diabetics with acute hepatitis and continuation of sulphonylurea treatment, or diabetics with liver cirrhosis dosed with sulphonylureas (DOLGER, 1956; SEIDLER et al., 1957; HOFSTETTER and RAMEL, 1958). Therefore, we can now say that BZ 55 and D 860 do not have any toxic effect even on the damaged liver. Against the application of D 860 and BZ 55 as therapeuticals in acute or chronic diseases of the liver, speaks besides the not very convincing previous experience, the unclear conceptions of the mechanism of "liver protection" (glycogen augmentation following sulphonylureas only appears in fasting conditions, not however, on food intake, comp. p. 46) and the danger of hypoglycaemia.

3. Epilepsy

KOLARIK and MIKULA surprisingly observed on changing over a diabetic suffering from grand mal attacks to BZ 55 (1.5 g daily) that the attacks ceased. This is not surprising when considering the fact that other urea derivatives are used as anti-convulsants. Further research is necessary to find out whether BZ 55 is superior to the known drugs, so that its application as an anti-epileptic drug, despite the dangers of low blood sugar in this condition, is justifiable.

4. Psychiatric shock therapy

Here (in the previously discussed effects on non-diabetic diseases undesired) the blood sugar decreasing effect of sulphonylureas is therapeutically used in non-diabetics. In several investigations, it was shown that the combined dose of insulin and BZ 55 (VOELKEL, 1956; VOELKEL et al., 1957; BAYREUTHER and SPECHT, 1956; BAYREUTHER, 1957) also D 860 (BAYREUTHER) given to attain hypoglycaemia in a psychosis can have certain advantages. According to VOELKEL the therapeutic risks (cerebral convulsions and delayed return to consciousness) is slighter and insulin can be reduced to 50%. BAYREUTHER found, besides an average insulin reduction of 30%, that sulphonylureas are especially indicated in patients who are relatively insulin resistant. Because here beneficial effects are found since the insulin reduction per. milligram sulphonylureas increases with the square of the strength of the individual insulin resistance. According to these authors, the sulphonylureas only support the insulin effect without any specific action on the psychosis. It is questionable whether this fact justifies the general use of sulphonylureas as hypoglycaemic therapy in psychoses. The combination therapy also does not seem to be much used, as no further papers have been published. When the insulin requirements are unusually high to cause hypoglycaemic coma, and in patients tending to convulsions under insulin (so-called early epilepsy), one can advise attempting the addition of sulphonylureas to the insulin treatment.

The findings of FROST, who saw a beneficial effect on the psychoses in 45 of 60 schizophrenics on administering BZ 55 for several weeks (1.5 g/day) without insulin, have not yet been confirmed. He especially indicated the euphorising and anti-hallucinatory effect of this therapy. As there was no blood sugar lowering, the mechanism of action found in a series of cases treated by FROST were not reinvestigated.

Above has been mentioned the beneficial effect of D 860 on *angina pectoris*, also found in the non-diabetic (comp. p. 63).

IV. Other clinically tested sulphonylureas

To conclude the discussion on the blood sugar lowering sulphonamide derivatives, some other sulphonylureas must be mentioned that have been clinically proven and are on the market, e.g. K 386 and chlorpropamide, or withdrawn owing to its side-effects, e.g. metahexamide. As is shown in the chapter on structure and effectiveness (comp. p. 7), countless combinations have been synthesised that have an equal or better blood sugar effect than BZ 55 and D 860. It would be theoretically possible to try many further sulphonylurea compounds in treating diabetes.

Against this, however, is to be warned. The effective principle of the whole group is probably the same, namely, the action on the β-cells and the influencing of various enzyme reactions especially in the liver. An unlimited increase in effect by raising the dose is not possible, as there is a dose-effect relationship which is linear only to a limited point. Therefore, it is of no advantage if some substances show the same effect with a lower dose or sometimes even a slightly better anti-diabetic effect than BZ 55 or D 860, because this is either attained by a longer half-life time, or by special affinity to the site of action, e.g. β-cells and/or, the liver cells. In both cases the danger of side-effects increases. This is so as either excretion is delayed or tissue binding increased. Thus the general toxicity is raised, or the stronger effect on the β-cells and liver can cause specific damage (exhaustion of insulin production, s. p. 37 respectively liver cell changes). The risk involved, despite the slight advantage of using low doses, does not justify the production of limitless amounts of drugs, nor does effectiveness in the few patients who do not, or incompletely respond to D 860. For here there is danger of the new substances not being as thoroughly tested as was the case with the first drugs. Then the more effective and more dangerous drugs (seen by experience to date) would not only be applied in the case of the few patients whose diabetes can only be compensated by them, but also in those of diabetics who respond satisfactorily to the less effective D 860 medication. Thus the damage caused by the frequent redundant treatment of diabetics with these drugs outweighs the advantage it has for the few. Following the principle of nil nocere, one should, on grounds of valuable experience with the less effective, but in every case the least dangerous sulphonylurea, try to make do principally with this drug. This is D 860 according to corresponding views. Thus this substance should be used as a standard of safety for all further sulphonylurea preparations. If no effect is reached with D 860, BZ 55 can under circumstances be used. A new sulphonylurea should be used only as a third resort.

If further sulphonylureas are introduced to practice, to allow patients this form of therapy, one must realise that according to the principle of action the number of patients treated will always be limited. They would consist of those with endogenous insulin reserves and there is always the danger when applying the more active compound, that the β-cytotropic effect transcends to a β-cytotoxic one (comp. p. 41). We cannot except real progress in oral diabetes therapy with some new sulphonylurea, but only with some substance with a different mechanism of action.

The discussion of other experimentally and clinically tested sulphonylureas, rather than BZ 55 and D 860, will be confined to a comparison of effect, mechanism of action, and side-effects.

a) 1-cyclohexyl-3-p-tolylsulphonylurea (K 386)

K 386 will be mentioned briefly as here only the butyl rest of D 860 has been replaced by a cyclohexyl rest (comp. Tab. 7). The compound has, like D 860, no bacteriostatic properties and only slight toxicity and also a stronger blood sugar lowering effect in animal experiments than D 860 (JANONO et al., 1957). The pharmacological tests were made by the firm Carlo Erba in Milan and put by them on the Italian market. The clinical investigations of JACONO et al. (1957), ANGELI and ALBERINI also MORSIANI and SERRAVALLI showed it to have good antidiabetic effect with only slight toxicity. MORSIANI and SERRAVALLI observed that in 106 diabetics treated with K 386, the indications and the rarity of side-effects corresponded to those following D 860. ANGELI and ALBERINI described one case of urticaria in 72 patients treated with K 386. The mechanism of action should not differ from that of the sulphonylureas.

b) N-propyl-3-p-chlorbenzoylsulphonylurea (chlorpropamide P 607)

There are a large number of publications on chlorpropamide; this is meanwhile, on the market in the USA (formula s. Tab. 7). Owing to chloride substituents at the benzol ring, there are also no bacteriostatic effects.

1. Methods of determination, distribution, and excretion in animals and man

For determining in the serum, a modification of the method developed by SPINGLER for D 860 was used (ROOT, SIGAL and ANDERSON, 1959), and a method by TOOLAN and WAGNER based on the ultra-violet absorption of this compound at 232.5 nm. This method is not applicable for determining chlorpropamide in the urine. Therefore, investigations on the half-life time were also made and excretion studies with ^{35}S-labelled chlorpropamide were performed in animals (SCHNEIDER et al.) and in man (JOHNSON et al.); absorption from the intestine is rapid. Excretion occurs practically only via the kidneys. Degradation of these substances was only found in the dog (ROOT, 1959). Here only 1/3 of the administered chlorpropamide was excreted unchanged. About 40% appears as p-chlorbenzoylsulphonylurea and in the remaining 16—24% the urea is also split off. In the rabbit, 80—95% was excreted unaltered (ROOT, 1959). Man mainly excretes unchanged chlorpropamide according to JOHNSON et al. ROOT (1959), however, also assumes for man 1 or 2 unidentified metabolites. In the dog, chlorpropamide can still be found in the serum 96 hrs after a single chlorpropamide dose. In the rabbit, there is only a very low plasma level after 24 hrs (ROOT, SIGAL and ANDERSON, 1959; SCHNEIDER et al.). The half-life time of chlorpropamide in man averages 35 hrs (JOHNSON et al., FORSHAM et al., KNAUF et al., 1959a; STOWERS et al., 1959; WEST and JOHNSON). According to JOHNSON et al. who worked with ^{35}S-labelled chlorpropamide, it was found that for 80% the half-life time was that of BZ 55 in man. The other fraction is much more slowly excreted (for approximately 16 days). The authors leave open whether here is a non-identified metabolite of chlorpropamide, or if the slowly excreted component is firmly bound to serum protein. This is so since they found the substance to show strong protein binding tendency. After dialysis for 48 hrs, 5—13% of the chlorpropamide added in vivo or vitro was still bound to serum protein. The absolute amount of bound substance increased with the rising chlorpropamide concentration. Also ESMANN et al., also CARLOZZI et al. emphasised the long time required for the total elimination of chlorpropamide (8—14 days).

The distributary space of chlorpropamide for man is only 10—13 liters (STOWERS et al., 1959; JOHNSON et al.). The same is true for D 860.

The necessary plasma level for successful chlorpropamide long-term treatment averages 10—20 mg-%. They found, in fact, values between 2.5 and 32 mg-% (ESMANN et al., STOWERS et al., 1959; BEASER, 1959; HADLEY et al.). CARLOZZI et al. stated that an effective plasma level could not be maintained with doses under 100 mg. chlorpropamide daily; with 250 mg daily, the plasma level was 10 mg-%, with 500 mg daily, 18 mg-%; and with 1 g daily, 32 mg-%. Thus, there is the danger of chlorpropamide accumulation in patients receiving larger doses. In the dog, this is the case only with doses of over 50 mg/kg (SCHNEIDER et al.).

2. Toxicity, acute blood sugar decrease and mechanism of action

Toxicity experiments were performed in rats, mice, cats, dogs and rhesus monkeys (ROOT, SIGAL and ANDERSON, 1959; SCHNEIDER et al., BÄNDER, 1959a). Greater toxicity was found here than either with BZ 55 or D 860. The DL_{50} for the mouse was according to SCHNEIDER et al. 1.7 g/kg, according to ROOT, SIGAL and ANDERSON (1959) only 0.7 g/kg; for the rat, according to SCHNEIDER et al., 2.4 g/kg, and according to ROOT, SIGAL and ANDERSON (1959), only 0.9 g/kg orally. SCHNEIDER et al., also ROOT, SIGAL and ANDERSON (1959) did not find any pathological organ changes during chronic toxic experiments. Only in pancreatectomised dogs chronically receiving chlorpropamide severe intestinal haemorrhages were seen following decrease in prothrombin values owing to general liver damage (ROOT, SIGAL and ANDERSON, 1959), as has also been described for D 860 and BZ 55 (comp. p. 15). BÄNDER (1959a), however, saw in rats receiving 250 mg/kg chlorpropamide and sometimes more daily, and also in dogs given 10—50 mg/kg chlorpropamide daily, fatty and degenerative changes in the liver and kidney. Some of BÄNDER's animals died during these doses that were well tolerated in rats in the chronic experiments of SCHNEIDER et al. also ROOT, SIGAL and ANDERSON apart from retarded growth. This discrepancy can be connected with the different animal strain or method of applying the substance (tube feeding by BÄNDER, addition to food by SCHNEIDER et al., also ROOT, SIGAL and ANDERSON). This explanation is not very satisfactory. However, SCHNEIDER et al. indicate that higher chlorpropamide doses lead in all species to muscular weakness and ataxia that could not be influenced by glucose. Similar symptoms have been described for the human being (s. p. 90).

The *blood sugar lowering* effect of chlorpropamide in rats and dogs is twice that of BZ 55, the doses being equal according to ROOT, SIGAL and ANDERSON (1959). SCHNEIDER et al. found in rats and dogs receiving the same doses of D 860 or chlorpropamide the same maximal blood sugar decrease that was however of longer duration following chlorpropamide. Only in the rhesus monkey did chlorpropamide depress the blood sugar more strongly *and* longer than D 860. Investigations in man do not definitely show that chlorpropamide has a stronger effect than D 860 following a *single* dose. FORSHAM et al., also WEST and CAMPBELL, however, found a doubly strong blood sugar lowering effect of chlorpropamide after an oral dose; this indicates better intestinal absorption whereby a higher plasma level is attained (WEST and CAMPBELL, WEST and JOHNSON, KNAUFF et al. 1959a). Following the equal i.v. dose, the blood sugar effect is of the same magnitude in both chlorpropamide and D 860 (CRAIG et al. 1959a, KNAUFF et al. 1959a, WEST and CAMPBELL, WEST and JOHNSON). TORNOW et al. even found in diabetics receiving an oral dose of 1 gram D 860 or chlorpropamide an almost identical blood sugar decrease. The various clinical reports stating the greater effectiveness of chlorpropamide in long-term therapy must therefore be based on its delayed excretion and, or, the stronger protein and tissue binding.

The *mechanism of action* of chlorpropamide does not differ to that of BZ 55 and D 860 as far as can be said from the sparse investigations. SCHNEIDER et al. found a degranulation of the β-cells following several days of chlorpropamide, a significant increase in liver glycogen 2 hrs following chlorpropamide application, severe hypoglycaemia in adrenalectomised animals, normal blood sugar decrease in hepatectomised, and ineffectiveness in alloxanised animals. The insulin and glucose tolerance of dogs treated for 1 year with 15—100 mg/kg chlorpropamide was also not significantly altered. However, BÄNDER (1959a) described for dogs and rats following chlorpropamide application for several weeks diabetic glucose tolerance. ROOT, SIGAL and ANDERSON (1959) found in pancreatectomised dogs and severely alloxanised rabbits 18 hrs following the last insulin dose, a significantly blood-sugar-lowering effect of chlorpropamide. This is also known for D 860 and BZ 55. GRANDE and MARTINEZ could even normalise the blood sugars of moderately mild alloxan-diabetic mice with chlorpropamide. RENOLD et al. (1959) achieved in vitro the same effect on the ketogenesis of liver slices with chlorpropamide, also on the glucose oxidation and lipogenesis of adipose tissue as with D 860 (comp. p. 19 and 20f.). FOA et al. (1959) found no significant blood sugar decrease following the injection of 5 mg/kg chlorpropamide into the pancreatic artery, but found, however, after injecting higher doses (50 mg/kg) into the femoral artery a non-insulin-like decrease in glucose, pyruvate, and lactate. This they believed to be caused by diminished hepatic glucose production.

Also in man there does not seem to be fundamental differences from BZ 55 and D 860 regarding the mechanism of action. Thus chlorpropamide was ineffective in totally pancreatectomised human beings (TINES et al., FORSHAM et al.). Also in juvenile patients suffering from a typical insulin deficiency diabetes no effect could be found (LOEWENTHAL et al., HEINSEN, DEHN and HAGEN 1958). However, in cases with an abnormally high insulin requirement (over 80 U) some insulin reduction was achieved when using chlorpropamide (DOBSON et al. 1959a). This observation also corresponds to the experiences with D 860 (comp. p. 58f.).

3. Permanent therapy and side-effects

The great effectiveness of chlorpropamide during permanent treatment of diabetes is uniformally acclaimed by the clinicians (MURRAY et al., FORSHAM et al., HEINSEN et al. 1958, KNAUFF et al. 1959a, SUGAR et al., BLÖCH and LENHARDT,

TORNOW et al., STEWART et al. 1959). The same group of patients respond to chlorpropamide as to D 860 and BZ 55. The daily maintenance doses are significantly lower—0.125—0.5 g. (rarely to 1 gram). It is not necessary to give the dose twice. From this we see that the greater effectiveness is due to the more constant plasma level. The question whether patients, not or unsatisfactorily responding to D 860, or if as secondary failures they have lost the initial response, can be treated with chlorpropamides, is of interest. UNGER, MADISON and CARTER (1959) only achieved satisfactory control with chlorpropamide in 12% of their insufficiently to D 860 responding patients. LEE et al., however, achieved good control with chlorpropamide in 11 from 12 diabetics ineffectively compensated with D 860. CAMPBELL (1959) achieved the same with 24 such patients. SUGAR et al. could successfully treat 20 from 31 secondary failures with chlorpropamide. Also, TORNOW et al. had some therapeutic success in secondary failures of the D 860 therapy or in the poorly controlled D 860 patients. Seen as a whole, the group of patients responding to chlorpropamide is not very large as also the secondary failures of the D 860 group are relatively rare (comp. p. 59 f.).

The *side-effects* of chlorpropamide are of significance. On them depends to what extent a change-over from D 860 to these more effective substances is justified. When compared to BZ 55 and D 860 these side-effects are much more severe. Statistically nothing can be proved as the reported number of patients treated with chlorpropamide is still relatively small. The most frequent and banal side-effect is a *gastro-intestinal* disturbance (sense of repletion, loss of appetite, sickness, nausea). Of 215 patients, 10.7% complained of these symptoms and ceased to, in most but not all cases, on reducing the dose (BLÖCH and LENHARDT). *Skin reactions* occur as frequently as with BZ 55 (3.5% of the 215 cases of BLÖCH and LENHARDT). STEWART et al. (1959) described a case of dermatitis exfoliativa. CAMPBELL (1960) saw a case of photo-allergy. He also observed *pancytopenia* following chlorpropamide. *Leucopenia* has only been seen once (SUGAR et al. 1959). *Hypoglycaemic* reactions appear remarkably often which is comprehensible when considering the cumulative tendencies with higher doses. This calls for careful individual control. LEE et al. saw among 32 patients 8, TORNOW et al. among 33 cases, 3 of hypoglycaemia. STEWART et al. (1959) observed among 50 patients 5 with blood sugar values between 45—60 mg-% without subjective symptoms of hypoglycaemia. A 66 year old female described by STEWART et al. had a blood sugar value of 42 mg-% without specific symptoms; several days later she was found dead at home. An autopsy was not made. COATES and ROBBINS observed in an 88 year old female patient receiving 2×250 mg chlorpropamide daily a hypoglycaemic shock with blood sugar values of 8 mg-%; death did not ensue. Also LINDEMAN described a case of severe chlorpropamide shock with a blood sugar value of 12 mg-% which could be overcome by high doses of glucose.

Most workers describe relatively often occurring side-effects, general muscle weakness, tiredness, vertigo, ataxia and nystagmus, not necessarily accompanied by low sugar values and are thus taken for direct effects on the *central nervous system*. They occur mostly at doses of 0.75—1 g daily and often disappear on reducing the dose (WALKER 1958, GREENHOUSE 1959, BEASER 1959). Such side-effects are practically unknown for D 860 and BZ 55; these weigh against the chlorpropamide therapy.

Finally, several cases of *cholostatic hepatosis* following chlorpropamide administration have been described, i.e. this kind of liver damage is generally thought to be a hypersensitive reaction and is well known as salvarsan early jaundice also found following doses of methyltestosterone and especially chlorpromazine. The intensity of this jaundice (biochemically characterised by the signs of obstructive jaundice) oscillates strongly. It depends largly on whether the condition has been recognized and the therapy momentarily discontinued. The jaundice ran a lethal course in one 61 year old female patient (DOBSON et al. 1959a). In this case the daily dose, exactly as in the cases of jaundice of STEWART et al. (1959), BROWN et al. (1959) and PALMAS, was only 0.5 g of chlorpropamide. Therefore, the avoidance of higher doses is no protection against this severe complication. It is difficult to assess the total number of observed cases of jaundice. HAMFF saw jaundice among 20 treated cases, 3 times, PALMAS among 110 cases, 4 times, BROWN et al. (1959), among 49 cases, 3 times. Other authors only saw single cases. However, this complication is so characteristic for the chlorpropamide therapy that weekly contrcl of the alkaline serum phosphatase and serum leucine-amino-peptidase, which in cholostatic hepatosis show elevation often before an increase in bilirubin, is necessary at least during the first 8 weeks of chlorpropamide treatment. Most cases of jaundice appear during this time (BROWN et al. 1959).

As final, more frequently than after D 860 or BZ 55, appearing side-effect, alcohol intolerance after chloropropamide will be mentioned (SIGNORELLI also SIGNORELLI and POSA, TCLOMELLI and BACCI, ESMANN et al., BLÖCH and LEN-HARDT). 11% of BLÖCH's and LENHARDT's 215 patients suffered spontanously from antabuse-like complaints. SIGNORELLI and POSA found alcohol intolerance in 8 of 23 cases. However following alcohol loading, all patients showed typical side-effects.

It has been repeatedly mentioned that many but not all side-effects depend on the dosage. GREENHOUSE reaches this conclusion despite the 30 cases from 50 showing side-effects that on administering lower doses, the side-effects would be minimal. PALMAS (17% side-effects among 110 cases) is more reserved in his views and WALKER (1958) (15 cases of intolerance among 43 patients) believes the general use of this substance to be questionable.

On looking through the present literature, we must come to the conclusion that the strong blood sugar effectiveness of chlorpropamide is combined with too great a toxicity. If the side-effects on lower dosage (0.25—0.5 g daily) are less frequent, then it must be said that the cases who only require these chlorpropamide doses can to a large extent also be controlled by 0.5—1.5 g D 860 or BZ 55. These latter having much larger therapeutic breadth and in which administration of twice or three times the dose has no dangers for the patient. Therefore, chlor-propamide should not be used as a substitue for the sulphonylureas which are known to be safe, but only in patients that respond unsatisfactorily to D 860 despite sufficient dietary control; experience with chlorpropamide has not been adequate. Only HEINSEN et al. (1958) reported of a secondary failure during chlorpropamide therapy to date.

c) N-(3-amino-4-methylbenzoylsulphonyl)-N'-cyclohexylurea (Metahexamide)

Metahexamide first promised to be a great success owing to its strong effective-ness in experiments and diabetics as is seen from the numerous publications (formula s. Tab. 7). It advantages were, however, alleviated by a series of severe liver damage, causing the clinical withdrawal of this drug (FORSHAM 1959). The most important data given for this substance will be discussed briefly because they throw light on the possibilities and dangers that the group of sulphonylureas still has to offer us.

1. Methods for determination, distribution, excretion in animals and man

For estimating metahexamide, the method of BRATTON and MARSHALL or a modification of this is suitable (FORIST 1959). Absorption from the intestine is rapid and excretion almost entirely by the kidneys. Acetylisation does not occur in the rabbit that usually acetylises especially well, probably because of the neighbouring methyl- and amino group at the benzol ring. 30—35% of the administered metahexamide is excreted unaltered in dogs and rabbits, the rest following splitting-off of the cyclohexyl rest and also partially of the urea rest (ROOT, ANDERSON and WELLES).

The half-life time in man is diversly indicated by different authors (between $5^1/_2$ and 26 hrs). This may be caused partly by the method, as here the plasma levels are much lower on administering therapeutic doses than in the previously discussed sulphonylureas, but finally only from these, conclusions are possible. In any case, the half-life time is longer than that of D 860 and significantly shorter than that of BZ 55 and chlorpropamide. SILVER et al. (1959) found an average half-life time of $5^1/_2$ hrs in the healthy subject, in the diabetic of 10 hrs; GRANVILLE-GROSSMAN et al. found in healthy subjects an average of 10 hrs in diabetics, 26 hrs. CREUTZFELDT, ANDREU- KERN and DISCHER reckoned an average half-life time of 7—9 hrs for healthy controls following i.v. dose of metahexamide. The fact that after single oral or i.v. dose, 70% of the applied metahexamide is found in the urine within 24 hrs and in the subsequent 24 hrs a further 18% (CREUTZFELDT, ANDREU-KERN and DISCHER) disapproves the correctness of some higher half-life time values proposed by some authors (MORGENSTERN and GARRETT, WEST and JOHNSON, HAMWI et al.) with 19 hrs, respectively with 26 hrs (KNAUFF et al. 1959 b). The distributary space was estimated at 12.7% of the body weight (GRANVILLE-GROSSMAN et al.), the clearance with 10 ml plasma/min (CREUTZFELDT, ANDREU-KERN and DISCHER). During long-term therapy of 100—200 mg metahexamide, the daily estimated plasma level was 3—4 mg-% during the day (HAMWI et al., GRANVILLE-GROSSMAN et al., CREUTZFELDT, ANDREU-KERN and DISCHER). In the morning before the tablet administration, very often only 1—2 mg-%. Thus, they attained only 1/5 of the average values found after other sulphonylureas.

2. Toxicity, acute blood sugar decrease and mode of action

The results of toxicity experiments in mice, rats, and dogs were published by ROOT, ANDERSON and WELLES. The acute toxicity is much lower than that of chlorpropamide (the DL_{50} on oral doses was 1.3 g/kg for mice, 1.4 g/kg for rats). In the chronic feeding experiments no organic changes in rats, rabbits and dogs were found by ROOT, ANDERSON and WELLES. However, in dogs receiving doses of over 10 mg/kg, anorexia and resulting fatty liver degeneration occurred. Pancreatectomised, insulinised dogs showed after chronic doses of metahexamide, exactly as after the other sulphonylureas, prolongation of the prothrombin time and severe intestinal haemorrhages (ROOT, ANDERSON and WELLES)). BÄNDER (1959a) believes the fatty liver degeneration, nephrotic changes and frequent deaths already found in normal rats and dogs (using the same metahexamide doses) to be caused by tube feeding or by using other animal strains: his explanations remain unsatisfactory, because the same author's same toxicity experiments with D 860 were negative.

The *blood sugar decreasing* effect of metahexamide in the acute experiment is much stronger when compared to the other sulphonylureas discussed above. Thus in rats receiving the same dose, a 4 times greater blood sugar decrease was found for metahexamide than for D 860. In dogs, 1/3 of the necessary plasma level for chlorpropamide was sufficient for achieving the same blood sugar decrease (ROOT, ANDERSON and WELLES). Also in man, a greater effectiveness was seen. WEST and JOHNSON found metahexamide 3—4 times as effective as D 860 on i.v. injection. CREUTZFELDT, ANDREU-KERN and DISCHER compared the minimal blood sugar lowering dose of metahexamide and D 860 and found a relation of 1:5; a corresponding relation was also seen when comparing the plasma level necessary for a blood sugar decrease. KNAUFF et al. (1959b) found that metahexamide, when measured by the blood level, is 4 times as effective as D 860 and chlorpropamide; when measured by the oral dose necessary for achieving a blood sugar decrease in the normal control, metahexamide is even 15 times more effective than D 860.

Thus, metahexamide differs from the above discussed sulphonylureas in that it is much more blood sugar active in the acute experiment in animal and man. Longer half-life time or firmer tissue binding plays no part in this. It is more likely that the substance has greater specifity; wherin this lies is not known as the entire mode of action has not yet been cleared. Orientation investigations as to the *mode of action* of metahexamide showed no differences from the other sulphonylureas. Thus was found a liver glycogen increase in fasting rats (ROOT, ANDERSON and WELLES; CREUTZFELDT, ANDREU-KERN and DISCHER), degranulation of β-cells in rats (CREUTZFELDT, ANDREU-KERN and DISCHER), rise in plasma insulin activity in man and rats (PFEIFFER et al. 1959b) and potentiation of the insulin effect in the pancreatectomised dog (ROOT, ANDERSON and WELLES). In diabetics the blood sugar curve following oral glucose loading remained diabetic after longer metahexamide therapy, as was also found after other sulphonylureas. It was only lower in relation to the fasting level (HAMWI et al.).

3. Long-term therapy and side-effects

The superiority of metahexamide to the other sulphonylureas found in man during the acute experiment was also present in long-term therapy of diabetes. With an average maintenance dose of 100 mg/day (POLLEN et al.) respectively 150 mg/day (MOSS and DE LAWTER) satisfactory control could be reached. OWEN (1959) determined the maintenance dose of different sulphonylureas in 11 diabetics and reported of an average demand of 1 g. D 860, 250 mg. chlorpropamide and 50 mg metahexamide in these patients. SILVER et al. (1959) were able to control their patients with a dose of metahexamide that was 1/10—1/20 of the previously necessary D 860 dose. These experiences correspond to those of numerous other authors who did not publish their results as the clinical trials were discontinued. The maintenance doses of DOBSON et al. (1959) also of HAMWI et al. of 200—300 mg/day are, compared to the above, unusually high.

Apart from the differences in the doses which in itself is of no special advantage (for the size of the tablet is unimportant), some authors were able to control patients with metahexamide who did not, or no longer respond to the other sulphonylureas (HAMWI et al., POLLEN et al.).

Among the *side-effects* was gastric intolerance (HAMWI et al., SILVER et al. 1959), skin reactions (HAMWI et al., SILVER et al.), vertigo (SILVER et al.) and liver damage (DREY, HAMWI et al., GRANVILLE-GROSSMAN et al., WELLER et al. 1959, DOLGER 1959, SILVER et al.). The skin reactions did not occur more frequently than during the other sulphonylureas, and the typical allergic reaction was independent of the dose. In a group of 883 diabetics treated with metahexamide by various workers, it was seen that the side-effects appeared with doses of under 200 mg/day in 6.4% and with doses of more than 200 mg/day in 21.7% of the cases (POLLEN et al.). A serious side-effect was *liver damage*. Partly only elevation of the alkaline serum phosphatase occurred (WELLER et al. 1959, SILVER et al., HAMWI et al.) respectively pericholangitis without jaundice (DREY et al.), partly, however, apparent jaundice. These cases of jaundice sometimes led to the biochemical and histological signs of cholostatic hepatosis (GRANVILLE-GROSSMAN et al.) as in the case of chlorpropamide. However, most cases displayed

hepatocellular damage with necrosis (HAMWI et al., DOLGER 1959, MACH et al.
1959) or post-necrotic cirrhosis of the liver (UNGER et al.). The clinical and histological picture is difficult to distinguish from a real virus hepatitis. It is identical
with the meanwhile well known liver damage through iproniazid (marselid)
(POPPER 1958, KAHN and PEREZ). Liver damage also appears more frequently
on daily doses of over 200 mg (4.4%) than on lower doses (0.5%) (POLLEN et al.).
The further tests on metahexamide have been wisely and welcomely discontinued
owing to these liver findings. This is also because the advantage of small tablets,
or the possibility of enabling the small number of additional diabetics to receive
oral treatment does not outweigh the risk of serious liver damage. From the
unpublished test report of the firms Upjohn (Dr. O'DONOVAN) and Lilly (Dr. KIRT-
LEY) is seen that among 7500 diabetics treated with metahexamide there were
99 cases of jaundice (among which 5 died of acute liver dystrophy), thus, in 1.3%.
In most cases there was hepatocellular damage in some, however, cholostatic
hepatosis.

Guanidine and guanidine derivatives

While the knowledge of the blood sugar lowering properties of the sulphonamide derivatives have been available for 20 years, the hypoglycaemic effect of
guanidine was already known before insulin was discovered. The attempt performed 30 years ago in troducing synthalin, a derivative of guanidine, in diabetes
mellitus therapy failed. Another derivative of guanidine—phenylaethylbiguanide
(DBI)—has been increasingly used in diabetes therapy especially in the States,
for the last 3 years.

A. Guanidine

a) Pharmacological and metabolic properties

In 1914, UNDERHILL and BLATHERWICK observed that experimental animals,
after parathyreoidectomy, displayed not only tetany, but also a depression of the
blood sugar accompanied by a disappearance in liver glycogen. Hypoglycaemia
appeared before tetany. Hypoglycaemia could always be alleviated by glucose
doses, but the appearance of convulsions was not influenced by these. Hypoglycaemia and tetany could be temporily prevented by calcium lactate injection
(UNDERHILL and BLATHERWICK).

WATANABE was the first who stated that the hypoglycaemia following parathyreoidectomy was due to the elevation of the blood guanidine content, and
attempted to produce the same by injecting guanidine in the rabbit. While
100 mg/kg guanidine injected s.c. had no effect, after 150 mg/kg in most of the
cases a slight or moderate blood sugar decrease occurred. Following the guanidine
injection, first hyperglycaemia, and only later (after about 7 hrs), hypoglycaemia
appeared. Animals showing hypoglycaemia died almost always within 24 hrs of
the injection. The blood sugar decrease was accompanied by a rise in anorganic
phosphorus in the blood and a slightly later appearing decrease in blood calcium
(WATANABE). After STARKENSTEIN had previously shown in the isolated muscle
that phosphate and also citrate causes muscular tremors through precipitation of
calcium, WATANABE stated that the cramps following guanidine application were
caused by the reduction in blood calcium. MINOT and CUTLER (1928) prevented
the decrease in blood sugar following guanidine by administering calcium. The
condition necessary for a protective calcium effect was a sufficiently high hepatic
glycogen content. The same authors (MINOT and CUTLER, 1930) found that the

glycogenolytic ability of epinephrine is connected with a sufficient blood calcium concentration. According to this, calcium would counteract a decrease in the blood sugar following guanidine by allowing an increased liver glycogenolysis through epinephrine. On the other hand, the blood sugar level could be normalised by glucose; the remaining toxic effects and lethal convulsion could not be prevented as is the case with calcium. Also the rise in the blood lactate level found by MINOT following guanidine failed to appear after calcium. MINOT showed besides, in later experiments, that calcium has also a certain protective effect on the guanidine intoxication if the liver glycogen is reduced. MINOT believed this effect to be caused by increased glycogen synthesis from lactate in the liver by the epinephrine beneficially influenced by calcium. But after recent findings, epinephrine only has a glycogenolytic action, and none for promoting glycogen synthesis (SOKAL and SARCIONE).

b) Acute toxicity

In the frog, clear fibrillary muscle twitchings appear after 2—3 mg.; 15—20 mg. are fatal (FÜHNER). Mice die after 4—5 mg. showing symptoms of motoric tremors and sudden twitches of the whole animal (FÜHNER; FRANK, STERN and NOTHMANN). Rats die after 15—30 mg. s.c. (FÜHNER). Rabbits show fascicular muscle twitchings after 300 mg/kg. The lethal dose is around 500 mg/kg s.c. and per os (FRANK, STERN and NOTHMANN). Dogs and cats die after 200—250 mg/kg s.c. (FRANK, STERN and NOTHMANN). Guinea-pigs showed tremor, tachypnoe, motoric unrest and diarrhoea on doses under 100 mg. 100—200 mg s.c. are fatal (FÜHNER).

c) Investigations on the mechanism of the blood sugar lowering by guanidine

CLARK (1923) found that the blood sugar lowering effect of guanidine was inversely proportional to the liver glycogen content. Besides there was no initial blood sugar increase following guanidine (rabbits, 100 mg/kg i.v.), if ergotamine had been given previously. Hypoglycaemia was increased here. From this CLARK concluded that guanidine first causes a stimulation of the sympathetic nervous system leading to hyperglycaemia if there is glycogen in the liver. Simultaneously the vagus is stimulated which, when the sympathetic effect has ceased, effects insulin liberation from the pancreas leading to hypoglycaemia. CLARK could support this by the early investigations of other authors (MCCORNICK and O'BRIEN) who by careful stimulation of the vagus saw an increased insulin secretion. CLARK believes he could support his theory of insulin secretion stimulation by guanidine, by another experimental set-up; he administered 3 mg. ergotamine tartrate to rabbits, one hour later, guanidine plus 0.15 mg. atropine sulphate were i.v. injected; now the strong hypoglycaemic reaction which usually appeared was not seen; the blood sugar remained normal or was only slightly depressed.

To explain the blood sugar lowering effect of guanidine also another mechanism of action is possible; WATANABE saw a rise in anorganic phosphorus in the blood. MINOT found an elevated blood lactate level. These findings indicate inhibition of respiration and increased glycolysis. Inhibition of muscle respiration in vitro could already be demonstrated in 1921 by MEYERHOF by 0.02 m guanidine solution. The mechanism of respiratory inhibition through guanidine was recently cleared to a great extent by HOLLUNGER. HOLLUNGER proved that guanidine inhibits electron transfer during the oxidation chain to O_2 at the level of cytochrome c. The inhibition of oxidation leads to increased glycolysis (inhibition of the Pasteur-effect) and thus to an increased glucose consumption. RANDLE and SMITH also MORGAN et al. proved that O_2 deficiency led to an unspecific increase of permeability in the muscle cells. With this increase in permeability is connected, among other processes, an elevated glucose uptake. One may assume that respiratory inhibition through guanidine leads to an increased uptake of glucose by the muscle. This glucose is immediately consumed by glycolysis. Besides this, guanidine causes a decrease in muscle glycogen; this is however, not as marked as the reduction in liver glycogen (WATANABE; MINOT).

B. Constitution and blood sugar lowering effect of various guanidine derivates

After the hypoglycaemic activity of guanidine was published, FRANK, NOTH-MANN and WAGNER (1926a) were the first who attempted, by systematically altering the guanidine molecule, to intensify the blood sugar lowering effect, respectively, to separate the toxic from the blood sugar lowering effect by suitable substitution. Subsequently, BISCHOFF, SAHYUN and LONG in Great Britian and SLOTTA and TSCHESCHE, together with HESSE and TAUBMANN in Germany systematically worked on this problem. SHAPIRO recently continued the research of the Germans in the USA.

All the results showed that a free guanidine rest, that can only be substituted at one nitrogen, is essential for a hypoglycaemic effect, i.e. all effective guanidine derivatives have the following general formula:

$$\begin{array}{c} H \\ R-N \\ \diagdown \\ C-NH_2 \\ \parallel \\ NH \end{array}$$

The effective derivates of guanidine can be subdivided into 3 groups.

        1. Monoguanidines
        2. Diguanidines
        3. Biguanides

1. Monoguanidines. This group is comprised of substances in which the guanidine molecule is substituted at the N by an alkyl-, or aryl rest or by another organic group. These substances were first investigated by FRANK, NOTHMANN and WAGNER (1926a). The alkyl derivative N_1-methyl-guanidine and N_1,N_1-dimethyl-guanidine proved to be totally ineffective on the blood sugar and highly toxic. Therefore, FRANK assumed first that the substituting group must have an amino group (analogous to the biogenic amines). From the synthesised compounds, following the general formula:

$$\begin{array}{c} R \\ \diagdown \\ N-(CH_2)_n-N \\ \diagup \qquad\qquad \diagdown \\ R \qquad\qquad\qquad C\cdot NH_2 \\ \parallel \\ NH \end{array}$$

only agmatin evinced

$$H_2N-CH_2\cdot CH_2\cdot CH_2\cdot CH_2-N \begin{array}{c} H \\ \diagdown \\ C-NH_2 \\ \parallel \\ NH \end{array}$$
$$\text{Agmatin}$$

as being clearly more effective than guanidine. From other monoguanidines with a lateral chain containing N, only guanylpiperidin has a slight blood sugar lowering effect (BISCHOFF, SAHYUN, and LONG).

$$\text{HN}\underset{\text{CH}_2-\text{CH}_2}{\overset{\text{CH}_2-\text{CH}_2}{\Big\langle}}\text{CH}-\overset{\text{H}}{\text{N}}-\underset{\underset{\text{NH}}{\parallel}}{\text{C}}\cdot\text{NH}_2$$

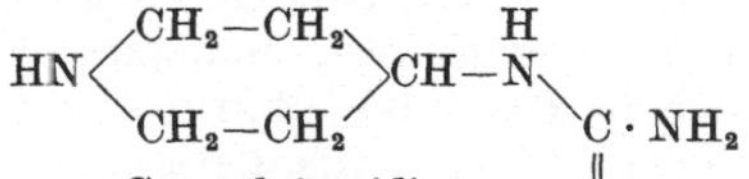

Guanylpiperidine

Further investigations showed, however, that an amino group in the lateral chain
was not really necessary. Thus galegine, found in the seed of the goats' clover
(galega officinalis), has a significant blood sugar lowering effect (MÜLLER and
REINWEIN). This substance was found to be isoamylene-guanidine by BARGER
and WHITE also SPÄTH and PROKOPP.

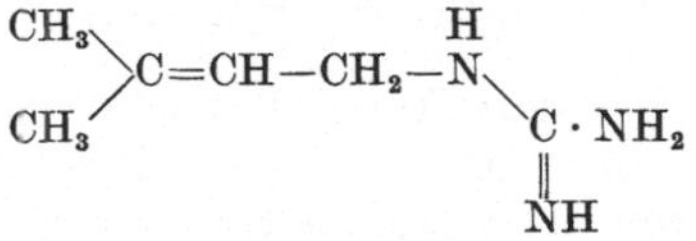

$$\underset{\text{CH}_3}{\overset{\text{CH}_3}{\Big\rangle}}\text{C}=\text{CH}-\text{CH}_2-\overset{\text{H}}{\text{N}}-\underset{\underset{\text{NH}}{\parallel}}{\text{C}}\cdot\text{NH}_2$$

Isoamylene-guanidine (Galegine)

4 mg/kg (i.e. 1/50 of the necessary guanidine dose) of galegine caused hypoglycaemia in the dog (MÜLLER and REINWEIN).

A further blood-sugar-lowering monoguanidine derivative without N in the
lateral chain, is β-phenylaethyl-guanidine (KRONEBERG and STOEPEL).

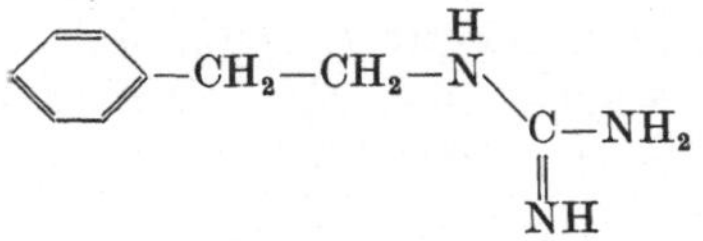

$$\bighexagon-\text{CH}_2-\text{CH}_2-\overset{\text{H}}{\text{N}}-\underset{\underset{\text{NH}}{\parallel}}{\text{C}}-\text{NH}_2$$

β-Phenylethyl-guanidine

However, the blood-sugar effect is not very strong. 25 mg/kg i.v. lead to a blood-
sugar decrease of 20—30% in the rabbit. Higher doses are ineffective, respectively
toxic.

BISCHOFF, SAHYUN and LONG proved that all fatty acid derivatives of guanidine
are completely ineffective. They are neither toxic nor do they lower the blood
sugar.

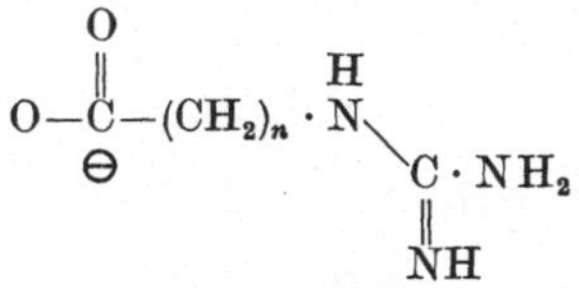

$$\underset{\ominus}{\text{O}}-\overset{\overset{\text{O}}{\parallel}}{\text{C}}-(\text{CH}_2)_n\cdot\overset{\text{H}}{\text{N}}-\underset{\underset{\text{NH}}{\parallel}}{\text{C}}\cdot\text{NH}_2$$

Guanidinecarbonic acid

BISCHOFF, SAHYUN and LONG relate the ineffectiveness of these guanidine
fatty acid derivatives to the negative charge of the lateral chain. This seems all
the more probable as the strongly basic derivatives of guanidine as e.g. N_1,N_1-
dimethyl-guanidine are exceptionally toxic.

From the series of the monoguanidines no substance has been used for diabetes
therapy, apart from the short experiments with galegine.

2. *Diguanidines*. These have the following common formula:

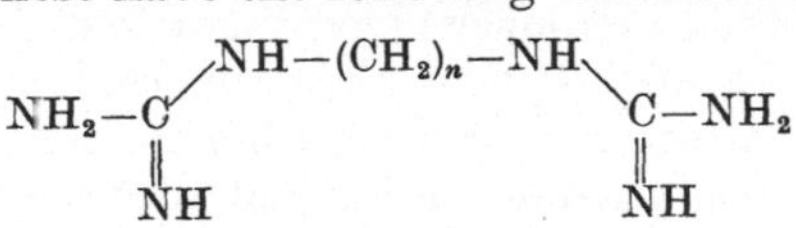

$$\text{NH}_2-\underset{\underset{\text{NH}}{\parallel}}{\text{C}}\underset{}{\overset{\text{NH}-(\text{CH}_2)_n-\text{NH}}{\Big\langle\quad\Big\rangle}}\underset{\underset{\text{NH}}{\parallel}}{\text{C}}-\text{NH}_2$$

Diguanidine gen. form.

Among the diguanidines, we find to date the most effective known blood sugar lowering guanidine derivatives. FRANK, NOTHMANN and WAGNER discovered the diguanidines. On attempting to synthetise, analogues to agmatine, these authors founds, evidently by chance (s. BISCHOFF, SAHYUN and LONG), extraordinarily strong blood sugar lowering substances—the diguanidines. Further investigations showed that the blood sugar lowering effect of the diguanidines increased proportionally to the lengthening of the aliphatic chain. Thus the pentamethylene-diguanidine

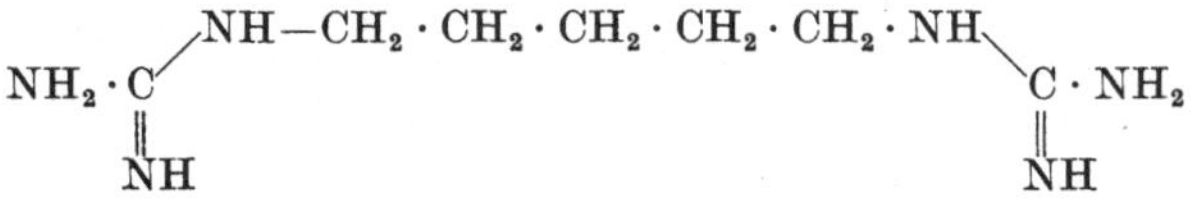

$$NH_2 \cdot C \underset{\underset{NH}{\|}}{\overset{NH-CH_2 \cdot CH_2 \cdot CH_2 \cdot CH_2 \cdot CH_2 \cdot NH}{\diagup}} \underset{\underset{NH}{\|}}{\overset{}{\diagdown}} C \cdot NH_2$$

Pentamethylene-diguanidine

is 3 times more effective than guanidine (BISCHOFF, SAHYUN and LONG). The effectiveness increases with the number of methylene-groups to decamethylene-diguanidine; this is about 150 times more active than guanidine.

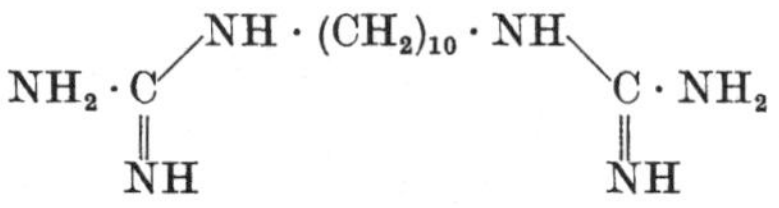

$$NH_2 \cdot C \underset{\underset{NH}{\|}}{\overset{NH \cdot (CH_2)_{10} \cdot NH}{\diagup}} \underset{\underset{NH}{\|}}{\overset{}{\diagdown}} C \cdot NH_2$$

Synthalin A

This substance as synthalin, respectively synthalin A, was used in diabetes therapy. Dodecamethylene-diguanidine, also introduced by FRANK to diabetes therapy (called synthalin B, or synthalin-neu), is already less effective than decamethylene-diguanidine (BISCHOFF, SAHYUN and LONG). FRANK, NOTHMANN and WAGNER (1926a) saw a decrease in toxicity with increasing blood sugar lowering effectiveness, i.e. increased dissociation of both the properties of guanidine. However, BISCHOFF, SAHYUN and LONG found that the blood sugar decreasing effectiveness of the diguanidines was parallel to the increase in toxic properties. This problem will be discussed in the paragraph on the pharmacological properties of the guanidine derivatives.

3. *Biguanides*. The biguanides which have been most thoroughly investigated have the following general formula:

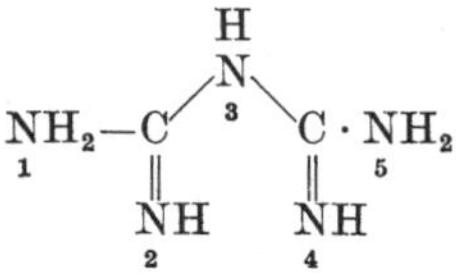

$$\underset{1}{NH_2} - C \underset{\underset{2}{\overset{\|}{NH}}}{\overset{\overset{H}{\overset{N}{\diagup}}{}^{3}\diagdown}} C \underset{\underset{4}{\overset{\|}{NH}}}{\overset{}{}} \cdot NH_2 \, {}_{5}$$

Biguanide

SLOTTA and TSCHESCHE synthesised numerous biguanides whose pharmacological properties were investigated by HESSE and TAUBMANN. Biguanide was similar in its blood sugar lowering effect to guanidine. 200 mg/kg biguanide sulphate lowered the blood sugar in the rabbit to 45 mg-% (HESSE and TAUBMANN).

Investigations of the biguanide derivatives show that substitution at the amino group (N_1) marked on 1 leads to stronger blood sugar lowering derivatives. Simultaneously substituting at N_1 and N_2 nitrogen only results in ineffective or toxic substances (HESSE and TAUBMANN). Substituting at the N_1 nitrogen leads to many substances with hypoglycaemic action not directly related to the chain length, as in the case of diguanidine.

SHAPIRO divided the blood sugar effective biguanides in 2 groups.

a) Derivatives of N_1-phenylpolymethylene-biguanide:

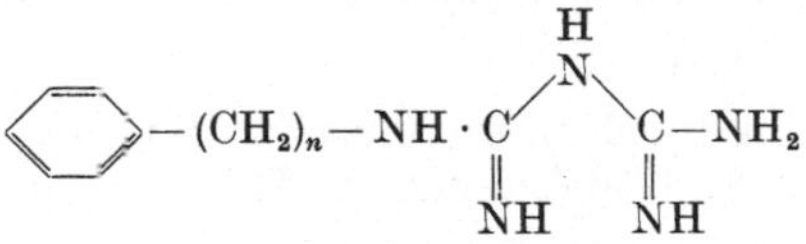

N_1-Phenylpolymethylene-biguanide

There is a relatively strong blood sugar decrease following benzyl-biguanide (SHAPIRO):

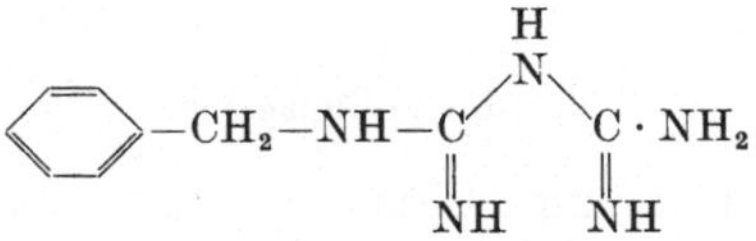

N_1-benzyl-biguanide

Even more effective is the derivative with 2 methylene groups, phenylethyl-biguanide.

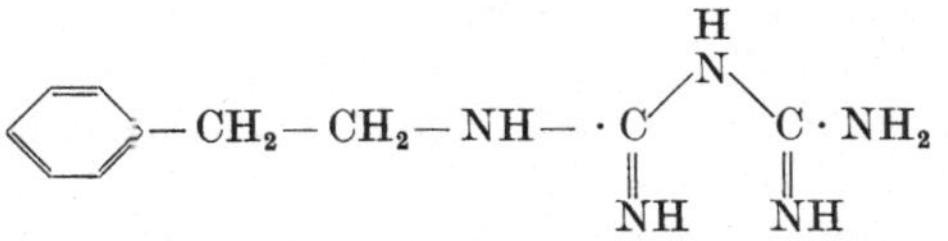

N_1-phenylethyl-biguanide (DBI)

UNGAR, FREEDMAN and SHAPIRO introduced phenylethyl-biguanide in 1957 in the USA to the diabetes therapy, and it is now on the market under the name of DBI. It is not principally different from the other biguanides as will be mentioned later. Among the derivatives of phenylpolymethylene-biguanides, in which also the second proton at the N_1-nitrogen is substituted, only N_1-methyl, N_1-benzyl-biguanide (DBC) was found to have a blood sugar lowering effect (SHAPIRO).

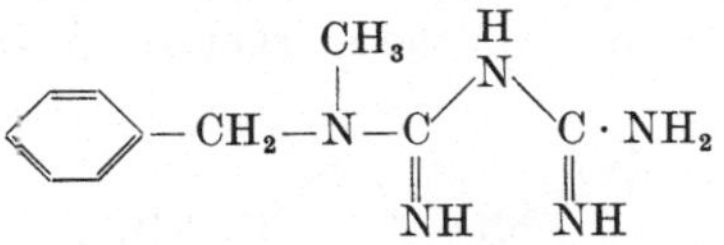

N_1-methyl, N_1-benzyl-biguanide

From the derivatives substituted at the benzol ring, the methyl derivatives were useless (SHAPIRO). While on introducing a methoxy-group in p-position, a good effect was seen (SHAPIRO). Also halogen substitution (chlorine, bromine and fluorine) in m- or p-positions were effective (SHAPIRO). If the phenyl ring is substituted by a pyridine-, thiophene- or furan ring, the blood sugar lowering effect is maintained. Complicated derivatives of phenylethyl-biguanide as indolin-biguanide or tetrahydroisochinoline-biguanide are almost completely inactive (SHAPIRO).

b) Alkylbiguanides:

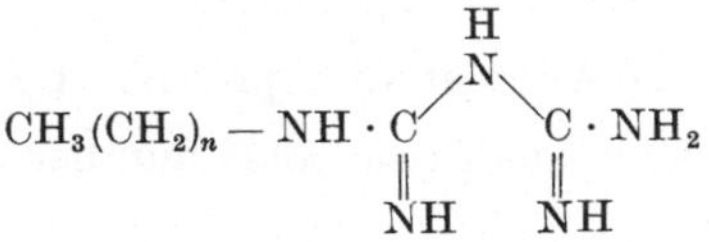

N_1-monoalkyl-biguanide

Many of the derivatives having only one proton at the N_1-nitrogen substituted
by an alkylrest, were clearly blood-sugar lowering. HESSE and TAUBMANN described N_1-allyl-biguanide. Doses of 50—100 mg/kg s.c. lowered the blood sugar
in the rabbit to shock values.

N_1-n-butyl-biguanide is much more effective (SHAPIRO; SÖLING and CREUTZ-
FELDT; SÖLING, WERCHAU and CREUTZFELDT). It is now on the market in Germany
as Silubin (W 37).

$$CH_3-CH_2\cdot CH_2\cdot CH_2\cdot NH\cdot C\underset{NH}{\overset{H}{\underset{\|}{N}}}C\cdot NH_2$$

N_1-n-butyl-biguanide

also N_1-n-amyl-biguanide (SHAPIRO; WILLIAMS, TANNER and ODELL)

N_1-n-amyl-biguanide N_1-isoamyl-biguanide

and N_1-isoamyl-biguanide (SHAPIRO; WILLIAMS, TANNER and ODELL). These
substances were almost as effective as the phenylaethyl-biguanide. Further
lengthening of the chain of alkyl rests to 6—8 C atoms led to a decrease in effectiveness. When the chain was lengthened to 10 C atoms, no blood sugar lowering effect
was found (SHAPIRO). Derivatives with branched alkyl rests have less effect than
the same n-alkyl derivatives (SHAPIRO).

Among the biguanides, where both protons are alkylised at N_1-nitrogen,
HESSE and TAUBMANN found a strong blood-sugar-lowering substance, N_1,N_1-
dimethyl-biguanide; 100 mg/kg s.c. of this drug led to hypoglycaemic convulsions
in rabbits. This substance is now on the market as glucophage:

N_1,N_1-dimethyl-biguanide

The corresponding N_1,N_1-diethyl-biguanide was completely ineffective (HESSE
and TAUBMANN). However, N_1,N_1-diallyl-biguanide had a slighter effect than
N_1-allylbiguanide (HESSE and TAUBMANN). Apart from N_1,N_1-dimethyl-biguanide,
the N_1-monoalkyl-biguanide is more effective than the corresponding N_1,N_1-
dialkyl-biguanides (SHAPIRO).

Simultaneous substitution at N_1 and N_2 nitrogen only results in blood-sugar-
lowering substances if two conditions are fulfilled:

1. Not more than 3 of the 4 replaceable protons should be substituted.

2. The alkyl rests must be small (the total number of C atoms of all 3 alkyl
rests should not exceed 5).

N_1-n-propyl, N_5,N_5-dimethyl-biguanide meets these conditions (SHAPIRO).

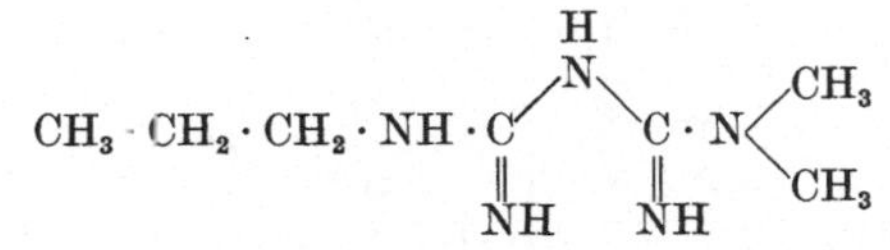

$$CH_3 \cdot CH_2 \cdot CH_2 \cdot NH \cdot C \overset{\overset{\textstyle H}{N}}{\underset{\underset{\textstyle NH}{\|}}{}} C \cdot N \overset{CH_3}{\underset{CH_3}{}} , \quad \underset{\underset{\textstyle NH}{\|}}{}$$

N_1-n-propyl, N_5, N_5-dimethyl-biguanide

This substance is of interest in so as far as it strongly decreases the blood sugar, parenterally, while being ineffective orally (SHAPIRO). In contrast to this, are the other mentioned blood sugar lowering biguanides, as they are both parenterally and orally effective. N_1-parachlorophenyl, N_5-isopropyl-biguanide (Paludrine) used in malaria therapy is among the biguanides substituted at N_1 and N_5.

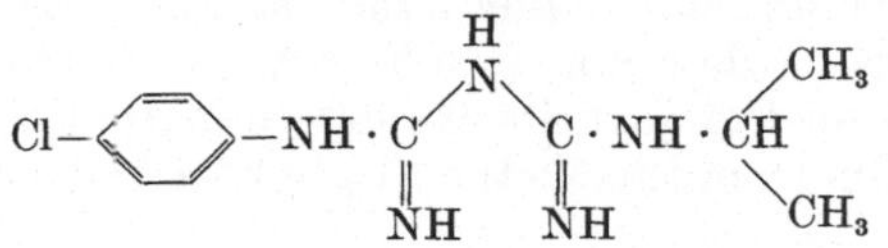

Paludrine

This compound has only very slight blood-sugar-lowering properties (SCHMIDT, HUGHES and SMITH; CHEN and ANDERSON).

SHAPIRO found that the biguanides under physiological p_H conditions probably appear in ring form as monobasic hydrophile cations with the following structure:

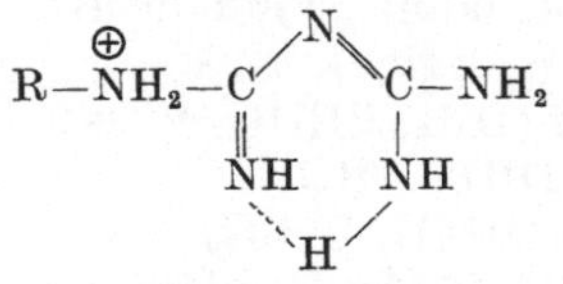

Monobasic form

It is assumed that many biguanide derivatives are ineffective because the substituents prevent ring formation. The named ring form is, on the condition of a strongly acid p_H as found in the stomach, in equilibrium with the corresponding di-basic non-conjugated cation (SHAPIRO):

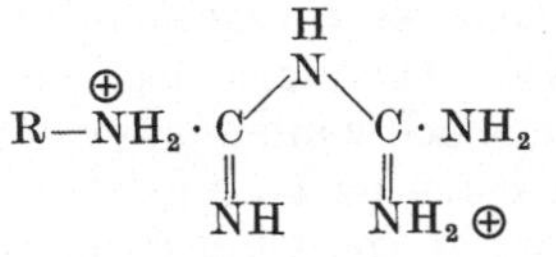

Dibasic form

The fact that the biguanides in the organism, following absorption, are present in the form of conjugated monobasic cations explains why cyclic biguanides

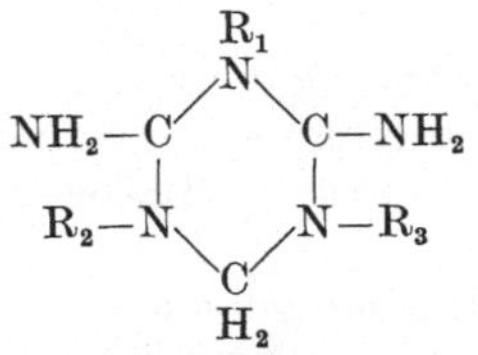

Cyclic biguanides

as have also been investigated by HESSE and TAUBMANN, are ineffective.

Also the ineffectiveness of di-biguanides observed already by HESSE and TAUBMANN

$$NH_2 \cdot C\!\!\begin{array}{c} \overset{H}{N} \\ \| \\ NH \end{array}\!\!C\!-\!N\!-\!R\!-\!N\!-\!C\!\!\begin{array}{c} \overset{H}{N} \\ \| \\ NH \end{array}\!\!C \cdot NH_2$$

Di-biguanide (gen. form.)

is probably caused by marking it impossible for the ring to close as described by SHAPIRO.

There are no investigations on the relation between structure and *absorption*, therapeutic plasma level and *elimination* of the guanidine derivatives. This is because no applicable methods for determination have yet been found. Only recently has a method been found for the quantitative determination of DBI (SHEPHERD and MCDONALD). No results from this method have been published.

C. Experimental research on various guanidine derivatives

This survey is limited to a discussion of those guanidine derivatives that have been or are used for a short or long time in diabetes therapy. To this group belong the following compounds:

1. Decamethylene-diguanidine (synthalin A)
2. Dodekamethylene-diguanidine (synthalin B)
3. Isoamylene-guanidine (galegine)
4. Phenylethyl-biguanide (DBI, PEDG, W 32)
5. N_1-n-amyl-biguanide (DBB, ABG)
6. N_1-isoamyl-biguanide (DBTU, IABG)
7. N_1,n-butyl-biguanide (W 37, DBV, silubin)
8. N_1,N_1-dimethyl-biguanide (La 6023, glucophage)

I. Pharmacology and toxicology

It had been shown for all 8 derivatives that the animal experimental results could only be transferred to the human being with certain limitations. The diversly examined animal species show extreme differences as regards sensitivity towards guanidine derivatives. Therefore, e.g. guinea-pigs receiving 20 mg/kg DBI s.c. show hypoglycaemic shock while rats even after 75 mg/kg scarcely show any reaction and dogs even react by an elevation in the blood sugar (UNGAR, FREEDMAN and SHAPIRO; SÖLING and CREUTZFELDT). The reaction is similar to the other guanidine derivatives. It has already been mentioned that for the cited substances no investigations have been made on the rate of absorption, plasma half-life time and detoxication. However, the pharmacological behaviour of all substances, and the resulting metabolic changes are so similar that they can be discussed together.

Synthalin differs only from the biguanides in that it causes clear histological changes, especially in the liver and kidney, and the biguanides only slight changes (CREUTZFELDT and MOENCH; LAZARUS, BRADSHAW and VOLK) or none at all (s. p. 104 f.).

The fate of blood-sugar-lowering guanidine derivatives in the organism has only been investigated by WICK and STEWART using DBI; rats given 100 mg/kg ^{14}C-labelled DBI, orally or i.p., excreted 90% of the radio-activity within 24 hrs in the urine while no $^{14}CO_2$ was found in the respiratory air. During the first hours following administration, the labelled substance was almost only concentrated in the intestine and liver. SHEPHERD and McDONALD (b) state that DBI is not bound strongly to the plasma protein.

a) Acute toxicity

In 1921, FRANK, STERN and NOTHMANN stated in a paper on guanidine tetany "that there seemed to be no guanidine dose efficax bene tolerata. Animals tolerate a fairly large amount of the poison without reaction: a slight increase in the dose and with the first symptoms death can be imminent, at least the course of further developments cannot be foreseen". This unpleasant characteristic is also preserved to a varying degree in the therapeutically used guanidine derivatives. Thus one finds in the dog, following s.c. application of 40 mg/kg DBI, neither a change in the blood sugar nor in the general condition. After 50 and 60 mg/kg s.c., strong hyperglycaemia preceeds death by paralysis of the respiratory centre (SÖLING and CREUTZFELDT). JUNKMANN found similar to be true for synthalin.

To judge the relation between toxic and blood-sugar-lowering effects in the guanidine derivatives, comparison with guanidine is of interest (s. p. 95).

1. Synthalin

Mice die after 50 mg/kg showing the symptoms of guanidine poisoning (JUNKMANN). No investigations have been made on acute synthalin toxicity in rats. From research done by CREUTZFELDT and TECKLENBORG is seen that dosage between 6 and 12 mg/kg can still be tolerated. Dogs tolerate 5 mg/kg s.c. without symptoms (JUNKMANN). After 10 mg/kg s.c., dogs first become apathetic, vomit and suffer from diarrhoea. After several hours paresis of the extremities and respiratory disturbances occur. Death results without convulsions. According to FRANK, NOTHMANN and WAGNER (1926b), dogs die after a single dose of 4 mg/kg within 3—4 days. Rabbits tolerate 1 mg/kg i.v. without symptoms. 5 mg/kg i.v. cause death showing hypoglycaemic symptoms (STAUB). Exact data is lacking on the acute fatal smallest possible dose for the rabbit. It is according to the various investigations (STAUB; BODO and MARKS; BLATHERWICK, SAHYUN and HILL; HUUSAKO; CREUTZFELDT and TECKLENBORG) approximately between 10—20 mg/kg s.c. Guinea-pigs die within 2—3 days when receiving a daily dose of 2—3 mg/kg s.c. After 12 mg/kg s.c., death occurs within a few hours under the signs of hypoglycaemia (CREUTZFELDT and TECKLENBORG).

2. Biguanides

In mice the DL_{100} for DBI and n-butyl-biguanide (W 37) is 300 mg/kg i.p. The DL_{50} of DBI for the mouse is 202 m 7.16 mg/kg i.p., for W 37 213 $\pm$ 9.18 mg/kg i.p. (SÖLING and CREUTZFELDT). Death occurred after DBI under signs of a guanidine poisoning, after W 37 under hypoglycaemic conditions. Rats tolerate 75 mg/kg DBI s.c. well, while 150 mg/kg cause death under hyperglycaemic symptoms (SÖLING, WERCHAU and CREUTZFELDT). Rabbits display no effect worth mentioning after 50—100 mg/kg given orally. 100 mg/kg DBI s.c. lead to definite apathy without lowering the blood sugar. Animals frequently die when the blood sugar is elevated. 150 mg/kg cause death preceeded by a biphasic blood sugar course often during hypoglycaemia, but sometimes only if the blood sugar has re-increased (CREUTZFELDT and FINTER 1959). 100 mg/kg s.c. of N_1,N_1-dimethyl-biguanide causes convulsions and death (HESSE and TAUBMANN). After the same dose, rabbits also die (often first after 24 hrs) when the blood sugar has been normalised by glucose injection (STERNE and DUVAL). Guinea-pigs die almost always in the

state of hypoglycaemia shock following 20 mg/kg DBI s.c. (SÖLING and CREUTZ-
FELDT). If guinea-pigs do not die during the hypoglycaemic shock they do so
later, after prolonged apathy without convulsions. W 37 differs from DBI only
in that guinea-pigs regularly show hypoglycaemic shock first after 25 mg/kg s.c.
In the dog, doses over 50 mg/kg DBI s.c. always cause death by paralysis of the
respiratory centre while the heart is still beating. Here the blood sugar is elevated
and death is mostly preceeded by vomiting and diarrhoea (SÖLING and CREUTZ-
FELDT). Lower doses have no effect either on the blood sugar or on the general
condition.

25 mg/kg i.v. of N_1,n-butyl-biguanide cause death in the anaesthetised dog
after $1^1/_2$—2 hrs. Here the blood sugar is decreased to shock values, and the blood
pressure is strongly reduced (SÖLING and CREUTZFELDT). In the monkey, 25 mg/kg
DBI given orally causes death during hypoglycaemic shock (UNGAR, FREEDMAN
and SHAPIRO).

3. Symptomatology of the acute poisoning

If animals are given acute lethal doses, they die independently from the method
of application, generally while the heart is still beating, from paralysis of the
respiratory centre. This is true for synthalin (JUNKMANN) and for DBI (SÖLING
and CREUTZFELDT). After smaller doses of synthalin, and also of DBI and W 37,
prolonged peripherally caused hypotonia is seen (JUNKMANN; SÖLING and CREUTZ-
FELDT). Simultaneously more shallow and accelerated respiration was seen. Also
"Traube-Herings' waves" often appear after both substances (JUNKMANN; SÖLING
and CREUTZFELDT). By experiments on the spinal cord animal, JUNKMANN could
show that the blood-sugar decrease following synthalin is caused by a peripheral
effect leading to dilation of the splanchnic vessels. A momentary re-increase of the
blood pressure and normalising of respiration is seen in the dog after injection of
100 mg. methylene blue i.v. Improvement lasts about 15 mins (SÖLING and CREUTZ-
FELDT). The side-effects on the intestinal tract (comp. p. 126 and 138) which occur
after all mentioned guanidine derivatives during the treatments of diabetes, can
also be demonstrated in the animal experiment (FRANK, NOTHMANN and WAGNER
1926a and b, UNGAR). Convulsions even appear if the blood sugar is normal or
elevated following synthalin administration (SIMOLA), and also after biguanides.
This is probably caused by an extraordinarily strong central nervous stimulation
as was shown by KRONEBERG and STOEPEL by experiments on the spinal cord
animal.

b) Chronic toxicity

After the appearance of jaundice in man following the application of synthalin
(s. p. 127), attention was paid to the toxic effect of synthalin. Then in the countless
animal experiments histological organ damage was described.

HORNUNG investigated the effect of the chronic feeding of synthalin (10 to
20—30 mg/day) in healthy dogs. Already after a short time, the typical signs of
guanidine poisoning were seen (anorexia, increasing cachexia) that disappeared
momentarily on discontinuing synthalin. In the third to fourth week, the phenol-
tetrachlor-sulphonephthalein test showed a significantly delayed excretion by the
liver. The autopsy performed after four weeks of synthalin feeding showed the
histological picture of necrosis and fatty liver degeneration. In one dog, kidney
damage was seen. KARR, BECK and PETTY found in dogs receiving synthalin in the
chronic experiments in doses corresponding to those used in the human being, a
rise in the non-protein nitrogen in the blood, also increased albuminuria and
cylinduria. The histological findings corresponded to those of HORNUNG. KLEE-

BERG investigated the comparative effect of guanidine (6×1 g/week) and synthalin (6×30 mg/week) on chronic administration in the dog. Two months after commencing feeding, an increase of urea in the blood could be proved after guanidine and also after synthalin that subsequently increased continuously. After 3 months, the animals showed signs of intoxication (apathy, scrubby fur). All animals were sacrificed after 4 months. Histological organ damage could only be found in the synthalin treated animals (fatty kidney degeneration, renal tubular damage, liver damage), despite the fact that the guanidine treated dogs also showed increased blood urea. HORNUNG and KLEEBERG saw massive iron depositions in the spleen.

VARELA, COLLAZO and RUBINO found after oral dose of 2—3 mg/kg/day of synthalin A in rabbits after 2—3 days a rise of the non-protein nitrogen in the blood and simultaneous polyuria. The post mortem examination showed histological necrosis of the liver (mainly in the centre of the lobulus) and necrosis of the renal tubules. BLATHERWICK, SAHYUN and HILL confirmed these findings. STAUB also saw in the rabbit, after acute synthalin application, necrosis in the liver and kidney. This corresponds to the findings of RUNGE (1954), CREUTZFELDT 1954, CREUTZFELDT and TECKLENBORG, also CREUTZFELDT and MOENCH, after acute synthalin poisoning in the guinea-pig and rabbit. After the acute synthalin poisoning, tubular necrosis in the sense of toxic nephrosis is also found in the guinea-pig (CREUTZFELDT and MOENCH).

The massive organ toxic effect of synthalin is not found in the case of the biguanides. UNGAR, FREEDMAN and SHAPIRO could not see in guinea-pigs orally treated for 2 weeks daily with 20 mg/kg DBI, either histological damage in the thorax or abdominal organs, or changes in the blood picture. Guinea-pigs show no histological damage or blood changes after 6 months of chronic feeding orally with 10—20 mg/kg DBI. The same is true for the rat receiving 50—100 mg/kg orally daily for the same length of time (UNGAR). A somewhat higher dose (15—25 mg/day s.c. for 3 days consecutively) can lead to mild liver cell necrosis and definite *tubular damage* of the kidney in guinea-pigs (CREUTZFELDT and MOENCH). Hereby should be appreciated that these doses lead to severe hypoglycaemia, while those doses used by UNGAR et al. in the chronic experiment only caused a weak, or no blood sugar lowering. Kidney damage (tubular degeneration) was also found in the rabbit 5—8 days after a twice daily dose of 25 mg/kg s.c. (LAZARUS, BRADSHAW and VOLK). They caused parenchyma degeneration and fibrosis on further treatment. GEORGII saw in rats orally receiving 50 mg/kg N_1,n-butyl-biguanide for 140 days, focal, fatty degeneration of the tubulus that disappeared on discontinuing the biguanide therapy. The chronic toxicity of N_1,n-amyl-biguanide (DBTU) was investigated by WILLIAMS, TANNER and ODELL. Young guinea-pigs received 10 mg/kg DBTU s.c. twice daily for $5^1/_2$ weeks. The weight increase of this group corresponded exactly to that of the control group. No tissue damage was seen in the histological examination of liver, kidney, pancreas, adrenals and muscle. The adrenals of the treated group had increased in weight. The authors conclude this to be due to the chronic stimulation of the adrenal medulla through hypoglycaemia. The strong activation of the adrenal medulla is shown by the vacuolation found in the adrenal medullary cells in rabbits and guinea-pigs during acute hypoglycaemia after synthalin (CREUTZFELDT and TECKLENBORG; CREUTZFELDT and MOENCH) and DBI (CREUTZFELDT and MOENCH). The increase in weight may also have been caused by the continuous stress of long-term medication. In the acute synthalin and DBI poisoning, there are clear histological signs of adrenal activation in the guinea-pig (CREUTZFELDT and TECKLENBORG; CREUTZFELDT and MOENCH).

STERNE and DUVAL found no histological damage in the internal organs or changes in the blood picture in rats chronically fed with 10 mg/kg/day N_1,N_1-dimethyl-biguanide orally for 1 year! The blood urea concentration was not elevated, blood phosphate activity was diminished. However, the applied dose is too small in comparison to the effective dose (200—800 mg/kg s.c.) to allow any valuable conclusions. A dog receiving 50 mg/kg s.c. N_1,N_1-dimethyl-biguanide daily for 1 year showed no changes in the blood values for urea, chlorine, sodium and potassium. Only a slight decrease of the blood calcium could be observed. (About α-cell damage in the pancreas through guanidine derivatives, s. p. 118.)

c) Comparing the effectiveness of guanidine derivatives and the sensitivity in different animal species

The effectiveness of the single derivatives varies greatly—clinically and experimentally. The most effective known guanidine compound, both in the various animal species and in the diabetic, is synthalin. In rabbits after 4—5 mg/kg given orally, it first has a blood-sugar-raising effect, then a definite blood sugar lowering action (FRANK, NOTHMANN and WAGNER 1926a and b). DBI first causes an average blood sugar decrease with doses between 20—40 mg/kg given orally (UNGAR, FREEDMAN and SHAPIRO). To cause the same effect, 100—200 mg/kg s.c. dimethyl-biguanide are necessary (STERNE and DUVAL). Also in the guinea-pig this can be demonstrated; 5 mg/kg s.c. synthalin are required for an average blood sugar lowering, 15—20 mg/kg s.c. DBI and 25 mg/kg s.c. W 37 (SÖLING and CREUTZFELDT).

Detailed investigations on the increase in sensitivity to the blood-sugar-lowering effect in the different animal species have been made for DBI (UNGAR, FREEDMAN and SHAPIRO; UNGAR). According to the results, the sensitivity of healthy animals to the blood sugar lowering effect of DBI increases in the following sequence: mouse, rat, rabbit, pigeon, cat, guinea-pig, rhesus monkey. The healthy dog and healthy human are resistant to the blood sugar decrease. Even if the corresponding findings for synthalin are more sparse, one must conclude that there are similar conditions, as the sensitivity increase is in the sequence—rat, rabbit, guinea-pig (CREUTZFELDT and TECKLENBORG).

There is no satisfactory explanation why the dog is completely resistant to the blood sugar lowering effect of DBI. The fact that there is a marked prolonged hyperglycaemia in the dog, speaks for a stronger stimulation of the sympathetic nervous system after this substance in the dog than in any other species. Probably the excretion and detoxication possibilities play a part in the different species. An allusion for this is given in that paludrine—also a biguanide (s. p. 101)—is 12 times more slowly degraded in the dog than in the rabbit (SCHMIDT, HUGHES and SMITH). In this connection it is worth mentioning that guinea-pigs, in contrast to dogs, show no hyperglycaemic reaction. A biphasic course (primary blood sugar rise, secondary hypoglycaemia) as is mostly seen in the rabbit is not found in the guinea-pig (SÖLING and CREUTZFELDT). Odly enough, dogs reacted to W 37 with a very strong blood sugar decrease not, or hardly, preceeded by an initial hyperglycaemia, while the other effects on the circulation and respiration are exactly as after DBI (SÖLING and CREUTZFELDT). Galegine can also reduce the blood sugar in the dog, however, with preceeding hyperglycaemia (MÜLLER and REINWEIN). N_1,N_1-dimethyl-biguanide has a similar effect on the dog (STERNE and DUVAL). FRANK, NOTHMANN and WAGNER, also READ and FODDEN saw, also, after synthalin in the normal dog a definite blood sugar lowering, while BERTRAM (1958a) described an almost total synthalin resistance.

Rats in which DBI in doses of 75 mg/kg only lead to a very weak and in-consistent blood sugar decrease, react to the same W 37 dose with a marked blood-sugar decrease (SÖLING, WEECHAU and CREUTZFELDT). An improved blood-sugar decrease was attained in the rat by N_1,N_1-dimethyl-biguanide, however with doses between 350—800 mg/kg s.c. (STERNE and DUVAL).

d) The guanidine-like properties of the guanidine derivatives

It is important to know if the application of guanidine derivatives is still accompanied by the signs of guanidine intoxication, or whether by changing the constitution insulin-like properties are produced.

FRANK, NOTHMANN and WAGNER (1926a) searched for new guanidine deriva-tives in order to separate the blood sugar lowering effect from the tetany pro-ducing respectively toxic effect of the guanidine. BLATHERWICK, SAHYUN and LONG already indicated that no success can be expected with synthalin in this direction. They believe that the increase in the blood sugar depressing effect was combined with a corresponding increase in toxicity.

The inhibitory action of guanidine on respiration has already been mentioned (comp. p. 95). This respiratory inhibition, apart from in how far it is responsible for the blood sugar lowering action, must be regarded as playing an important part in the toxic effect. By in vitro experiments can be shown that the ability of in-hibiting cell respiration is increased in the therapeutically applied guanidine derivatives; e.g. DBI inhibits muscle respiration in concentration of 2×10^{-3} mol (HERNANDEZ; UNGAR), while MEYERHOF required for this a guanidine con-centration of 2×10^{-2} mol.

After MARTENSSON had shown that in rabbits synthalin does not only produce an elevation of anorganic phosphorus but also of citrate in the blood, one is justified in directly connecting the reduction in ionised blood calcium with the inhibiting metabolic effect. The rise in citrate, and also to a lesser degree, of phosphate, leads to the formation of corresponding badly dissociable calcium salts, followed by a decrease in ionised calcium and an increased convulsion tendency. CRAIG, MILLER and WOODWARD showed that also DBI led to an elevation of the citrate level in man. In the animal experiment, the increase of anorganic phos-phorus following synthalin was seen by SIMOLA, following DBI, by UNGAR, and also by SHEPHERD and McDONALD. A decrease in the blood calcium was described after synthalin by SIMOLA, following DBI, by UNGAR. If one compares the applied guanidine doses with the same synthalin doses causing a similar effect on the blood calcium and inorganic phosphorus, one reaches the conclusion that in fact not only the blood sugar decreasing, but also the blood calcium depressing effect of synthalin has been greatly augmented. Further indications show that the toxic effects of guanidine have been maintained by its derivatives, at least in the animal experiments. This is especially true for the changes in carbohydrate meta-bolism accompanying the blood-sugar decrease that differ greatly from the insulin effect (see the following paragraphs).

e) Action of glucose in the hypoglycaemic shock

While insulin hypoglycaemia can be overcome by glucose administration, the animals treated with guanidine died despite glucose application (WATANABE). The same is true for the guanidine derivatives. FRANK, NOTHMANN and WAGNER (1926a) already indicated this property of synthalin which was also confirmed by CREUTZFELDT and TECKLENBORG. The same was described for the biguanides by HESSE and TAUBMANN. This is one reason why the authors rejected the use of biguanides in the diabetic therapy. The same is true also for the newer biguanides, DBI and W 37 (SÖLING, WERCHAU and CREUTZFELDT). JANSEN and BAUR called attention to the difference in the hypoglycaemic shock following insulin and that after synthalin: while in animals in the insulin shock, there are greater pauses between the single attacks and death occurs only after a longer period, even after hours; animals in synthalin shock mostly die within 30 mins without there being a significant interval during the cramps. This observation has been confirmed for the shock in the guinea-pig by CREUTZFELDT and MOENCH, also SÖLING and CREUTZFELDT.

Most workers who reported of the unsuccessfulness of the glucose therapy state that a momentary improvement of the shock state may occur following glucose, but that the animals relapse into a coma and often die after some time despite this. One reason for FRANK, NOTHMANN and WAGNER (1926a and b) assuming that synthalin acts like insulin was their observation that the pancreatectomised dog in shock condition caused by synthalin rapidly recovered after glucose dose. Despite this fact, these dogs mostly died within 24 or 48 hrs after the synthalin injection, while the controls lived for much longer.

f) Initial hyperglycaemia, epinephrine secretion, the effectiveness of epinephrine and glucagon

The biphasic blood sugar course, typical for guanidine, following blood-sugar-lowering doses of its derivatives is remarkable, especially in the rabbit. This effect was described for synthalin by many authors (BODO and MARKS; SIMOLA; JANSEN and BAUR; HUUSAKO; DAVIS 1952, CREUTZFELDT and TECKLENBORG), for galegine by MÜLLER and REINWEIN, for different biguanides by HESSE and TAUBMANN, for the N_1,N_1-dimethyl-biguanide, especially by STERNE and DUVAL, and for DBI by CREUTZFELDT and FINTER. Contrary to SÖLING and CREUTZFELDT who saw a significant blood sugar increase after s.c. dose of DBI in the dog, UNGAR saw no such increase in this animal.

CLARK was able to prevent the initial hyperglycaemia in his guanidine experiments by premedicating with ergotamine. From this he concluded there to be an increased *epinephrine secretion* through guanidine. MÜLLER and REINWEIN could also inhibit the initial hyperglycaemia after galegine, FRANK, NOTHMANN and WAGNER (1928), after synthalin B with ergotamine. MÜLLER and REINWEIN do not explain this effect by epinephrine mobilisation, but by an epinephrine-like action of galegine. This hypothesis has not been proved. HUUSAKO could definitely show that synthalin leads to a very strong epinephrine release by determining the epinephrine content of the supra-renals in untreated rabbits and those treated with synthalin. Moreover the hyperglycaemia, following synthalin, could not only be inhibited by ergotamine (STAUB; FRANK, NOTHMANN and WAGNER 1928), but also by cutting the splanchnic nerves (HUUSAKO). KRONEBERG and STOEPEL showed that the guanidine derivatives do not promote epinephrine liberation by a direct effect on the adrenal cortex, but by central nervous stimulation. Neither glucagon nor epinephrine led to a blood sugar increase if they were given sometime after the application of guanidine derivatives in blood-sugar-lowering quantities. In respect to synthalin, this fact was published by BODO and MARKS for epinephrine and CREUTZFELDT and TECKLENBORG for glucagon. HESSE and TAUBMANN indicate that in the case of the biguanides the hypoglycaemic shock is not influenced by epinephrine, in contrast to the insulin shock. NIELSEN, SWANSON, TANNER, WILLIAMS and O'CONNELL found for DBI that neither 30 γ

epinephrine nor 20 γ glucagon given s.c. could abolish hypoglycaemia in the guinea-pig. The impossibility of raising the blood sugar by epinephrine or glucagon if it has already decreased on the administration of guanidine derivatives, can be understood as the liver glycogen content is greatly reduced at the time of the blood sugar decrease. In contrast to these experiments epinephrine prevented or delayed the blood sugar lowering effect of DBI in guinea-pigs when given before the application of the biguanide (SÖLING, WERCHAU, ARENS and CREUTZFELDT).

g) Liver glycogen

Depletion of liver glycogen was found during the hypoglycaemia following parathyreoidectomy (UNDERHILL and BLATHERWICK), after guanidine dose by (WATANABE; CLARK; MINOT), synthalin (STAUB; BODO and MARKS; SIMOLA; KAUFMANN; HUUSAKO; RATHERY et al. 1928; CREUTZFELDT and TECKLENBORG; RUNGE), N_1-amyl-biguanide (HESSE and TAUBMANN), N_1,N_1-dimethyl-biguanide (HESSE and TAUBMANN; STERNE and DUVAL; SÖLING, WERCHAU and CREUTZFELDT), DBI (UNGAR, FREEDMAN and SHAPIRO; NIELSEN, SWANSON et al.; STEINER and WILLIAMS 1958, WILLIAMS, TYBERGHEIN et al.; CREUTZFELDT and MOENCH; SÖLING, WERCHAU and CREUTZFELDT) and W 37 (SÖLING, WERCHAU and CREUTZFELDT). BISCHOFF, SAHYUN and LONG had already stated in 1928 that the disappearance of liver glycogen and the blood sugar lowering effect are connected in all guanidine derivatives which are effective in this direction.

Contrary results are few; in 1958 KRONEBERG and STOEPEL described an unusual increase in liver glycogen in the guinea-pig following i.p. injection of 140 mg/kg N_1,N_1-dimethyl-biguanide; here the blood sugar decrease was 40—50%. In accordance with these findings, they saw a definite hyperglycaemia after an s.c. injection of 150 γ/kg. epinephrine The epinephrine was administered at the point where the blood sugar decrease was most marked. The reason for the inconsistence of these findings with those of HESSE and TAUBMANN, STERNE and DUVAL also SÖLING, WERCHAU and CREUTZFELDT remain unclear.

FRANK, NOTHMANN and WAGNER, also ARNDT, MÜLLER and SCHEMANN observed that higher doses of synthalin led to a glycogen reduction while small synthalin doses led to a glycogen increase in the liver of dogs and rabbits. UNGAR indicates that the glycogen reduction in starving experimental animals is more marked than in animals who have had enough to eat. The investigation of STAUB indicates that several factors are responsible for the liver glycogen reduction. STAUB found that also in the isolated perfused dog's liver, synthalin causes a stronger glycogen reduction than in the controls. HUUSAKO saw in splanchni-ectomised rabbits treated with synthalin a stronger blood-sugar decrease and a diminished, but still clear, liver glycogen reduction. Also in adrenalectomised rats, a definite liver glycogen reduction is seen after W 37 (SÖLING, WERCHAU and CREUTZFELDT). TYBERGHEIN and WILLIAMS even found in vitro, glycogen reduction in the liver slices of guinea-pigs after adding DBI. WILLIAMS refers to the findings of KREBS and FISCHER where in vitro the so-called PR-enzyme, which catalyses the change of muscle phosphorylase from the active a-form to the inactive b-form, is inhibited by DBI (inhibition is almost 80% at a DBI concentration of 1×10^{-2} m). In how far the reaction is of significance is unclear, as the PR-enzyme can be inhibited by many unspecific substances. Besides DBI had no influence in vitro, either on the activity of the a-form or on the b-form of the phosphorylase. Also the activity of the enzyme that changes the b- into the a-form remains untouched.

II. Animal experiments on the mechanism of blood sugar lowering through guanidine derivatives

a) Investigations with synthalin

FRANK, NOTHMANN and WAGNER believed after their investigations that synthalin had a similar effect to insulin. This was supported by their own findings that synthalin leads to a blood sugar decrease in the pancreatectomised dog (comp. p. 119) and an increase in the peripheral glucose uptake. (In the canine experiment after injection of synthalin into the femoral artery a definite increase in the arteriovenous glucose difference in the same extremity occurred, reaching a maximum of 22 mg-% after 2 hrs).

The view stated by FRANK, NOTHMANN and WAGNER that synthalin had a similar effect to insulin was made doubtful by the knowledge of the respiratory inhibitory action of guanidine. It was discussed that the blood-sugar decrease following the administration of guanidine derivatives was only a real guanidine effect, decreasing the blood sugar by inhibition of respiration and increasing anaerobic glycolysis.

This view could be experimentally supported by STAUB. He proved, using the synthalin doses necessary for depressing the blood sugar, that O_2 consumption of the animals was strongly reduced while simultaneously the blood lactic acid increased. In the eviscerated, hepatectomised and decapitated animals (Dale preparation), an increased glucose uptake was effected by synthalin. STAUB could prove, using balance experiments, that the amount of increased metabolised glucose reappeared in the form of lactate. Besides, he was not able to procure the synthesis of liver glycogen in experiments with synthalin by glucose or lactate application. In complete contrast to insulin, synthalin does not cause increased carbohydrate utilisation, but an increased carbohydrate reduction in the organism. The results of STAUB were completely confirmed in 1928 by BODO and MARKS. STAUB could also prove respiratory inhibition caused by synthalin in microorganisms (bacteria). Already with a synthalin concentration of 10 mg-% in the nutrative medium, a significant inhibition of growth was seen. Also the accelerated development of snail and toad larvae through thyroxin doses was retarded by low synthalin concentrations (GESSNER). SIMOLA found that the synthalin amounts that effected a blood sugar decrease in the healthy animals (sheep) lead to a rise in the blood lactate level and the anorganic blood phosphate level. The elevation in the blood citrate level in the rabbit observed by MARTENSSON following synthalin has already been mentioned (s. p. 107). STAUB assumed on grounds of NEGELEIN's reports of glycogen increase after respiratory inhibition through cyanide, that the site of synthalin action must be in the respiratory chain. The correctness of this assumption was proved by HOLLUNGER. Guanidine and synthalin inhibit electron transport via the respiratory chain at the cytochrome c level (comp. p. 95).

b) Investigations on the biguanides

1. Investigations in vitro

α) **Glucose uptake.** A definite increase in glucose uptake is found in the isolated rat diaphragm when adding DBI to the incubation medium (WILLIAMS, TYBERGHEIN, HYDE and NIELSEN; TYBERGHEIN and WILLIAMS; STEINER and WILLIAMS 1958; HERNANDEZ; FORBATH and CLARKE 1959a and b; UNGAR, RAFFAELSEN). The DBI concentration in the incubation medium was between 1.75 and 2.5×10^{-3} m in these experiments (synthalin increases the glucose uptake according to RAFFAELSEN at concentrations of 1.1×10^{-4} m). The glucose uptake of brain slices increased after DBI application to the same extent as in the diaphragm (HERNANDEZ). In contrast to these findings DITSCHUNEIT, PFEIFFER, and ROSSENBECK saw no significant effect of DBI on the glucose uptake by the rat diaphragm. They used however a lower concentration of DBI $(5 \times 10^{-4}$ m).

In the diaphragm of alloxan diabetic rats, the increased glucose uptake through DBI is more definite. Here the increase under DBI is about the same as that in the diaphragms of untreated non-diabetic rats (FORBATH and CLARKE 1959).

WICK and LARSON saw during investigations on the rat diaphragm and on isolated adipose tissue, no increase in the ^{14}C activity in the corresponding organ after a supply of ^{14}C-labelled glucose. As the assimilated glucose by the EMDEN-MEYERHOF pathway is rapidly degraded to lactate and in this form eliminated from the cell, no accumulation of ^{14}C-activity can be expected in the cell. DITSCHUNEIT et al. who observed no increasing effect of DBI on the glucose uptake by the rat diaphragm, found an increased glucose uptake by the rat adipose tissue. The increase was 138% when the DBI concentration was 1×10^{-4} m. A higher concentration $(5 \times 10^{-4}$ m) had no additional effect.

β) Glucose output from liver tissue, the glycogen content of liver slices and diaphragm. No significant increase in the glucose output was found in liver slices incubated with DBI $(2.5 \times 10^{-4}$ to 2.5×10^{-3} m) (TYBERGHEIN and WILLIAMS). Both in liver slices and also in the isolated rat diaphragm incubated with DBI $(1-2 \times 10^{-3}$ m) a definite decrease in the glycogen content is seen (TYBERGHEIN and WILLIAMS; FORBATH and CLARKE 1959a and b; RAFFAELSEN). Also in the diaphragm of alloxan diabetic rats there is a definite glycogen reduction (FORBATH and CLARKE 1959a and b). The absence of a glycogen increase in the diaphragm is the fundamental difference between the biguanide and the insulin effect.

γ) Oxygen consumption. The O_2 consumption of the isolated rat diaphragm is clearly diminished by DBI $(2.5 \times 10^{-3}$ m) (TYBERGHEIN and WILLIAMS; STEINER and WILLIAMS 1958a and b; HERNANDEZ). STEINER and WILLIAMS indicate that the decrease in O_2 consumption already commences before an increased glucose uptake is realised. The respiration of heart muscle homogenate (UNGAR) and of brain slices (HERNANDEZ) is also increased.

The liver slices of guinea-pigs $(1 \times 10^{-3}$ m DBI) and rats $(2.5 \times 10^{-3}$ m DBI) likewise showed inhibition of respiration of 29% respectively 36% (STEINER and WILLIAMS 1958a and b). UNGAR saw under the same conditions inhibition of respiration of 69% $(2 \times 10^{-3}$ m DBI) in liver homogenates. The liver slices and liver homogenates of animals receiving DBI in blood sugar lowering doses before sacrifice displayed a slightly less marked respiratory restriction (10—20%) (STEINER and WILLIAMS 1958b; UNGAR).

Heart muscle homogenate shows no significant respiratory restriction under these condition (UNGAR).

However, adipose tissue exhibits a definite restriction of respiration at 2×10^{-3} m DBI, measured by the oxidation of glucose acetate and succinate (WICK, LARSON and SERIF). The respiratory inhibition is directly proportional to the DBI concentration. The oxidation of acetate is still inhibited 30% at concentrations of 6.75×10^{-5} m DBI. These data can be completed by the recent experiments of DITSCHUNEIT et al.: while DBI $(1 \times 10^{-4}-5 \times 10^{-4}$ m) had no significant effect on the $^{14}CO_2$ formation from C_1-labelled glucose in the rat adipose tissue under normal conditions, the increased glucose oxidation via the hexose-monophosphate shunt performed through insulin could be nearly completely suppressed by the same concentrations of DBI.

δ) Glycolysis. There is an increase in anaerobic glycolysis under the action of DBI in muscle (rat diaphragm) (TYBERGHEIN and WILLIAMS; STEINER and WILLIAMS; FORBATH and CLARKE 1959), also in liver slices (TYBERGHEIN and WILLIAMS). This is recognized by augmented lactate and phosphate output. Increased lactate synthesis commences only when respiration is reduced (STEINER and WILLIAMS 1958 b); this speaks for there being a direct connection in the sense of an abrogation of the Pasteur effect. In contrast to these findings, UNGAR does not see an increase, but a decrease in lactate output compared to controls in the liver *homogenates* despite the fact that the respiration in these experiments was restricted to 31%. According to UNGAR's investigation on muscle homogenates, there is only also a maximum increase in lactate output of 23% despite reducing O_2 consumption 70—80%. However, TYBERGHEIN and WILLIAMS saw augmented lactate output at the same DBI concentration (2×10^{-3} m) in the isolated rat's diaphragm of about 265%. For this question cellular homogenate does not seem suitable, for as is well known the enzymes of glycolysis are present in the cytyplasm and those of the tricarbonic acid cycle and the respiratory chain in the mitochondria. It is important in such a complex mechanism as the abrogation of the Pasteur effect that the spatial relationships should be intact as LYNEN recently indicated again. UNGAR himself seems to have reached similar conclusions as he will repeat his experiments on liver *slices*.

ε) Cellular permeability for glucose and other sugars. CLARKE and FORBATH (1959, 1960) did not only investigate in the isolated rat diaphragm the DBI effect on glucose uptake, but also the uptake of fructose and other pentoses. Here the DBI effect was compared to the action of insulin and 2,4-dinitrophenol. According to these findings, not only glucose, but also fructose uptake is increased by DBI (2×10^{-3} m), not however, the pentose uptake. Should one assume the increased glucose or fructose uptake to be the result of direct guanidine action on the permeability of the cell membrane, then it is not comprehensible that there is no effect on the pentose penetration, if respiratory inhibition is the basis of the biguanide effect. This is so because it was recently shown by MORGAN, HENDERSON, REGEN and PARK that the uptake of d-arabinose definitely increased under O_2 deficiency. After 2,4-dinitrophenol (2.5×10^{-3} m), CLARKE and FORBATH (1960) also find augmented pentose uptake. In their comparative experiments, insulin, as was expected, led to an increased uptake of glucose, fructose, d-arabinose and d-xylose. CLARKE and FORBATH did not examine the galactose uptake. UNGAR, however, saw no increased galactose uptake in the eviscerated cat after DBI as was described for insulin by LEVINE et al. DEUTICKE and CREUTZFELDT also failed to find an effect of W 37 (DBV) on the galactose distribution in the eviscerated and nephrectomised rat. There is no proof that the guanidine derivatives which showed marked inhibitory metabolic effects in the above experiments lead to a specific increase in the efficiency of an active transport mechanism in the cell membrane. Considering the findings of CLARKE and FORBATH also of UNGAR, augmented glucose uptake could not be satisfactorily explained by an unspecific increase in permeability owing to respiratory inhibition as this should have been connected with an increased pentose or galactose uptake. On the other hand the fact that DBI—under O_2 deficiency conditions—does not increase glucose uptake in the rat diaphragm, speaks for the implication of respiratory inhibition (STEINER and WILLIAMS 1958, 1959).

The theoretic possibility remains that the concentration gradient for glucose between the extra and intracellular space has been greatly raised, the cell membrane being intact. There is no proof for this. However following DBI (contrary to insulin that produces a reversed effect) there is a reduction in the amount of free glucose in the muscle (CLAEKE and FORBARTH 1959, 1960). This reduction remains under 20%. It must remain open whether this is a sufficient explanation for the observed increased glucose uptake. At present there is no satisfactory explanation why there is no DBI effect on the pentose respectively glucose uptake.

ζ) **Investigations on the localisation of the biguanide effect in the intermediary metabolism.** STEINER and WILLIAMS (1958b) saw with DBI concentrations of over 1×10^{-3} m an increasing inhibition of succino-oxydase (rat liver). Succino-dehydrogenase was also inhibited by higher DBI concentrations (over 3.3×10^{-3} m). The above authors took this inhibition to be unspecific, as N_1,n-amyl-biguanide (ABG), that in vivo depresses the blood sugar as strongly as DBI, has a much weaker inhibitory effect on the named enzymes.

Inhibition of cytochrome c oxydase was investigated by 2 different methods by STEINER and WILLIAMS (1958b): measuring the oxidation of reduced cytochrome c spectrophotometrically, and measuring ascorbate oxidation. The first method only showed inhibition at very high concentrations of DBI or ABG ($1-2 \times 10^{-2}$ m), the second method already at lower DBI concentrations ($1-3 \times 10^{-3}$ m).

Neither WICK, LARSON and SERIF, nor UNGAR, PSYCHOYOS and HALL could demonstrate inhibition of cytochrome oxydase through DBI concentrations in which already restriction of succinate oxydation was proved (2×10^{-3} m). UNGAR, PSYCHOYOS and HALL proved inhibition of all DPN depending oxidation steps in the tri-carbonic acid cycle, while other oxidation processes (e.g. Wood-Werkmann reaction, synthesis of phospho-enol-pyruvic acid [Utter reaction]) was not inhibited (WILLIAMS, HYDE and NIELSEN). Also glucose-6-phosphate-dehydrogenase was not inhibited.

WICK, LARSON and SERIF could abrogate the inhibition of succinate oxidation by adding ascorbate; this indicates that succino-dehydrogenase itself is not inhibited. UNGAR, PSYCHOYOS and HALL also excluded this possibility.

KRUGER, SKILLMANN and HAMWI, also UNGAR, PSYCHOYOS and HALL were able to abolish partially, the restricted cell respiration caused by DBI, by adding uncoupling substances (2,4-dinitro-phenol, salicylate, dicumarol). These results are confirmed and supplemented by HOLLUNGER using guanidine (s. p. 95). HOLLUNGER had concluded there to be block at the level of cytochrome c on the grounds that uncoupling substances (e.g. 2,4-dinitro-phenol) partially, or totally abolish the respiratory inhibitory effect of guanidine. During cytochrome oxydo-reduction, intermediate compounds appear that are rich in energy and whose structure is still unknown. They have an inhibitory action on respiration. This effect is normally not important as these intermediate compounds, rich in energy, are rapidly split while transporting energy to a phosphate bond. Thus ATP is formed from ADP (s. LEUTHARD p. 498). 2,4-dinitro-phenol restitutes inhibited respiration, probably by hydrolytically splitting the inhibitory intermediary compound. Inhibition of the ATPase through guanidine could lead to an insufficient supply of ADP and accumulation of the intermediate metabolites that inhibit oxidation. HOLLUNGER saw this only in the case of Mg^{++} deficiency and in aged mitochondria preparations. It is more probable that guanidine respectively guanidine derivatives, lead to accumulation of the respective inhibitory intermediate compound in a different way.

It can be understood that in UNGAR's organ preparation all steps dependent on DPN in the Kreb's cycle are inhibited. This is because the electron transportation necessary for DPN-H-oxidation also enters the oxidation chain via the diaphorase at the level of cytochrome b, or possibly also at the controversial Slater factor; in any case however below cytochrome c. UNGAR, PSYCHOYOS and HALL do not conform with the conception of HOLLUNGER, despite ample proof. They believe the guanidine derivatives to cause competitive displacement of DPN at the various enzymes. If one considers the many inhibited metabolic stages and the relative concordance as to the strength of inhibition (especially the complete correlation of UNGAR's own findings with those of HOLLUNGER, also of WICK et al.) then UNGAR's conception of the competitive DPN displacement is not sufficient for refuting the fact that the guanidine derivatives have toxic effects on cell respiration.

UNGAR, PSYCHOYOS and HALL have further arguements against the belief that the blood-sugar lowering in animal experiments is caused by inhibition of respiration. Their investigations showed that DBI (50 mg/kg s.c.) led to a blood sugar decrease in the pigeon while an inhibitory effect on mitochondria preparations from pigeon's heart, liver or muscle could not be proved. The glycolysis theory could be questioned without doubt, should this finding be confirmed. The same authors investigated 15 different biguanide derivatives whereby often no correlation between the blood-sugar decrease and respiratory inhibitory action could be proved. The experiments on respiratory inhibition were only performed on the liver and not on muscle mitochondria preparations, in which perhaps a better relationship might have been found. Besides as admitted by the authors, under in-vivo conditions (hypoglycaemia experiments), absorption and permeability also play a different part. Finally it can be proved that the three examined preparations that most strongly depress the blood sugar (DBI, N_1,n-amyl-biguanide, synthalin A) also inhibit the O_2 consumption most strongly, even in those experimental conditions that are viewed critically. Besides in these 3 preparations, the strength of the blood-sugar-lowering effect is proportional to that of respiratory inhibition even if the relation for both factors does not correspond. UNGAR believes that inhibition of respiration, respectively of the Kreb's cycle, found in vivo is of an unspecific nature, and is not actually concerned with the actual mechanism of action. UNGAR indicated that many other substances inhibiting the tri-carbonic acid cycle or the oxidative phosphorylation do not cause hypoglycaemia. At first this does not seem to be of significance because this point has not been investigated at all for most of these substances, or as other drugs (e.g. salicylate) mentioned by UNGAR even cause hypoglycaemia (comp. p. 141 f.). STAUB reminds us that CLAUDE BERNARD already some decades ago, could produce hypoglycaemia in an animal through oxygen deficiency. VAN MIDDELSWORTH, KLINE, and BRITTON observed in rats that had been starved for 12 hrs, a definite hypoglycaemia if the O_2 tension in the respiratory air was reduced to 256 mm-Hg. This hypoglycaemia, similar to that following guanidine application, was preceeded by hyperglycaemia. HANDLER reached principally the same conclusion, after treating rabbits with cyanide or azide.

Finally the unpublished findings of SIPERSTEIN and MADISON (cited from MADISON and UNGAR 1959) shall be mentioned. They stated in contrast to the findings of other authors (TYBERGHEIN and WILLIAMS; FORBATH and CLARKE; WICK and LARSON) that in the liver slices of normal rats, DBI promotes (2—3 times) increased glucose oxidation by way of the hexosemonophosphate shunt (Horecker cycle).

η) Potentiation of the insulin effect in vitro. BOLINGER, McKEE and DAVIS (1960) found that an increase in glucose uptake by the isolated rat diaphragm first occurs above a DBI concentration of 1×10^{-3} m in the incubation medium. A maximum effect is found at a DBI concentration of 2×10^{-3} m. When the concentrations are over 2.5×10^{-3} m the increase in glucose uptake is decreased in proportion to the maximum effect. This corresponds well to the findings of STEINER and WILLIAMS (1958b) also UNGAR. DBI concentrations of (5×10^{-5}

to 1×10^{-4} m) that alone are ineffective, lead to a definite augmentation of glucose uptake through the isolated rat diaphragm if this has been pre-incubated with insulin. The glucose uptake on pre-incubating with insulin (5×10^{-4} U/ml medium) attains its maximal value at a DBI concentration of 5×10^{-5} m (compared with controls that were only incubated with insulin). No further increase in the glucose uptake could be reached by raising the DBI concentration under the same conditions to 2×10^{-3} m.

Thus there is the possibility of a potentiation of the insulin effect, especially with regard to the clinically much smaller amounts of biguanides used than in the animal experiments. The experiments of DEUTICKE and CREUTZFELDT show that this effect could also play a part in vivo in eviscerated and nephrectomised rats infused with glucose. Here premedication with W 37 (DBV) potentiated the blood sugar-lowering effect of small insulin doses. In the rat adipose tissue pre-incubated with insulin (1000 μ U/ml), DBI (1×10^{-4}—5×10^{-4} m) had only an additive, but no potentiating effect on the glucose uptake (DITSCHUNEIT, PFEIFFER, and ROSSENBECK).

2. Investigations on the non-diabetic animal

α) Glucose uptake. NIELSEN, SWANSON et al. performed experiments on eviscerated, nephrectomised guinea-pigs. The liver was eliminated by ligaturing all connections. Of these animals, the blood-sugar decrease in the controls after 60 mins was 19 mg-% (compared to the 62 mg-% in the animals s.c. treated with 20 mg/kg DBI). Following glucose doses, the controls showed a blood-glucose rise of 70 mg-% after 3 hrs; while the DBI treated animals displayed a decrease of 54 mg-%. These results correspond to those of STAUB also BODO and MARKS using synthalin in the Dale animals.

In contrast to this, WICK and LARSON found in the eviscerated nephrectomised rabbit no increase in peripheral glucose uptake through DBI. The authors find no satisfactory explanation for this. They mentioned the possibility that DBI has an effect mainly on the liver and leads there to an increase lactate formation besides inhibiting fat synthesis. The lactate released by the liver should then reach the muscle cell via the blood and be oxidised there. DEUTICKE and CREUTZFELDT found in eviscerated and nephrectomised rats, with and without adrenals, no significant increase in glucose uptake through W 37 (DBV) alone. Only the effect of a sub-optimal insulin injection was slightly potentiated through biguanides.

β) Glycolysis. After the administration of biguanides in blood-sugar-lowering doses, there is a significant elevation of blood lactate (TYBERGHEIN and WILLIAMS; CREUTZFELDT 1959b; UNGAR; SÖLING and CREUTZFELDT; SÖLING, WERCHAU and CREUTZFELDT). Also citrate (UNGAR) and pyruvate (CREUTZFELDT 1959b, SÖLING and CREUTZFELDT; SÖLING, WERCHAU and CREUTZFELDT) are increased. The increase of lactate is proportional to the administered DBI doses (SÖLING and CREUTZFELDT). The blood lactate level commences to rise before a blood-sugar decrease can be seen (TYBERGHEIN and WILLIAMS; SÖLING and CREUTZFELDT). This speaks for a causal connection between the blood-sugar decrease and increased glycolysis, under these conditions. The mostly simultaneously commencing percentual rise in lactate and pyruvate concentrations in the blood (SÖLING and CREUTZFELDT) indicates a preponderately increased *aerobic* glycolysis.

WILLIAMS, TYBERGHEIN, HYDE and NIELSEN could correspondingly find in guinea-pigs, receiving 20 mg/kg DBI s.c., no reduced CO_2 output. The portion of $^{14}CO_2$ of the entire CO_2 remained unchanged after administration of ^{14}C-labelled glucose.

8*

γ) **Hepatic glucose output.** NIELSEN, SWANSON et al. saw in the guinea-pig receiving DBI (30 mg/kg s.c.) a definite decrease in the glucose difference between the inferior caval vein and the hepatic vein. They conclude from this that the liver has a reduced glucose output. This conclusion, is however only possible if one simultaneously measures the blood flow, as theoretically the hepatic blood flow can be greatly increased following DBI administration as has been proved by TRANQUADA, KLEEMAN and BROWN (1959c).

δ) **Effect on gluconeogenesis.** The liver glycogen augmentation following injection of 2 gm/kg d,l-alanine in the guinea-pig is not found if 30 mins previously 50 mg/kg DBI were administered. Instead, the same reduction in liver glycogen occurs as is also normally seen after DBI (WILLIAMS, TYBERGHEIN, HYDE and NIELSEN). This is assumed to indicate inhibition of gluconeogenesis through DBI. Inhibition seems to take place at the deamination level of amino acids as STEINER and WILLIAMS were able to exclude inhibition of arginase (unpublished, cited from STEINER and WILLIAMS 1959). Investigations on the nitrogen balance did, indeed, show a greatly reduced nitrogen excretion in the urine of guinea-pigs receiving DBI. This could not be sufficiently explained by the increase in blood nitrogen also present (WILLIAMS, TYBERGHEIN, HYDE and NIELSEN). As there is also a greatly delayed increase in blood nitrogen in nephrectomised animals receiving DBI in contrast to the controls (TYBERGHEIN and WILLIAMS), inhibition of gluconeogenesis through guanidine derivatives must be regarded as proven. Inhibition of gluconeogenesis in the rabbit through synthalin was already seen by BLATHERWICK, SAHYUN and HILL in 1927. They found that injected glycine after synthalin was more slowly assimilated than in the controls. Also in these experiments, the simultaneously found kidney damage dit not promote this. Independent from the question of gluconeogenesis, was apparent that in the old synthalin and new DBI experiments, blood urea increased despite reduced gluconeogenesis; this indicates a disturbance in renal function (comp. p. 105).

ε) **Inhibition of insulin degradation.** Inhibition of insulin degradation in the liver through DBI as was found in vitro WILLIAMS, TYBERGHEIN, HYDE and NIELSEN, must be regarded as unspecific inhibition of proteases. Likewise, glucagon degradation was inhibited in their experiments. Besides, no inhibition of insulin degradation could be proved in vivo (WILLIAMS, TYBERGHEIN et al.).

ζ) **Combination with insulin and tolbutamide.** A combination of insulin and DBI in the guinea-pig leads to a definite increase in the blood sugar raising effect. Hereby the reduction in liver glycogen, also the elevation of blood lactate and pyruvate is not as marked as on administration of the same DBI doses alone (ANDREU-KERN, SÖLING and CREUTZFELDT).

The combination of DBI and D 860 (tolbutamide) leads to no additive effect on the blood sugar. The metabolic changes (abrogation of the increased glycogen storage induced by D 860, comp. p. 46 f., increase in blood lactate and blood pyruvate) show that the DBI effect is established in the first place under these conditions. D 860 alone does not significantly change the concentration of blood lactate and pyruvate in the guinea-pig (ANDREU-KERN, SÖLING and CREUTZFELDT).

η) **The effect of methylene blue on the blood sugar decrease.** In guinea-pigs and rats, the blood-sugar decrease can be partially or completely inhibited after DBI and after W 37 (depending on biguanide doses) if 30 mins previously and 1 hr after biguanide application, methylene blue (100—150 mg/kg total dose s.c.) has been given. Abrogation of the blood sugar decrease can also be demonstrated in the adrenalectomised rat. The protective effect only lasts 2—4 hrs owing to the rapid excretion of methylene blue. A similar effect could be reached by giving

100 γ/kg s.c. epinephrine instead of methylene blue. Gluthathion has no effect on the blood sugar lowering (SÖLING, WERCHAU, AHRENS and CREUTZFELDT).

ϑ) Indirect metabolic changes caused by epinephrine release. There is still the question to be answered in how far the metabolic effects in the animal experiments are caused by the epinephrine liberation that is always initiated by guanidine derivatives.

HUUSAKO showed in 1940 that synthalin leads to stronger hypoglycaemia in the adrenalectomised rabbit with simultaneously reduced lactacidaemia. The increase of lactate and pyruvate formation through epinephrine has been known longer. SÖLING, WERCHAU and CREUTZFELDT could confirm HUUSAKO's findings in the adrenalectomised rat. The significance of epinephrine for the speed of the initial glycogenolysis in the liver has already been discussed. It is known that epinephrine inhibits the glucose uptake of the diaphragm in vivo that is instigated by insulin (GROEN et al.). This finding could be confirmed for the eviscerated, hepatectomised rat by DEUTICKE and CREUTZFELDT. Increased peripheral glucose uptake stimulated by DBI is not at all, or only in very high concentrations (0.1 mg-%), affected by adrenalin (BOLINGER, MCKEE and DAVIS 1959). By increasing the DBI concentration, it is also possible to abolish the slight inhibition of glucose uptake caused by very high concentrations of epinephrine. The part played by epinephrine in the metabolic changes observed in vivo following guanidine derivatives varies without doubt greatly in the different animal species. Therefore, in the guinea-pig the absence of any hyperglycaemic reaction (even in very high doses) and the great sensitivity to the blood sugar lowering effect speaks for a relatively slight epinephrine liberation. In correlation to this, are the findings of SÖLING and CREUTZFELDT, namely that in the guinea-pig the blood sugar decrease is directly proportional to the blood lactate increase (comp. p. 115). The same experiments showed that 2 biguanides of different effectiveness (DBI and N_1,n-butyl-biguanide) administered to guinea-pigs in equal blood sugar lowering doses lead to an elevation in blood lactate of the same degree. Such parallelity is unexpected should the adrenal medulla play an important part. That it is different in the rabbit can be seen from the above mentioned experiments (p. 108) of HUUSAKO. In the dog showing no blood sugar decrease, and often an increase after DBI, the stronger rise in blood lactate and pyruvate (SÖLING and CREUTZFELDT) is due to the epinephrine effect.

ι) Stimulation of insulin secretion. On the grounds of recent experiments performed in vitro with DBI, the blood sugar decrease is explained almost solely by the increasing effect the guanidine derivatives have on anaerobic glycolysis. But there are some metabolic effects which are not consistent with this theory (s. p. 113f., 121f.). Moreover, there are investigations that speak for the fact that guanidine derivatives also stimulate insulin secretion.

CLARK's investigations (1923) have been mentioned during the discussion on guanidine. They showed the probability of vagal stimulation of insulin secretion (comp. p. 95). The same question has been thoroughly investigated by ZUNZ and LA BARRE for synthalin A and was answered positively.

Synthalin doses were used that were so low (1—2 mg/kg i.v.) that they only caused a blood sugar decrease in the adrenalectomised dog. In the first series of experiments the greater pancreatic vein of an adrenalectomised donor dog was connected with the jugular vein of a second adrenalectomised recipient dog. The cross-connection remained closed until the synthalin had been distributed in the donor dog. After opening the connection in all experiments, it was seen that within 30—60 mins there was an excessive decrease in the blood sugar of the recipient dog, while the blood sugar in the donor dog remained unchanged. No blood sugar decrease, even in the recipient dog, was found in the controls (dogs without synthalin). When the same experiment was again performed (this time cutting both vagal nerves in the donor dog before administering synthalin) no effect was seen in the recipient dog. In a 3rd. experimental set-up, the head of the donor dog (A) was severed from the trunk, the vagal nerves being intact. This head received its blood supply from the trunk of a 3rd. decapitated dog (C). (Both dogs, A and C, received artificial respiration). As in the previous experiment, cross-circulation was made via the pancreatic vein between the adrenalectomised donor dog (A) and the adrenalectomised recipient dog (B). Synthalin was injected i.v. in dog C. Thus, synthalin had no contact with the circulation in dog A and B. Following synthalin injection, there was a moderate blood sugar decrease in dog C. This decrease is understandable as de-capitated animals, owing to the absence of the hyperglycaemic counter-regulation, show a blood sugar decrease more easily than intact animals (KRONEBERG and STOEPEL). Dog A showed no change in the blood sugar. Dog B, the recipient dog, displayed a marked blood sugar decrease that was not found in the controls (sodium chloride injection).

These findings can only be explained by the fact that synthalin stimulation of the vagus leads to an increased insulin liberation from the pancreas. MÜLLER and REINWEIN also BERTRAM already discussed this possibility in 1927. BERTRAM hereby had observed that small concentrations of parasympathetic drugs (e.g. pilocarpine, acetylcholine, choline, physostigmine) had a blood sugar lowering effect while only large doses elevated the blood sugar. Both effects could be abolished by atropine (BERTRAM 1927).

Also the findings of RALLI and TIBER speak for the fact that a pancreatic rest, capable of secreting insulin, plays a part in the metabolic effect of guanidine derivatives; in totally pancreatectomised dogs no blood sugar decrease could be achieved after glucose dose through synthalin; in the partially pancreatectomised dog, this was possible. Reduction of the blood amino acid nitrogen through glycocoll administration was possible in the partially pancreatectomised not, however, in the totally pancreatectomised animals.

One may also discuss whether the findings of RALLI and TIBER state that when insulin is not found in the organism, the effective guanidine dose must accordingly be higher.

From the research of ZUNZ and LA BARRE, it seems possible at first that besides other effects, that of insulin mobilisation plays a role in the blood sugar lowering effect of the guanidine derivatives. The absence of a significant β-cell degranulation, which was impressively found for all species following application of β-cell active sulphonylureas (comp. p. 29 f.), in the usually very sensitive guinea-pig following synthalin and also DBI application, speaks against this conception (CREUTZFELDT and MOENCH). The fact that STUHLFAUTH et al. on perfusing the isolated canine pancreas with DBI, failed to find a rise in the insulin content in the perfusate (present after BZ 55 and glucose) does not totally speak against the possibility of a stimulation of insulin secretion. As in the above mentioned investigations, this effect depends on an intact nervous supply.

ϰ) **α-cell changes following guanidine derivatives.** DAVIS described degranu-lation and hydropic degeneration of the α-cells of the pancreas in the rabbit receiving a dose of synthalin A. This could be confirmed by many authors for normal and alloxan diabetic rabbits (FODDEN; FODDEN and READ; v. HOLT, KRÖNER and KÜHNAU; CREUTZFELDT and TECKLENBORG). Also in the guinea-pig, synthalin A (RUNGE 1954; CREUTZFELDT 1954; CREUTZFELDT and TECKLENBORG; KORP and LE COMPTE) leads to degranulation and vacuolation of the α-cells; the same is also true for synthalin B and DBI (CREUTZFELDT and MOENCH). Normal and alloxanised rats show the same after synthalin A, namely degranu-lation and vacuolation of the α-cells (v. HOLT, v. HOLT, KRÖNER and KÜHNAU; CREUTZFELDT and TECKLENBORG). In 1954, these findings were interpreted as being the cause for the blood sugar lowering effect of synthalin (v. HOLT, v. HOLT, KRÖNER and KÜHNAU; v. HOLT and FERNER also FERNER and RUNGE). Such an effect should be caused by a deficiency or reduced production of glucagon. This view po int is based on the assumption that glucagon plays an important part in regulating the blood sugar level; there is no proof of this (comp. the review by CREUTZFELDT, 1957). In the partially pancreatectomised dog only retaining the duodenal part of the pancreas containing only β-cells, no glucagon deficiency syndrome appears (BENCOSME). DAVIS saw in the rabbit receiving synthalin B, also a blood sugar depressing drug, no α-cell damage. FODDEN had already mentioned in 1953 that cobaltous chloride damages the α-cells at least to the same extent as synthalin A, without the appearance of hypoglycaemia. Besides, first there is no parallelity between the extensive α-cell damage and hypoglycaemia effects, and secondly, it is not possible to prevent the synthalin shock by continuously injecting glucagon (CREUTZFELDT and TECKLENBORG). The discrepancy between the extent of α-cell damage and the blood sugar lowering effect is even greater for DBI (CREUTZFELDT and MOENCH). After DBI (15 to 25 mg/kg s.c. for 3 days), the α-cell changes in the guinea-pig are far less and more inconstant than following synthalin despite the fact that severe hypoglycaemia is regularly observed. According to the named investigations, the hypoglycaemia following the application of guanidine derivatives is with certainty not due to α-cell damage.

The cause of the α-cell damage has not been fully cleared (v. HOLT, v. HOLT, KRÖNER and KÜHNAU; v. HOLT and FERNER, also FERNER and RUNGE). These authors assume a direct α-cytotoxic effect of synthalin. DAVIS also CREUTZFELDT and TECKLENBORG explain the changes as secondary degeneration due to exhaustion. Here it is not very probable that the excessive glucagon production occurs following hypoglycaemia, as the extent of the blood sugar lowering would be parallel to the degree of the histological changes. They must be regarded as a more or less specific reaction of the α-cells to the changes in the metabolism. CREUTZFELDT and TECKLENBORG also CREUTZFELDT and MOENCH indicated the relation between histological liver damage and α-cell changes in the guinea-pig.

λ) **Effect on the glucose absorption from the intestine.** READ and FODDEN investigated the effects of synthalin A on the glucose absorption of alloxan diabetic and pancreatectomised dogs. While glucose absorption from the intestine in both types of diabetes could not be influenced by insulin, a dose of synthalin A (10 mg/kg s.c.) led to a strong inhibition of glucose absorption. In the non-diabetic animal, glucose absorption was not influenced by synthalin A. In how far this effect also plays a part in the blood sugar decreasing guanidine effect, must remain open. Corresponding investigations with the biguanides have not yet been published. BOL, SÖLING and CREUTZFELDT investigated the influence of N_1,n-butyl-biguanide on the absorption of instilled glucose in the isolated small intestine left in situ, of the rat. No significant influence of the biguanides on the glucose absorption was found either on s.c. or enteral application. The same was found in corresponding experiments using synthalin; synthalin could also not abolish the inhibition of glucose absorption caused by phlorizin (BOL, SÖLING and CREUTZFELDT).

3. Experimental diabetes

α) **Diabetes following pancreatectomy.** According to FRANK, NOTHMANN and WAGNER (1926), synthalin also depresses the blood sugar in the pancreatectomised dog (10 mg/kg s.c. or 20—30 mg/kg orally). This finding could not at first be confirmed by HEDON and VERTZMANN; RATHERY, KOURILSKY and GILBERT also RALLI and TIBER. MÜLLER and REINWEIN also saw no satisfactory blood-sugar decrease in the pancreatectomised dog given galegine. However, probably these controversies can be explained by the different doses. Because the synthalin doses used by RATHERY et al., also RALLI and TIBER (2—4 mg/kg orally) lowered the blood sugar inconstantly even in the normal dog. READ and FODDEN (1954) found just as FRANK, NOTHMANN and WAGNER a strong blood sugar decrease in the pancreatectomised dog receiving 10 mg/kg synthalin A. The same appears to be true for the pancreatectomised guinea-pig given DBI (NIELSEN, SWANSON et al. 1958). No effect either of N_1,n-butylbiguanide or of synthalin could be observed in the pancreatectomised, hepatectomised rat (DEUTICKE and CREUTZFELDT).

β) **Alloxan diabetes.** Synthalin also lowers the blood-sugar in the alloxan diabetic rabbit and rat (FODDEN 1953; v. HOLT, v. HOLT, KRÖNER and KÜHNAU; CREUTZFELDT and TECKLENBORG). DBI is said to have a blood-sugar-decreasing effect in alloxanised rats, rabbits and rhesus monkeys (UNGAR, FREEDMAN and SHAPIRO). The same is said for N_1,N_1,dimethyl-biguanide in the alloxanised rat (STERNE and DUVAL). Both groups of research workers do not mention the experimental set-up. SÖLING, RAUH and CREUTZFELDT saw no blood-sugar decrease in chronically alloxanised rats through N_1,n-butyl-biguanide. Even prolonged treatment with W 37 led to no improvement in the i.v. and oral glucose tolerance. Decreased glucosuria could with certainty, be traced back to delayed food intake and also to reduction of the glomerular filtration rate. MEIER and YERGANIAN found that DBI lowered the blood sugar of chinese hamsters with spontaneous hereditary diabetes only in mild cases which also responded to D 860. If D 860 was ineffective, DBI was too.

FODDEN observed, after applying synthalin A (6 mg/kg s.c.) to alloxan diabetic rabbits, definite ketosis even before the blood sugar decrease had reached its maximum. "Lipaemic turbidity" appeared simultaneously with ketonaemia and ketonuria. The alloxanised animals displayed no ketosis before synthalin. In normal animals synthalin led to a complete disappearance of glycogen without appearance of ketosis. FODDEN suspects that the $α$-cell damage caused by synthalin prevents metabolisation of the increased products of fat metabolism found in diabetes, thus causing ketosis. It is more probable that the combination of liver damage through synthalin with the disturbance of liver metabolism, directly and/or indirectly (through diabetes) caused by alloxan, leads to the break down of fat metabolism. To this is added inhibition of the liver glucose oxidation through synthalin. SKILLMAN, KRUGER and HAMWI (1959b) found in the rabbit with mild alloxan diabetes after DBI (100 mg i.v. per animal) a slight increase in ketonaemia from 7.3 to 13.7 mg-%. This increase occurred simultaneously with the maximum blood sugar decrease. FODDEN's experimental findings are most striking because relatively high doses of the more strongly liver toxic synthalin were used in animal experiments. Both investigations show that in the animal experiment, the blood sugar decrease is by no means connected with improvement in the diabetic metabolism. Rather there is an increased disturbance in fat metabolism. In the same sense speaks also the reduction in the alkali reserves found in the case of a stronger blood sugar lowering in the healthy dog given synthalin (HORNUNG).

γ) **Phlorhizin diabetes.** Synthalin has a very strong influence on phlorhizin diabetes (STAUB and KÜNG; STAUB and JEZLER; ÖSTERREICHER and SNAPPER), biguanides as far as have been investigated, however, do not (HESSE and TAUBMANN). Phlorhizin diabetic dogs recover within hours after synthalin administration even of they are already in pre-coma condition. Here glucosuria regresses, simultaneously also lactaciduria and acetonuria. In the phlorhizin diabetic dog, the blood sugar that is usually normal, does not decrease (ÖSTERREICHER and SNAPPER; STAUB and KÜNG). In this case, synthalin seems to act on the lower renal threshold for glucose instigated by phlorhizin. As an increase of the T_m glucose strongly reduced by phlorhizin is hard to imagine as being caused by synthalin, the change in the renal threshold can more easily be explained by a reduction of the glomerular filtration rate and thus, of the glucose loading.

Possibly the decamethylene chain of synthalin also plays a part. This could be so, owing to the fact that dicarbonic acids with long chains can also reduce glucosuria in the phlorhizin diabetic animal (BAER and BLUM). Acidosis, respectively ketosis, accompanying phlorhizin diabetes in the dog is rapidly improved by synthalin (ÖSTERREICHER and SNAPPER; STAUB and KÜNG). This improvement can be adequately explained by regression of glucosuria as the presence of sufficient amounts of glucose is enough to normalise the reactively increased fat degradation and elevated gluconeogenesis. There is no real metabolic disturbance apart from the lower renal threshold for glucose, in the phlorhizin diabetes. In contrast to the beneficial influence of synthalin on phlorizin diabetes in the dog, SÖLING, RAUH and CREUTZFELDT saw no significant improvement of the phlorhizin diabetes of the rat after synthalin or N_1,n-butyl-biguanide.

III. Investigations on the mechanism of action in man

a) Theory of glycolysis

STAUB, who was the first to prove that the blood sugar lowering in the animal experiment was mainly caused by abrogation of the Pasteur effect with the resulting elevation in anaerobic glycolysis, refutes this as causing a blood sugar decrease in man (STAUB and JEZLER). STAUB bases this on the fact that in man there is no noteworthy increase in lactaciduria after synthalin even if a definite blood sugar lowering occurs. This has also, meanwhile, been found to be true for DBI. CRAIG, MILLER and WOODWARD observed a strong recession of glucosuria without nearly the corresponding increase in lactic acid excretion in the urine. The same was found for DBI and N_1,n-butyl-biguanide (W 37) by SÖLING, WERCHAU and CREUTZFELDT. Only KAUFMANN-COSLA and VASILCO saw in diabetics treated with synthalin despite complete dissipation of glucosuria, an unchanged high total carbon excretion in the urine. They conclude from this that there is no increased glucose utilisation but only a transformation to other metabolites that are also excreted in the urine. There are controversial statements as to an elevation in blood lactic acid in man following the administration of guanidine derivatives. HIRSCH-KAUFFMANN and WAGNER did not find a rise in serum lactate and pyruvate in diabetics receiving synthalin, and TRANQUADA et al. (1959b, 1960), after DBI. However, CRAIG and MILLER (1960) found an increase in lactate and citrate after DBI. SÖLING, WERCHAU and CREUTZFELDT also found in diabetics treated with DBI or W 37 an increase of the enzymatically determined blood lactate and pyruvate to about twice or three times that of the normal values. No increase was found in patients treated with insulin. FAJANS, MOORHOUSE et al. (1960) saw no rise in blood lactate following DBI but, however, a delayed decrease of the blood lactate and pyruvate level increased by pyruvate infusion.

The observation of LUBLIN speaks for a certain respiratory restriction. The respiratory quotient in patients treated with synthalin rises mainly by reducing the O_2 intake. Nevertheless an increase in *anaerobic* glycolysis as causing blood sugar decrease in man given tolerable amounts of guanidine derivatives is not possible. TRANQUADA, KLEEMAN and BROWN (1959, 1960) could find no changes in the O_2 consumption by the liver after DBI. In this connection, the fact that no blood sugar decrease can be achieved in the healthy human being, receiving tolerable amounts of biguanides is of significance (WILLIAMS; FAJANS and MILLER; SÖLING, WERCHAU and CREUTZFELDT; OTTO 1960; GÜTSCHE, MICHEL). MICHEL even saw a slight blood sugar increase in non-diabetics receiving 200 mg DBI.

He could also find in some cases of diabetes an initial blood sugar increase (up to 40% above the starting value) after loading with 200 mg DBI. Loading with 400 mg N_1-n-butyl-biguanide led to a very impressive initial blood sugar rise in non-diabetics and diabetics lasting for approximately 2 hrs. 400 mg DBI produced no such definite effects.

This makes it probable that the biguanides also have an initial stimulating effect on the adrenergic system in man even if this is not always visible. The increase in anorganic phosphorus and the decrease of calcium in the blood, typical for the animal experiment, was hardly investigated in man. ODELL et al. could find no changes in the serum phosphorus or serum calcium when compared to controls. No significant results have been obtained from experimentally improving synthalin tolerance by administering calcium (comp. p. 127).

b) Liver-glucose output and peripheral glucose utilization

BERINGER, HUPKA et al. found on investigating diabetics by hepatic catheterisation, a diminished glucose output through the liver. This had been found in the animal experiment by NIELSEN, SWANSON et al., TRANQUADA, KLEEMAN and BROWN (1959b, 1960) who, however, investigated fasting diabetics in the post-absorptive state using a similar method, found no change in the liver glucose output despite the fact that the hepatic blood supply was increased through DBI. Both research groups found correspondingly augmented lactate and pyruvate uptake by the liver following DBI. These findings also speak against there being increased anaerobic glycolysis in the liver of human subjects receiving DBI. BERINGER, HUPKA et al. found besides this, in the liver of diabetics treated with DBI (therapy lasting 4 months), no reduction in the histochemically found glycogen seen in the animal experiment, but an augmented glycogen reaction. This latter, was however, not as strong as after tolbutamide. Combination with insulin led to further increase in liver glycogen (BERINGER and THALER). However, a significant glycogen decrease was seen in the muscle after DBI treatment (BERINGER, HUPKA et al.).

Only few investigations are found on the peripheral glucose uptake following DBI therapy in man. Besides they do not correspond. BUTTERFIELD, FRY and HOLLING saw an increase in the peripheral glucose uptake after DBI, but only in those cases who responded well to oral anti-diabetic therapy.

MADISON and UNGER (1960) found no increase in the glucose uptake by the muscle. They suggest that augmented glucose uptake takes place through the adipose tissue and the liver. This could explain their findings of increased glucose utilization by the whole organism (about 26 mg/min in addition).

c) Other endocrine organs

The absence of blood sugar response to glucagon in the animal given DBI is not found in man. FAJANS, MOORHOUSE, DOORENBOS, LOUIS and CONN (1960) found absolutely no difference in healthy subjects between controls and those treated with DBI with respect to the glucagon response. In diabetics receiving DBI, the blood sugar increase following glucagon was even slightly stronger than in diabetics not given DBI.

Investigations of the adrenal cortical function by estimating the steroid excretion in the urine did not indicate any influence of DBI. This was shown by BERGEN and NORTON for the 17,21-dihydroxy, 20 keto-steroids, and by FAJANS, MOORHOUSE et al. (1960) for the 17-keto and 17-hydroxy steroids (comp. also BERGEN, HILTON and NORTON).

No investigations have been made on the influencing of gluconeogenesis in the diabetic receiving DBI. TRANQUADA et al. (1959 b, 1960) found that DBI administered to the diabetic did not lead to a change in liver urea production.

LAMBERT (1958) described a transitory reduction of ^{131}I uptake in the thyroid during DBI treatment. This finding could not be confirmed by SKILLMAN, KRUGER and HAMWI (1959).

d) Stimulation of insulin secretion

Already at the beginning of the synthalin era, the poor response of juvenile diabetics to synthalin was apparent. For this reason, MÜLLER and REINWEIN and also BERTRAM (1928) assumed that the blood sugar decreasing effect of the guanidine derivatives must be at least partly caused by a stimulation of the insulin secretion.

On the indication of CLARKS' animal experiments mentioned on p. 95 on rabbits, BERTRAM investigated the effect of atropine on the blood sugar course in 4 diabetics receiving synthalin; in 2 of these patients, the blood sugar decrease through synthalin was not very strongly diminished by atropine, while the other 2 with typical maturity-onset diabetes showed hardly any blood sugar decrease after atropine through synthalin. In these patients, synthalin alone showed a clear reduction of the blood sugar.

The investigations of BERTRAM showed a certain parallelity to a recent publication of JORDAN in which the blood sugar lowering properties of a choline esterase inhibitor are described (neoeserine). BUTTERFIELD, FRY and HOLLING also suspect that the effect of DBI is partially bound to the presence of insulin. They base this on the fact that increased peripheral glucose uptake after DBI as also after D 860 is found only in those patients showing a sufficient blood sugar response. The findings of BERGEN and NORTON are similar, namely that the non-esterified fatty acids in the blood of diabetics receiving DBI were only reduced and therefore reacted as after insulin (GORDON and CHERKES) if the blood sugar responded well to DBI.

e) Conclusion

If one considers the results found in humans treated with guanidine derivatives, the following conclusion is reached: the doses used in the animal experiments are so much higher than those clinically used or tolerated by the healthy, or diabetic person that no final conclusion can be reached from the findings in vitro and in the animal on the mechanism of the blood sugar decrease in the diabetic. According to the present investigations in man, it is unlikely that increased anaerobic glycolysis is the main mechanism of action. By this the existence of the guanidine effect even in man is not refuted. It is possible that it is responsible for many of the pathological clinical findings, especially intolerance (s. p. 126 and 138). Several observations show the possibility of a potentiation of the effective endogenous and/or exogenous insulin (BOLINGER et al., s. p. 114). One can also discuss a stimulation of insulin secretion as being partly responsible for the anti-diabetic effect of the guanidine derivatives especially in the mild maturity-onset diabetes. This is admittedly less probable than for the sulphonylureas. As in the latter, the blood sugar decreasing effect is the stronger, the greater the functional capacity of the β-cells is. Therefore, the strongest acute blood sugar decrease is in normal man and it decreases with increasing severity of the diabetes. However, the guanidine derivatives only have a blood sugar effect in the diabetic, but not in the healthy subject. The same is true for the spontaneous hereditary diabetes mellitus in the chinese hamster (MEIER and YERGANIAN). The blood sugar effective dose for these animals was half that of the effective dose for non-diabetic chinese hamsters (s. p. 124).

It must here be emphasised that the relevance of all previously mentioned findings from the animal experiment and in vitro, can only finally be discussed in relation to this mechanism of the anti-diabetic effect in man if we have results on plasma and tissue levels for the human.

D. Clinical experiments with various guanidine derivatives

I. Synthalin

a) Dosage

FRANK, NOTHMANN and WAGNER (1926) commenced dosing in the adult with 30—50 mg/day divided in 2 single doses with one day of abstinence after 3—4 days. In 1928, FRANK made a dosage scheme whereby 40 mg daily were maximally administered and always after 3 days, one of abstinence. His doses were later discounted by other authors as being too high. UMBER used an individual dosage whereby, with or without insulin, synthalin was only given every 2 days. The dose was between 10—80 mg/day. Doses over 50 mg/day were only exceptionally administered. EISMAYER gave maximally 3×10 mg/day with one days abstinence after 3 days, also a 1—2 weeks pause after 4—6 weeks of treatment. ADAM applied synthalin even more cautiously, in all only 10 mg daily, in many (to 6) single doses. BERTRAM (1928) saw no sufficient synthalin effect on using doses of 12 mg/day. He saw the best results with doses of about 20 mg/day. JACOBI and BRÜLL, who suggested individual dosage, emphasised the importance of treating with slowly increasing doses to attain a suffcient blood level with the lowest incidence of intolerance.

FRANK (1928), imagining synthalin to be a substance similar to insulin, attributed a certain insulin equivalent to synthalin. According to this, one unit of insulin corresponds to 1 mg of synthalin. The reference standard was based on the effect both substances had on glucosuria in diabetes. Later clinical experience showed that the conception of a standard insulin equivalent for synthalin was not possible. It differs from case to case and is not feasible in patients responding well to insulin and not at all to synthalin.

b) Effect of synthalin on the diabetic metabolic state

1. Glucosuria and hypoglycaemia

Reduction in glucosuria is the most prominent effect on the diabetic metabolism. FRANK, NOTHMANN and WAGNER reported of reduction in the daily sugar excretion to 50 gm/day. UMBER reached a reduction to 30 gm/day on long-term therapy. The effect of synthalin on the blood sugar is not so characteristic. The observation has been made by numerous research workers that synthalin leads to aglucosuria while the blood sugar is only slightly, or not lowered (UMBER; BERTRAM 1928; MORAWITZ; JACOBI and BRÜLL). This finding, together with the results of the synthalin investigations on phlorhizin diabetic dogs (s. p. 120), speaks for a rise in the renal glucose threshold instigated by synthalin as partly causing the reduction in glucosuria.

2. Ketoacidosis

FRANK, NOTHMANN and WAGNER (1926) used the good effect of synthalin on ketosis and acidosis of the diabetic as a strong arguement for its insulin-like properties. A reduction in acetonuria, and also in the excretion of β-hydroxy-butyric acid and acetoacetic acid has been confirmed by many clinicians (UMBER; MORAWITZ; STRAUSS). Such improvement of ketosis could only be achieved in relatively mild diabetes. BERTRAM (1928) even did not find it in these latter cases. If the diabetes was moderate to severe, most clinicians observed deterioration in the metabolism after administering synthalin. BERTRAM (1928) always found, after treating moderately severe juvenile diabetics with synthalin, deterioration in metabolism that persisted after discontinuing synthalin and recommencing insulin therapy. According to BERTRAM (1928), the moderately severe diabetes could change to a severe diabetes through synthalin. KLEEBERG found after discontinuing synthalin therapy because of metabolic decompensation or intolerance, higher insulin requirements than before synthalin treatment. Other authors repeatedly found unchanged or increased ketosis, respectively acidosis, after synthalin even if glucosuria and blood sugar were improved or normalised (HIRSCH-MAMROTH and PERLMANN; MORAWITZ; JANSEN and BAUR; JACOBI and BRÜLL). Even if insulin was slowly replaced by synthalin, sometimes ketosis occurred despite the fact that the metabolism—measured by the glucosuria—seemed to be normalised (JANSEN and BAUR).

c) Indication range

FRANK, NOTHMANN and WAGNER (1926) only saw a contra-indication of synthalin therapy in the presence of a diabetic pre-coma, respectively coma. The fact that synthalin therapy was not allocated to certain forms was not primarily due to the conception of "severe" and "mild" diabetics being classed according to their insulin requirements and less to the total metabolic changes. Clinical experience, however, showed that in maturity-onset diabetes, without ketoacidosis, was the real domain of synthalin therapy; while in insulin deficiency diabetes, the response was proportional to the own insulin production. FRANK had already confirmed that the insulin equivalent of insulin was less favourable in juveniles and children (FRANK, NOTHMANN and WAGNER 1926). According to PRIESEL and WAGNER, synthalin without simultaneous insulin dose is completely ineffective in the diabetic child. Synthalin also had no effect in a case of bronze diabetes (MORAWITZ). BERTRAM believed for these reasons that the pancreas must have a certain ability for insulin production for synthalin to be effective. Perusing the published therapeutical results on synthalin, shows that the duration of the existence of the diabetic metabolic state is irrelevant, for the success of the synthalin therapy. The therapeutical success depends, of course, primarily on the individual tolerance to a certain synthalin dose. On account of this, the possibility of a sole synthalin diabetes therapy was limited; only the maturity-onset diabetic controlled dietetically, or by small amounts of insulin is suitable for a pure synthalin therapy (BERTRAM 1928; EISMAYER). In all other cases synthalin had to be administered in combination with insulin (UMBER). The necessary insulin dose was often reduced when given together with synthalin. UMBER proceeded thus: he slowly reduced the insulin requirements by administering 2.5 mg synthalin on every second day (maximally about 4 U/day), in this way up to 50 U insulin could be saved. The insulin reducing effect was measured by the blood sugar lowering and the degree of glucosuria. Complications that led to metabolic decompensation (e.g. infection) could not be counteracted by increasing the synthalin, but only by raising the insulin dose (UMBER).

While the value of this partial insulin substitution through synthalin, only on the grounds of reducing insulin, was questioned, combination in some cases was expedient as achieving more success than by one of the drugs alone. This was

especially found in the case of juvenile diabetics who oscillate between acidosis
and hypoglycaemia. In these cases, today termed as brittle diabetics, a certain
stabilisation of the metabolic state was achieved. UMBER saw, e.g. in a three year
old child with brittle diabetes requiring insulin an improvement in the metabolic
state, that is aglucosuria and cessation of hypoglycaemia by additional synthalin
dose of 5 mg every second day.

A combination of synthalin with insulin has proved to be effective in all cases
with primary or secondary *insulin resistance* (FRANK, NOTHMANN and WAGNER
1926; UMBER; NISSEL and WIESEN).

Summarising we find that the success of the synthalin therapy depends on the
presence of exogenous or endogenous insulin. Insulin is necessary because synthalin
only acts on the diabetic symptoms (glucosuria, hyperglycaemia), while the basic
metabolic disturbances (not omitting the disturbed fat metabolism) are not
affected. Possibly the ability of synthalin to inhibit cell respiration found in the
animal experiment causes an increase in the already present acidosis tendency
in the diabetic. BERTRAM (1928a and b) believes this to be so on the grounds of
clinical investigation.

d) Toxic effects of synthalin in man

1. Acute toxic symptoms

α) Symptomatology. Hypoglycaemia after synthalin therapy alone was not seen.

From the beginning, synthalin treatment was affected by unpleasant side-
effects (FRANK, NOTHMANN and WAGNER 1926b). They were usually comprised
of gastric symptoms: nausea, vomiting, metallic taste, pressure in the epigastrium
and diarrhoea. To this appeared such general symptoms as loss of appetite, discomfort and adynamia and mental depressions and diphoria (UMBER) recently
characterised by WILLIAMS (for DBI) as "lack of pep".

FRANK, NOTHMANN and WAGNER (1926a), in their first publications on these
symptoms, indicated their similarity with those found in cats after guanidine
poisoning (FRANK, STERN and NOTHMANN), and assumed there to be a central
rather than a local cause. This was also indicated by the appearance of symptoms
in cats given guanidine parenterally. Similar to this is also the appearance of side-
effects not effecting the gastro-intestinal tract directly, as e.g. sweating, headaches
and functional heart complaints (UMBER). The observation that synthalin treated
patients could not tolerate fatty foods led ADLER to suspect that the side-effects
were symptoms of a toxic liver effect. KAUFMANN also SZCEKLIK made the same
suggestion. This assumption seemed to be supported by the liver damage following
chronic synthalin treatment, as will be discussed later (s. p. 127). The recent
experiences with the biguanides indicate, however, that the side-effects are of
central nervous origin. The side-effects observed in the biguanide therapy are the
same as those appearing after synthalin, but previous investigations do not
include proof of liver damage (s. p. 140).

The *frequency* of the side-effects varies according to each research worker, not
only because the indication for synthalin treatment varied. Thus PRIESEL and
WAGNER saw symptoms of intolerance in all their cases (children). MORAWITZ also
JANSEN and BAUR observed toxic side-effects in most patients. JACOBI and BRÜLL
saw such symptoms only in about 1/3 of the patients. UMBER, who has the greatest
experience in synthalin treatment (more than 200 cases), described intolerance
in 49% of all treated patients. Sickness, vomiting and loss of appetite were the
most frequent symptoms. The patients then often eat even less than usual. Thus
the juvenile ketosis tendency is fostered. Synthalin B showed no clinical difference
from synthalin A (FRANK, NOTHMANN and WAGNER 1928).

β) **Measures for preventing symptoms of intolerance.** The most successful measure is without doubt the immediate discontinuation of synthalin treatment already indicated by FRANK, NOTHMANN and WAGNER (1926b). This usually causes all symptoms to subside within 48 hrs.

The appearance of symptoms showing intolerance can often be avoided by slowly increasing the dose and retaining relatively low permanent therapeutic doses. Considering the good effect calcium application had in cats poisoned by guanidine derivatives, UMBER tried to counteract the toxic side-effects of synthalin by administering calcium salts. Success varied and no certain conclusion could be reached. STRAUSS reported of increased synthalin tolerance following administration of calcium carbonate in a diabetic with tuberculosis.

ADLER, believing the side-effects to be signs of liver intoxication, administered 0.5 g decholine to patients with each synthalin dose. Not only were the side-effects removed by this, but also the synthalin dose could be increased. Other cholates were also recommended (degalol, cholactol) (ADLER; MORAWITZ). But only those authors who introduced the cholates found them to be of value. Others (UMBER) had no success.

2. Toxic symptoms during long-term synthalin treatment

Today extensive clinical investigations on the possible toxicity of a new substance is a matter of routine (red and white blood pictures, liver or kidney function tests or biopsies). In the synthalin era, this was not the case. As a result only clear clinical symptoms indicated possible organ damage caused by synthalin.

α) **Liver damage.** ADLER concluded from the fact that diabetics often showed intolerance to fat after synthalin treatment, also confirmed by others (STAUB and JEZLER), a disturbance in the liver function. His conclusion was supported by the frequent appearance of urobilinogenuria following synthalin treatment. Even if other authors did not find this (HIRSCH-KAUFFMANN; STAHL and BAHN; UMBER; FRANK 1928) the appearance of jaundice in diabetics receiving synthalin seemed to confirm ADLER's view. ADLER reported on an observation of a colleague (case HOLZWEISSIG) who saw a severe case of jaundice preceeded by days of gastric disturbances in a patient who prior to synthalin treatment had normal liver function. MORAWITZ described the appearance of painful liver swelling with subsequent jaundice in a patient treated for 3 months according to FRANK's scheme (3 days of treatment, one of abstinence) with 45 mg. synthalin daily. This patient was, however, a potator; therefore, previous liver damage could not be excluded. FRANK himself reported of 2 cases with jaundice. In both, relatively high synthalin doses were continued despite increasing gastric complaints lasting for days and weeks. Both patients recovered after some time when the drug was discontinued. One of BERTRAM's (1928a) female patients died during synthalin treatment of acute liver dystrophy. She had continued taking synthalin for 2 weeks after the appearance of jaundice and was only delivered to the clinic in the state of hepatic coma. SZCEKLIK reported of a case of jaundice in a female patient receiving synthalin. In this case, however, previous liver damage was probable. JACOBI and BRÜLL published a case with no liver history where mild jaundice appeared on synthalin application. BERTRAM (1928a) mentions further cases published only in the form of discussion remarks on the appearance of liver function disturbances and jaundice. Liver complaints following synthalin treatment, without the appearance of jaundice, have also been observed (BERTRAM 1928a). Contrary to the above mentioned findings, DAVID saw no delay in the recovery of a juvenile diabetic in whom synthalin treatment was commenced during hepatitis.

The findings of a liver toxic synthalin effect in man seem to be strongly supported by the animal experiments discussed above where histological liver damage after synthalin A and B could be proved (comp. p. 104 f.). As the dose applied in animal experiments greatly exceeds that used clinically, the above argument is not really valid. Furthermore, it must be realised that the number of synthalin treated patients complaining of ensuing liver damage is relatively small when compared to the total number of diabetics receiving synthalin (at least several thousand). Perhaps some patients only suffered from virus hepatitis as diabetics are more susceptible to hepatitis than non-diabetics (comp. the review of CREUTZFELDT 1959 d).

β) **Kidney damage.** In the animal experiments, synthalin in doses high enough to cause liver damage also led to kidney changes (tubular necrosis, comp. p. 105). Clinical investigations on this point are sparse. In BERTRAM's (1928 a) case, who died in an hepatic coma following synthalin treatment, histological investigations showed necrosis of the renal tubules. However, tubular necrosis often accompanies hepatic coma, and in the above mentioned case are probably not caused by a direct synthalin effect on the kidney. FRANK, NOTHMANN and WAGNER (1926 b) and also STRAUSS reported of single cases in which oliguria was seen following synthalin. In a case described by STRAUSS, definite oedema of the eyelid and ankle was seen accompanying this.

The cases of jaundice, and the frequent symptoms of intolerance added to the restricted application range, have shown the inadviseability of using synthalin in diabetic treatment. Some clinicians refused to use it at all. The production and sale, however, continued until 1945 in Germany and was only stopped for external reasons.

II. Galegine

Galegine was not further used clinically, although REINWEIN (1927) reported of general better tolerance of this substance than of synthalin after a galegine trial in 35 diabetics. Admittedly in single cases there was greater intolerance. Using galegine, it was possible to eliminate sugar excretion of 25 g respectively replacing up to 30 U of insulin (REINWEIN). There are no publications on the chronic toxicity of galegine in animals and man.

III. Biguanides

When the synthalin therapy was relinquished, much of the clinical experience was forgotten. As a result, findings gained from the biguanides were unimpaired by previous experience with synthalin. We will, however, see that as in the animal experiments mentioned above on the mechanism of action, the clinical results also show no great difference between synthalin and the biguanides.

a) The effectiveness of the biguanides
on the blood sugar in the healthy human subject

There are few investigations of this subject. From them can be assumed that the blood sugar in man is not affected by biguanides in tolerable doses. FAJANS, MOORHOUSE, DOORENBOS, LAWRENCE and CONN (1960) saw no blood sugar decrease within 8 hrs after DBI (100—400 mg) administration, even after several weeks of a diet poor in calories. Similar experiences were made by WILLIAMS. W 37 also did not affect the blood sugar in healthy controls (SÖLING, WERCHAU and CREUTZFELDT). The same observations were also made by OTTO (1960). MICHEL saw even a slight blood sugar rise in healthy subjects receiving 200 mg DBI. He could see in several cases of diabetes, after loading with DBI (200 mg.), an initial blood sugar elevation (to 40% over the initial value). Loading with 400 mg. N_1,n-butyl-biguanide caused an impressive initial blood sugar increase in diabetics and also in healthy subjects. This increase lasted for about 2 hrs and was clearer than after 400 mg. of DBI. The blood sugar rise after glucose loading or injection of glucagon was not changed through DBI in healthy controls (FAJANS, MOORHOUSE et al. 1960).

b) Results of the biguanide therapy in diabetes mellitus

The early clinical experiences with synthalin were hardly ever compared to those of the biguanides, while the different properties of the sulphonylureas and biguanides have been extensively discussed. In contrast to the sulphonylureas, biguanides are said to be effective in all types of diabetes (POMERANZE, FUJIY and MOURATOFF). However, after some experience, it was seen that the above assumption was not totally correct. Should treatment be successful using the biguanides alone, the same criteria must be fulfilled as for treatment with sulphonylureas.

1. Investigations on the controllability of diabetes with biguanides alone

Body weight. Over-weight obese patients show a definitely better response to biguanide therapy than those of normal or under-weight (SKILLMAN, KRUGER and HAMWI 1959, LISBOA et al. [21 patients]; McKENDRY et al.; SCHILLING; AZERAD and LUBETZKI).

Insulin doses. The success of the biguanide therapy is inversly proportional to the insulin requirement. The average upper dose is 20—30 U. The above was observed by all clinicians who investigated the problem [KRALL and BRADLEY (173 patients); ODELL et al. (61 patients); SKILLMAN, KRUGER and HAMWI (29 patients); McKENDRY, KUWAYTI and RADO (58 patients); SCHILLING (80 patients); AZERAD and LUBETZKI (118 patients)].

Length of diabetes. According to KRALL and BRADLEY, the chance of successful DBI treatment is the greater, the shorter the existence of diabetes is. This was confirmed for DBI by SKILLMAN, KRUGER and HAMWI (1959), and for N_1,N_1-dimethyl-biguanide by AZERAD and LUBETZKI. SCHILLING (1959a) does not believe the duration of diabetes to be important, but indicates also that patients whose diabetes is of shorter duration respond better.

In contrast to these findings, ODELL et al., also TRANQUADA, KLEEMAN and BROWN (1959a) saw no connection between success of treatment and the length of diabetes.

Age of manifestation of diabetes. The effectiveness of the biguanide therapy increases with rising manifestation age. This connection was first seen by KRALL and BRADLEY from experience gained (173 patients) and has since been confirmed many times (LISBOA et al.; McKENDRY, KUWAYTI and RADO; SCHILLING; WALKER).

This makes it probable that the biguanides, also in man, cause an initial stimulation of the adrenergic system even if this cannot always be seen. POMERANZE and GADEK refuse the existence of such connection. However, if one measures their findings by the same criteria used by KRALL and BRADLEY also SCHILLING, there is here also a certain dependence on the age of manifestation. POMERANZE and GADEK could change over 39 from 81 patients to DBI alone whose diabetes had started after the age of 30, and in 6 cases he could decrease the insulin dose to 50% or more. From 17 unstable juvenile diabetics, not one could be changed over to DBI alone, while in 10 cases insulin could be reduced by 50% or more. Also AZERAD and LUBETZKI found no connection, in 118 diabetics treated with N_1,N_1-dimethylbiguanide, to age. ODELL et al. also SKILLMAN, KRUGER and HAMWI found the same for DBI. Unfortunately all these authors only considered the actual age which was comprised of both the length of diabetes and also the age of manifestation.

Despite these contradictory results, one can see a certain parallelism in the controllability with biguanides and the results of sulphonylurea therapy (comp. p. 53 f) in which the conditions were much clearer. The most important criteria for controllability seemed to be similar as those for sulphonylureas: insulin requirement and age of manifestation. This is impressively seen on comparing SCHILLING's published diagrams (diagram 2) with a corresponding diagram for the sulphonylureas by MOHNIKE, ULRICH and JUTZI (comp. diagram 1, p. 55).

2. Effectiveness in different forms of diabetes

The effectiveness is judged very differently. While POMERANZE (POMERANZE, FUJIY and MOURATOFF; POMERANZE; POMERANZE and GADEK) counts every blood sugar decrease after DBI and also any reduction in insulin, as a therapeutic success, SCHILLING only considers treatment a success if the patient can be completely changed over to biguanides. One should, however, consider both; whereby insulin reduction through biguanides should only be valued as a therapeutic success if the insulin requirement was abnormally high previously, or if the metabolic state was simultaneously improved (s. below).

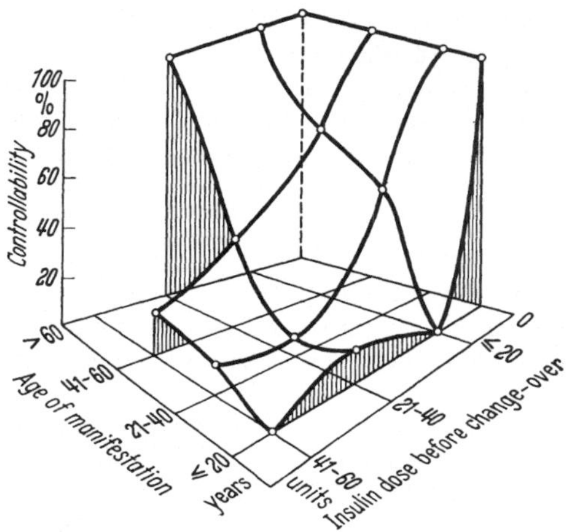

Fig. 2. Controllability of diabetics with DBI (in %) in relation to the age of manifestation of the diabetes (in years) and to the insulin requirement (in units). After SCHILLING (1959a)

α) **Stable diabetes in the adult.** The stable maturity-onset diabetic without ketosis tendency often responds well to biguanide therapy alone. These are patients who could previously be controlled by diet or small doses of insulin (KRALL and BRADLEY; LISBOA et al.; SCHILLING; POMERANZE and GADEK; DEUIL; STERNE). The biguanide doses necessary are mostly less (50—150 mg. DBI/day) than for other forms of diabetes (WALKER). As a result, symptoms of intolerance appear less frequently improving the chances of a long-term treatment. In stable maturity-onset diabetics not satisfactorily controlled by biguanides alone, a small addition of insulin is often enough to control metabolism (WALKER; KRALL and BRADLEY). Only exceptionally can over 40 U of insulin be replaced by biguanides in maturity-onset diabetes (SCHILLING). SKILLMAN, KRUGER and HAMWI (1959) never achieved success if the insulin requirement prior to DBI treatment exceeded 26 U. In patients who could be completely changed over to biguanide therapy, there was never a hypoglycaemic reaction (ODELL et al.; WALKER; TRANQUADA, KLEEMAN and BROWN 1959a) SCHILLING's case (1959a) exhibiting clinical shock after treatment with 150 mg. DBI alone, is not convincing, as hypoglycaemic blood values were not present.

As a whole, the therapeutic success in this group corresponds to that seen after the sulphonylureas, as is repeatedly indicated (KRALL and BRADLEY; WALKER;

SCHILLING; DOBSON; DEUIL). Biguanides are often effective in primary or secondary sulphonylurea failures. SCHILLING saw among 10 tolbutamide failures, 4 times a good, 4 times a moderate and twice no success with DBI; while 6 patients who responded well to tolbutamide could all be successfully treated with DBI. OTTO (1958) reached corresponding conclusions. McKENDRY et al. (1959) were, however, only able to change-over 3 to DBI from 7 patients controlled succesfully with tolbutamide; conversly of all primary tolbutamide failures 4, of 4 secondary tolbutamide failures 1 responded well to DBI. The authors conclude from these observations that there is a different mechanism of action and a different indication for both substances. KRALL was able to control 34 of 39 diabetics, not or no longer, responding to sulphonylureas with DBI respectively DBB alone (see also KRALL and BRADLEY). Also DE LAWTER et al. were able to control 55% of their secondary failures of response to D 860 with DBI.

β) **Mild juvenile diabetes.** The success of a biguanide therapy in this already very small group is not as great as in the stable diabetes of the adult. However, it is sometimes also possible here to change patients over to biguanides (POMERANZE; POMERANZE and GADEK; KRALL and BRADLEY; SCHILLING; WALKER). These are usually patients who have been controlled by diet or with small amounts of insulin, and who theoretically could have been treated with sulphonylureas. KRALL and BRADLEY found that diabetics in this group relatively often showed spontaneous remission of their diabetes and cannot be counted as therapeutic successes (comp. also KRALL, WHITE and BRADLEY). WHITE and KRALL saw, e.g. of 38 DBI treated children, 20 (equals 55%) in the remission phase of their diabetes. Only these children could be controlled with DBI alone. The other 18 children were unstable diabetics requiring insulin.

γ) **Insulin deficiency diabetes of the juvenile and adult.** In cases of insulin deficiency diabetes, a change-over to biguanides alone is not possible. However, in many cases, insulin can be reduced if insulin and biguanides are given together. Especially in the moderately severe forms, the insulin amount can often be reduced by more than 50% (POMERANZE and GADEK; KRALL and BRADLEY; MEHNERT and SEITZ 1958a; OTTC; SEYDL and SCHULLERI; SCHILLING; AZERAD and LUBETZKI). When judging the mechanism of action of the biguanides on the diabetic metabolism, the fact that reduction of the insulin dose has limits, is decisive. If this is exceeded, then metabolic decompensation occurs with ketoacidosis also in the not very severe diabetes (KRALL and BRADLEY; SCHILLING; WALKER; SKILLMAN et al.). KRALL and BRADLEY and also SCHILLING reported of cases where the previously high insulin doses could be extensively reduced under DBI, but that a residual insulin amount of 10 U or less was necessary. The questionable value of insulin reduction, especially if it concerns only a few units, will be discussed later. Only TRANQUADA, KLEEMAN and BROWN (1959a) report of successful change-over of insulin deficiency diabetics to DBI alone. These results are contradictory to the experience of most other authors. Diabetics who displayed ketosis on commencing the biguanide therapy, or who have coma history, are practically resistant to biguanide therapy alone, whether juvenile or maturity-onset diabetics (SKILLMAN et al.). If insulin is reduced in these cases by simultaneously administering biguanides, ketosis can appear or be increased if a certain limit is exceeded, even if control, measured by blood sugar and glucosuria, appears to be good (KRALL and BRADLEY; KLEEFIELD; SKILLMAN, KRUGER and HAMWI 1959, 1960; WALKER; OTTO 1958; SCHILLING). The biguanide therapy of the diabetic with ketoacidosis tendency, with the exception of the unstable cases (s. below), is today therefore inadviseable (OTTO; SKILLMAN, KRUGER and HAMWI;

9*

SCHILLING) or is only to be used with restraint (WALKER and LINTON; KRALL, WHITE and BRADLEY).

In the typical brittle diabetes, biguanides often lead to a decrease of the metabolic oscillations. The hypoglycaemia, characteristic for this type of diabetes, appears less frequently. The biguanides have this "smoothing effect" on the diabetic metabolism, even if little or no insulin can be reduced. The biguanide dose necessary for stabilising unstable diabetics is often lower than that required for a blood sugar decrease in the same patient. Improved controllability of unstable diabetes is described by many authors (KRALL and CAMERINI-DAVALOS; WILLIAMS, TANNER and ODELL; KRALL and BRADLEY; MEHNERT and SEITZ; OTTO 1958; WALKER; McKENDRY et al.; KLEEFIELD; PEARLMAN; PERKIN; KRALL, WHITE and BRADLEY; WHITE and KRALL; SCHILLING; STERNE; DEUIL). The value of treating unstable diabetics with biguanides does not lie in the saving of insulin, but in reducing metabolic oscillations. As most unstable diabetics tends towards ketoacidotic decompensation, reduction in the insulin dose is not adviseable (OTTO 1958; SCHILLING). The astonishing insulin reduction in severe diabetes, partly even in the ketotic state (POMERANZE; KRALL and BRADLEY; SCHILLING; TRANQUADA, KLEEMAN and BROWN 1959a), are exceptions that cannot be generalised. WALKER and LINTONS' experience show that too great a reduction in the insulin treatment, even if metabolism appears to be controlled, can lead to severe ketosis or even acidosis within a very short time (s. p. 134).

δ) Rare, special forms of diabetes. *Diabetes following pancreatectomy.* CREUTZFELDT, KÜMMERLE and KERN saw in a pancreatectomised diabetic sub-optimally controlled by insulin, recession of glucosuria and acetonuria after 200—250 mg. DBI without certain effect on the blood sugar. During the insulin witheld experiment in another pancreatectomised diabetic, the blood sugar course under DBI (100—250 mg.) differed only slightly compared to that without DBI. However, glucosuria was reduced under DBI, and the appearance of acetonuria delayed and the rapid decrease in the alkali reserve was absent. However, the DBI effect on the metabolism was in no way comparable to that of insulin. BERGEN and NORTON had to discontinue DBI treatment in a pancreatectomised diabetic owing to symptoms of intolerance despite that at first, part of the insulin could be replaced by DBI without increased glucosuria. SKILLMAN, KRUGER and HAMWI (1959) could not reduce the insulin dose despite daily treatment with 225 mg. DBI over 1 week. 3 of TRANQUADA, KLEEMAN and BROWN'S (1960) eight diabetics were pancreatectomised. For various reasons, 3 of the 8 patients were not included in the final examination; it is not clear whether pancreatectomised patients were among the three. The mean value of the arterial glucose concentration of the 5 investigated patients shows a maximal reduction of 20% after 4 hrs. There are no reports on the individual blood sugar course; thus, nothing certain can be deduced from this concerning a possible blood sugar elevation in the pancreatectomised diabetic.

From the limited investigations on pancreatectomised patients the following conclusion is reached to date: DBI has no similar metabolic effect to insulin; the metabolic disturbance resulting from the insulin deficiency is only, if at all, delayed through DBI and not avoided.

Bronze diabetes. In 2 cases of bronze diabetes, BERINGER (1960) could achieve a definite insulin reduction. In one case, the insulin dose could be reduced from 90 U to 40 U. McKENDRY et al. (1959) treated a case of tolbutamide resistant bronze diabetes with DBI. The outcome of treatment was not published. STERNE, who doubted the therapeutic success of treating bronze diabetes with biguanides, reported of successful treatment with N_1,N_1-dimethyl-biguanide in 2 cases of insulin resistant bronze diabetes.

Diabetes with acromegalia. In the case of a 38 year old insulin resistant diabetic suffering from acromegalia for 10 years, the biguanides were very effective. The patient who required 600 U insulin per day could, after transient treatment with insulin and N_1-isoamyl-biguanide (IABG) (4×200 mg/day), respectively N_1,n-amyl-biguanide (ABG) (4×125 mg/day), be controlled by DBI (4×100 mg/day alone). Glucosuria vanished having been 300 gm/day. BERINGER (1960) also described a beneficial effect of DBI in 2 patients with acromegalia. Here an increase in the glycogen content of the liver was found.

In an own case of a 53 year old female patient with acromegalia for 6 years and with diabetic symptoms of 3 months standing, we also saw a clear biguanide effect.

Glucosuria, apparent at the beginning of 120—150 g/day with slight acetonuria, did not respond at first to a single dose of W 37. After metabolism was recompensated through insulin (48 U), a satisfactory control was reached with 250 mg W 37 without additional insulin. An ACTH test performed in this phase (40 mg long-acting ACTH) immediately caused acute metabolic decompensation with glucose excretion of 115 grams. Therefore, further treatment was carried out with 48 U of insulin.

Condition following hypophysectomy in the juvenile diabetic. SKILLMAN, KRUGER and HAMWI (1959, 1960) tried to change-over a diabetic, hypophysectomised because of severe progressive retinitis proliferans, to DBI. Despite the fact that the insulin requirement had dropped from 80 to 14 U through hypophysectomy, not even four units could be spared through DBI. In a case described by BERINGER (1960) of a hypophysectomised diabetic with a Kimmelstiel-Wilson syndrome, the necessary insulin dose could be reduced from 24 to 8 U by application of W 37. The biguanide therapy was discontinued owing to symptoms of intolerance.

Nothing has been published on the therapeutical results with *Cushing's disease* and with *hyperthyroidism.* STERNE saw a good effect in *steroid diabetes* with N_1,N_1-dimethylbiguanide. In two own cases of prednisone induced steroid diabetes we saw a good effect with W 37 (200 mg/day), while in a third case the biguanide therapy was interrupted because of side-effects.

3. *Metabolic observations in diabetics treated with biguanides*

α) Daily blood sugar profile, glucose tolerance, insulin and glucagon loading. *Daily blood sugar profile.* SCHILLING investigated the effect DBI had on the daily blood sugar profile (9 blood sugar values in 24 hrs): the blood sugar curve of 10 patients requiring insulin, being controlled by diet alone at the time of examination, was smoothed by DBI. The blood sugar curve of patients who were changed over from tolbutamide to DBI corresponded with all characteristic daily oscillations to that during tolbutamide therapy; the blood sugar values were only lower. In insulin treated patients, who could successfully be changed to DBI, the course of the daily blood sugar profile was smoothed. Especially those oscillations caused by food were reduced. In a group of 9 diabetics, receiving in addition DBI, the insulin dose could be reduced (measured by the urine sugar excretion) by more than 50%. However, the blood sugar profile showed a definite rise in the blood sugar during the night, not present with insulin alone, and indicating the short half-life time of DBI in man.

Glucose tolerance test. FAJANS, MOORHOUSE et al. (1960) did not find any change in the height or the duration of hyperglycaemia after glucose loading in 5 patients after successful DBI treatment. SCHILLING (1959 b) also CRAIG, MILLER and WOODWARD published a similar finding. POMERANZE, FUJIY and MOURATOFF saw in a case of mild diabetes treated with DBI a greatly changed blood sugar curve with smaller peaks and a more rapid decline. In a case of severe diabetes, published by the same authors, no noteworthy change with or without DBI is seen. GUTSCHE also saw no significant influence on the glucose tolerance in 24 diabetics and in healthy subjects. This is also true for 2 diabetics satisfactorily controlled with W 37.

Insulin tolerance test. The i.v. insulin loading (0.05 U/kg) in 2 diabetics, with and without DBI, produced an identical blood sugar course (FAJANS, MOORHOUSE et al. 1960). SCHILLING comparatively investigated in 12 patients the effect of an i.v. insulin loading (8 U) under insulin, tolbutamide, diet and DBI treatment. The maximal blood sugar decrease was the same in time and extent under the different conditions.

According to these findings, the sensitivity to exogenous insulin was not increased through DBI. However, clinical observations indicate that increased insulin sensitivity under DBI does occur in single cases (KRALL and BRADLEY).

Glucagon test. FAJANS, MOORHOUSE et al. (1960) saw following i.v. injection of 1 mg glucagon before and after DBI treatment in 2 cases with stable diabetes, in 1 patient no changes, and in the other a slight increase of the hyperglycaemic reaction through DBI.

β) **Biguanide therapy and ketosis.** The biguanides have a very limited effect on the ketotic metabolic disturbance in the diabetic. This was already mentioned in the discussion of the biguanide effect on the labile diabetic (s. p. 131).

Even if the cause of diabetic ketosis is not clear in every detail, it can be considered as a fact that one cause of this metabolic decompensation is an accumulation of active acetic acid (acetyl-S-CoA) with consecutive increase in acetoacetic acid condensation. Despite the fact that not all the metabolic processes leading to this block are known, the following can be said: besides inhibition of fatty acid synthesis, a deficiency of reduced nucleotides (DPNH, but especially TPNH) resulting from a decreased glucose oxidation is one of the main causes (comp. the review of WIELAND, also SIPERSTEIN). If the biguanides have an anti-ketogenic effect, then increased glucose oxidation should occur. No such effect of the biguanides has been proved in diabeties, while in nondiabetic animals an increase in the rate of aerobic glycolysis could be demonstrated (SÖLING and CREUTZFELDT). But an increase in the direct glucose oxidation via the hexose-monophosphate-shunt which is necessary for an antiketogenic effect has never been proved. In alloxandiabetic rabbits the blood sugar decrease after DBI was accompanied by an increased ketonaemia (comp. p. 120).

Diabetics whose insulin has been successfully replaced by biguanides frequently display, after some time, increasing insulin requirements (WALKER) or metabolic decompensation (SKILLMAN, KRUGER and HAMWI; WALKER and LINTON 1959b). SKILLMAN et al. even described the appearance of ketosis under combined insulin and biguanide therapy in 2 juvenile diabetics previously not showing ketosis. Also in 2 patients of WALKER and LINTON (1959b), suddenly severe ketoacidosis occurred with a strong decrease in the alkali reserve, while the blood sugar was not elevated. One of these patients could not be saved. Meanwhile many authors described the appearance of ketosis under biguanide therapy with normoglycaemic and no, or slight, glucosuria (POMERANZE and GADEK; HALL et al.; WALKER and LINTON 1959a and b; WALKER; BERGEN and NORTON; McGAVAK). WALKER and LINTON (1959b) saw ketonuria even appear in 1/3 rd., and the occurrence of acidosis in 10% of their diabetics receiving DBI.

These observations correspond to the findings in alloxan diabetes (comp. p. 120). The biguanides lack an effect promoting direct glucose utilization.

In addition there is a certain loss of carbohydrates owing to the excretion of intermediate products of carbohydrate metabolism in the urine (CRAIG, MILLER and WOODWARD; SÖLING, WERCHAU and CREUTZFELDT; WALKER and LINTON 1959b). The elevation of blood organic acids promotes the diabetic acidosis tendency. Thus, the decrease in the alkali reserve following exercise is greatly increased under DBI (WALKER and LINTON 1959b). The appearance of ketosis, with or without acidosis, in the normoglycaemic only seems to differ from the real insulin deficiency ketosis that is usually accompanied by hyperglycaemia. In both cases, ketosis is the expression of an intra-cellular carbohydrate deficiency. In the case of hyperglycaemia, the reduced glucose utilization is a major issue; in the case of normoglycaemia, under biguanides, there is an additional substrate deficiency (e.g. deficiency of oxidisable glucose). Responsible for this, besides a relative deficiency in carbohydrates in the diabetic diet, is *reduced food intake* due to loss of appetite, i.e. hunger ketosis (POMERANZE and GADEK; WALKER). This should not hide the fact that the main cause for that is the summation of insulin deficiency and an acidosis promoting effect of the biguanides themselves.

The presence of exogenous and endogenous insulin is the fundamental condition for every biguanide therapy (KRALL and BRADLEY). Therefore reduction of the insulin dose, or even extensive replacement by the biguanides, is a therapeutic risk. This is so because the diabetic controlled thus practically lives with an insulin minimum. The risk is even greater as exclusive investigations of the blood sugar and glucosuria used as criteria for the whole metabolic state are relatively useless in this case.

Therapy of biguanide ketosis. Carbohydrate depletion is the basis of this metabolic disturbance. Therefore, the most important measure, besides a sudden complete discontinuation of the biguanide therapy, is an increased administration of carbohydrates. Insulin should only be applied with the greatest care, if at all (POMERANZE and GADEK), as the biguanide ketosis is usually accompanied by normoglycaemia or only mild hyperglycaemia. The case of ketoacidosis after DBI, described by WALKER and LINTON, ended fatally despite the following therapy: carbohydrate administration, reduction of the DBI dose and additional insulin. Possibly the insulin addition was too high and the reduction of the DBI dose too slight. Therefore POMERANZE and GADEK advise a large carbohydrate intake during DBI therapy. 1800 calories are the minimum caloric requirement.

4. Indication and contra-indication, treatment

α) **Indication and contra-indication.** The indication range of the biguanide therapy was discussed with the controllability of different diabetics. As compared with the sulphonylureas, clinical experience with the biguanides is limited and no final judgement can be given.

Biguanides seem to be *indicated* in cases of primary or secondary sulphonylurea failures in maturity-onset diabetes. It is sometimes possible to control diabetes in these cases without additional insulin dose. Further indication for a biguanide trial is given by the labile insulin deficiency diabetic. In such cases, metabolic stabilisation can be achieved by the additional administration of biguanides. Biguanide therapy can also be tried in the cases having abnormally high insulin requirements, and if other measures (insulin change and desensibilisation, sulphonylurea therapy) were unsuccessful. In some cases of maturity-onset diabetes not controllable with sulphonylureas, or technically difficult to treat with insulin, one must often be satisfied with a sub-optimal control by biguanides alone.

We believe the biguanides *not to be indicated* in patients who are well controlled by sulphonylureas. Also no indication is given in the cases of diabetics of the insulin deficiency type. Finally, when ketoacidosis tendency is present, a biguanide trial is not advisable.

Sufficient experience has not been gained on the question whether control is adequate in the case of operations or infections with biguanides alone, or whether change-over to insulin is indicated. With such complications, the danger of ketosis is increased; the greatest care is necessary in any case. KLEEFELD reported of his experience with 11 *tubercular* diabetics receiving DBI. No difference was found compared to the treatment of non-tubercular diabetics.

It is also not known if diseases of the *circulatory system*, especially arteriosclerotic changes, are contra-indications (comp. p. 138). As, however, the dangers of hypoglycaemic reactions are not very great, the biguanide therapy may be better in the case of arteriosclerotic changes than insulin. No experience has been made with the effectiveness of biguanides in the diabetic vascular, respectively, organ changes *(retinopathia diabetica, Kimmelstiel-Wilson syndrome)*. The same is true for diabetic neuritis. One should refrain from using biguanides in the case of nephropathies on grounds of the toxic nephrosis found in guinea-pigs (CREUTZFELDT and MOENCH), also rabbits (LAZARUS, BRADSHAW and VOLK 1960) receiving DBI. Also if acute or chronic liver disease is apparent, biguanides should be applied with discretion. SCHILLING also KRALL and BRADLEY report of treating some patients with liver diseases (mostly cirrhosis of the liver). No signs of deterioration in the liver function were apparent. If biguanide therapy is attempted in diabetics with liver disease, the liver function should be controlled with the greatest care.

We think that *pregnancy* is an absolute contra-indication for the biguanide therapy owing to its metabolic effects. There are no publications on pregnant diabetics treated with biguanides.

β) Combined treatment with insulin and sulphonylureas.

Biguanides and insulin. This combination has already been discussed in relation to the different forms of diabetes. Combination is not justifiable owing to the unclear mechanism of action only on the grounds of reducing insulin, when the requirement is not abnormally high.

The brittle diabetes, difficult to control, indicates, as seen from clinical experience, a biguanide trial. Here combination therapy can often smooth the strong oscillations of the blood sugar, However, combined insulin—biguanide therapy can cause hypoglycaemia (ODELL et al.; TRANQUADA, KLEEMAN and BROWN 1959a; SCHILLING 1959a). KRALL and BRADLEY advised care when insulin is added during biguanide therapy, as a strong blood sugar decrease can occur within a few hours.

Biguanides and sulphonylureas. Such a combination was first tried by BERINGER (1958) in 2 cases of secondary failures to sulphonylurea therapy. It was proved advantageous in as far as the necessary biguanide dose could be kept low enough to prevent symptoms of intolerance. Withheld experiments of each of both components, indicated an additive action. MEHNERT and SEITZ (1958b) also used a combination of DBI, respectively W 37 and D 860 in primary sulphonylurea resistant diabetics (13 patients). First they tried to control with D 860 alone. If this was insufficient, biguanides were given in addition. Using this combination, satisfactory control was reached with biguanides in doses not causing symptoms of intolerance. These positive results have been confirmed in a larger number of patients (BEASER 1960, DOLGER 1959, 1960, UNGER, MADISON and CARTER 1959, GRANVILLE-GROSSMAN et al.; MEHNERT and KRALL 1960, F. STEIGERWALD 1960).

In 25 patients showing primary sulphonylurea resistance and 75 secondary failures, DOLGER could achieve satisfactory control with 50 mg DBI/day if in addition, the maximum effective sulphonylurea dose was administered. Combined DBI-chlorpropamide treatmnet was also effective in some cases (KRALL). Also combined N_1,N_1-dimethylbiguanide-sulphonylurea therapy was successful (AZERAD and LUBETZKI). Good results even in cases of severe ketoacidosis are reported by BOULET, MIROUZE and SCHMOUKER with a combined N_1,N_1-dimethylbiguanide-chlorpropamide therapy.

γ) **Therapeutical measures in control and dosage.** As the individual intolerance dose oscillates strongly, the highest still tolerable dose cannot be predicted. At the beginning of the biguanide era, a relatively high dose was used (150—200—300 mg DBI); this was not beneficial. It is better to start with small amounts (e.g. 50 mg DBI) and to increase the dose slowly until the therapeutic aim is reached or side-effects appear (POMERANZE and GADEK; McKENDRY et al. 1959). POMERANZE and GADEK advise in building up the guanidine therapy a 4—7 day pause between the single stages. However, through this, the control of the diabetic with biguanides is a very lengthy process; the chances of success cannot be foreseen. Reducing the insulin dose must be done with as great care as the increasing of the biguanide dose. In brittle diabetes, the insulin dose should remain unchanged at first, and be reduced later. According to POMERANZE and GADEK, it is therefore advisable to leave a pause of several days between each increase in the biguanide dose, as a therapeutic effect sometimes does not appear until several days after commencing treatment. This was confirmed by SKILLMAN, KRUGER and HAMWI who saw the first blood sugar decrease on the second day of treatment, and an optimal effect was never seen before the 3rd. day. In one case, the maximum effect was not seen until the 6th. day. The daily dose should be given in 3—4—5 single doses after meals so that the gastro-intestinal side-effects are kept at a minimum. The change-over to biguanides should only be performed on hospitalised diabetics (KRALL and BRADLEY; SCHILLING), as the effectiveness of a certain biguanide dose can be as little foreseen as the appearance of side-effects. Symptoms of intolerance like nausea and anorexia can lead to uncontrollable changes in the caloric intake. Especially in the juvenile diabetic, there is the additional danger of biguanide ketosis, often not seen by checking urine or blood sugar (comp. p. 134 f.). LISBOA et al., who controlled 21 diabetic out-patients with biguanides, reports of one such case.

Even if the change-over has been done in the hospital, blood and urine sugar and ketone bodies must be regularly controlled after discharge. If the patient has symptoms of intolerance, he should see a doctor (KRALL and BRADLEY). The ambulatory, long-term biguanide treatment requires special cooperation from the diabetic (KRALL and BRADLEY; LISBOA et al.).

N_1-*phenylethyl-biguanide* (DBI, PEDG, W 32). DBI is the most frequently used anti-diabetic biguanide to date, and is already on the market in the USA. The commencing dose is 50 mg/day. In the adult, sometimes 300 mg/day are still well tolerated, but generally the limit is 150 mg. Doses above this lead to signs of intolerance in 50% of the cases.

N_1,n-*amyl-biguanide* (DBB, ABG). ODELL et al. reported of clinical experience in 31 patients. The blood sugar lowering effect is slightly less than with DBI. ODELL's dosage was between 100 and 600 mg/day. Signs of intolerance appear as frequently as with DBI, but are said to be milder and disappear sooner. The limit between effectiveness and intolerance is not significantly displaced when compared with DBI. KRALL and BRADLEY also used DBB, but did not publish any details.

$N_1,isoamyl$-*biguanide* (IABG, DBTU). The effectiveness is definitely less than that of DBI. ODELL et al. have reported of clinical experience using this drug in 24 patients. Doses between 50—900 mg/day were administered. Taking the smaller blood sugar lowering effect into consideration, the frequency of side-effects with DBTU correspond to those with DBI.

N_1,n-*butyl-biguanide* (DBV, W 37, Silubin). Clinical experience with this derivative has been published by MEHNERT and SEITZ (1958b). KRALL also mentions treating some cases with DBV (s. also MEHNERT and KRALL). The blood sugar decreasing effect is only half that of DBI. The administered dose is between 150—400 mg/day. Clinical findings to date indicate better tolerance of DBV in relation to the effective dose. Own experience also speaks for this. It must be considered that trials with DBV were first undertaken when some experience had been gained from DBI application, especially for preventing side-effects and the best therapeutic dosage. This substance is on the German market as Silubin.

$N_1,methylbenzoyl$-*biguanide* (DBC). KRALL and BRADLEY mention the application of this derivative without giving any details. The effectiveness seems to be slightly less than that of DBI.

$N_1,N_1,dimethyl$-*biguanide* (La 6023, glucophage). AZERAD and LUBETZKI reported of clinical experience with 88 patients, GRANVILLE-GROSSMAN et al. in 8, and STERNE in 30 patients (s. also DEUIL). Its effectiveness is only about 10—15% that of DBI. The commencing dose was 2—3 g/day, the maintenance dose, 0.5—3 g/day. The frequency of signs of intolerance on applying a therapeutic dose correspond to those seen after DBI application. Severe side-effects are said to occur less often than after DBI. This substance is on the French market as Glucophage.

5. *Symptoms of intolerance and toxicity of the biguanides in man*

α) Symptoms of intolerance and their treatment. Biguanide therapy in man, similar to synthalin treatment, is handicapped by the frequent appearance of signs of intolerance. Intolerance corresponds to that found with guanidine intoxication (comp. p. 103 and 136). In almost all publications on the clinical use of biguanides, these symptoms of intolerance are cited as "side-effects" and contrasted with the toxic effects—meaning histologically, demonstratable organ damage. This is as impermissible, from a pharmacological viewpoint, as is the bagatellisation of bigeminus in the course of digitalis treatment as a side-effect. The side-effects appearing in the course of biguanide therapy must be regarded as an expression of biguanide intoxication—irrespectively whether organ damage can be proved in addition.

Gastro-intestinal complaints are in the foreground, the most frequent being: loss of appetite, nausea, discomfort and/or pain in the region of the stomach. These complaints are often preceded by a "metallic taste". When the disturbance is severe, vomiting and diarrhoea occur. Besides this, there are other symptoms that influence the general condition; frequently occurring weakness, adynamia and drowsiness, also headaches and vertigo. Some authors (LAMBERT 1958; TRANQUADA KLEEMAN and BROWN 1959a) described the appearance of pectanginose complaints under biguanide treatment. In 3 cases, LAMBERT could find corresponding changes in the ECG. Their connection with biguanide therapy is, however, not certain. SCHILLING did not see poorer tolerance in patients with signs of cardiac decompensation.

It is justified to view the side-effects as an expression of biguanide intoxication because the intolerance in some cases can be so increased that situations threatening life can arise. An example for this is given by a case described by SCHILLING (1959a).

In a 61 year old diabetic (of 12 years' standing) with a very labile metabolism (12—14 U long-acting insulin), it was possible on the 2nd. day of treatment to spare 10 U of insulin by administering 100 mg DBI. On the 4th. day of treatment, loss of appetite occurred, on the 5th. day (200 mg DBI and 10 U insulin), vomiting and progressive apathy. On the 6th. day, the patient was too apathetic to rise; then DBI was discontinued. Despite this, the picture of severe metabolic disturbance appeared: excessive adynamia with elevation of the plasma potassium concentration to 24.8 mg-%, vomiting of gall, rise in non-protein nitrogen to 148 mg-%, increased glucosuria from 18 grams to 81 grams/day, blood acetone rise to 16 mg-%, leucocytosis (16,800/mm³). The condition was improved within 3 days on the discontinuation of DBI, and with corresponding treatment.

Nothing is known about the cause of these symptoms of intolerance. No investigations have been performed using parenterally applied biguanides in diabetics. S. c. synthalin injection, causing similar symptoms (comp. p. 126), were believed to have a central nervous origin. Clinical experience with synthalin and biguanides indicate that the side-effects are related to the metabolic state. Several factors speak for this:

1. The side-effects can progressively change to severe metabolic decompensation (s. the above case of SCHILLING).

2. The biguanide ketosis is usually introduced by the normal symptoms of intolerance (metallic taste, loss of appetite, nausea) (POMERANZE and GADEK).

3. Diabetics poorly responding to the biguanides, thus especially the juvenile diabetics, more frequently show side-effects than patients responding well to biguanides (SKILLMAN, KRUGER and HAMWI 1959). This discrepancy is only partly explained by the higher dose required by poorly responding patients.

4. UNGER (1960) states that after vitamin K (or K_1) dose, the tendency to, vomit instigated by the biguanides in animals, ceases also in those cases where the blood sugar decrease is not affected. As vitamin K is implicated in the electron transportation via the respiration chain, the following can be deduced: the diminished nausea can be correlated to an improvement of the electron flow in the respiration chain instigated by vitamin K.

ODELL et al. noticed the so-called "late" side-effects (loss of weight, weakness, lethargy and hypochondria). These were first apparent during the later course of the biguanide therapy. These late side-effects are not only caused by a chronically reduced caloric intake, they can also appear if the food intake is normal and if there is no glucosuria. ODELL mentions the possibility of a chronic loss of metabolites which are rich in energy, in the urine.

The *frequency* with which side-effects appear is diversely indicated in the single clinical reports—between 30—60% of the treated cases. These discrepancies are not only caused by a difference in the dosage but also by the subsequent treatment (carbohydrate content of the diet, extent of the insulin reduction, type of patient, etc.). Symptoms of intolerance can appear during any therapeutic dose (e.g. with DBI from 50 mg/day). In every case, a further increase in the dose leads to an increase of symptoms.

Discontinuation of the therapy, on grounds of the side-effects, is only necessary in some cases. Very often the complaint can be improved or avoided by suitable measures. KRALL and BRADLEY only had to discontinue therapy because of side-effects in 43 from 173 patients receiving biguanides; the total number of patients with side-effects was much greater. The frequency of side-effects was higher at the beginning of the biguanide era. Meanwhile more careful dosage and therapeutic principles (comp. p. 136) have been made. When the symptoms of intolerance are mild, it is often enough to reduce the dose and thus also the complaint. After a pause of several days, it is sometimes possible, by carefully increasing the dose, to attain the commencing dose without the reappearance of the side-effects (KRALL and BRADLEY; POMERANZE and GADEK). If these measures are not successful, or if the symptoms of intolerance increase, the biguanides should then be discontinued. The side-effects nearly always disappear within 24 hrs. Sufficient carbohydrate intake is necessary (POMERANZE and GADEK). When the complaints have completely disappeared, a new trial can be made using slowly increasing biguanide doses. However, symptoms of intolerance can precede ketosis (compl. p. 139). For this reason, especially in the insulin deficiency diabetes, doses of insulin should only be increased with the greatest care on discontinuing the biguanides (comp. p. 135).

Several authors attempted to treat the gastro-intestinal complaints symptomatically. The simplest measure is to administer biguanide tablets only after meals (WALKER; AZERAD and LUBETZKI). SCHILLING suggests doses of hydrochloric acid in patients suffering from loss of appetite, while AZERAD and LUBETZKI administered the drug together with antacida. SEYDL and SCHULLERI saw no improved tolerance when giving digestive enzymes or antihistamines in addition. Assuming that symptoms of intolerance are caused by a biguanide effect on the central nervous system, drugs with a specific central nervous effect are advised; KLEEFIELD suggests compazine (a phenothiazine derivative) and PEARLMAN, dexedrine (dextroamphetamine sulphate) to combat the side-effects. SEYDL and SCHULLERI reported of using a combination of DBI and p-oxypropiophenone (200 mg p-oxypropiophenone, 50 mg DBI), but it was not more successful. The frequency of signs of intolerance corresponds to those seen by the other authors with DBI alone.

β) **Hypersensitivity reaction and organ changes.** TRANQUADA, KLEEMAN and BROWN (1959a) saw in a patient after 2 weeks of DBI treatment the appearance of a generalised *urticaria and angioneurotic oedema* that disappeared on discontinuing the DBI. BOECKH (1960) also saw the appearance of urticaria in a diabetic after W 37 that disappeared on discontinuing medication. We observed recently a severe anaphylactic shock (generalised urticaria, Quincke-Oedema, severe vasomotoric collapse) after 7 days of medication with W 37. This could be remedied only with high doses of prednisolone and infusions with nor-epinephrine. 36 hours after discontinuation of the biguanide-therapy the symptoms disappeared. The intradermal test with W 37 showed an immediate type reaction (KERP and CREUTZFELDT). KOOPMANN (1960) and also BOECKH (1960) each described a case suffering from a severe Menière syndrome following biguanide administration. The complaints receded on discontinuing the therapy.

The clinical, and especially animal experimental experiences regarding organ damage following synthalin administration, suggest that the problem of the clinically applied biguanides should be handled with care. The many investigations for more than 3 years on several thousand diabetics treated with biguanides do not show any reason for believing the biguanides (DBI especially) to have any damaging effect on the organs.

Liver function. Investigations on the liver function using modern methods showed no changes (KRALL and BRADLEY; KRALL; ODELL et al.; McKENDRY et al. 1959; TRANQUADA, KLEEMAN and BROWN 1959a; POMERANZE and GADEK; WALKER; SKILLMAN, KRUGER and HAMWI; MEHNERT and SEITZ; SCHILLING; STERNE and others). The biguanide therapy did not cause any deterioration in already existing liver disease (SCHILLING; KRALL and BRADLEY). The biopsy findings of BERINGER (1959) confirm this.

Changes in the blood picture. OTTO (1958) described a case where massive intestinal haemorrhages occurred parallel to a decrease in thrombocytes; in all other cases no damage to the bone marrow function could be found (KRALL; KRALL and BRADLEY; McKENDRY et al.; WALKER; AZERAD and LUBETZKI;

POMERANZE and GADEK; MEHNERT and SEITZ; SCHILLING; WELLER and McCAU-LAY).

Kidney function. No impairment of renal function could be found. Non-protein nitrogen and blood urea nitrogen are not elevated, urine is normal (KRALL; KRALL and BRADLEY; WILLIAMS, TANNER et al; MEHNERT and SEITZ; SCHILLING; WELLER and McCAULAY and others). No systematic renal function tests were published (clearances, phenol red excretion, concentration experiments, T_m estimations). In RADDINGS' investigations on the blood electrolytes, no direct relationship was found to the DBI therapy.

Autopsy findings. Autopsy and histological organ examination of patients who died during DBI therapy from causes not directly connected with diabetes (e.g. apoplexia), showed no damage through the biguanides in the liver, kidney or haematopoetic system (WELLER and McCAULAY; BRADLEY).

6. Comparison between synthalin and biguanide therapy in diabetes

Previous experience speaks for the fact that the biguanides do not have the organ damaging effect observed for synthalin in animal experiments and in single cases, also in man. In this respect, the change to biguanides is a real advance. The shorter time of effect, in comparison to synthalin, can be seen both as an advantage (reduced danger of accumulation), and as a disadvantage (irregular effect level).

If one judges the progress by 2 other criteria, namely the relation of effective dose to tolerance and the range of therapeutic use, the comparison is less favorable. The statements of BLATHERWICK, SAHYUN and LONG in 1928 have more or less been confirmed: *The blood sugar decreasing effect of the guanidine derivatives is closely correlated to the dose causing intolerance.*

The therapeutic effective synthalin dose is 20—50 mg/day, that of N_1,N_1-dimethyl-biguanide at 500—3000 mg/day, for DBI (150—200 mg/day) and for DBV (200—400 mg/day) it is between these. Despite this great difference in effectiveness, the frequency of symptoms of intolerance is in all cases nearly the same. Therefore, in *this* respect, the introduction of the biguanides indicates no measurable progress.

The range of therapeutic use of the guanidine derivatives has, in comparison to synthalin, not been increased by the introduction of the biguanides. This could be expected as the mechanism of action seems to be the same.

Regarding the fact that in all guanidine derivatives the blood sugar effectiveness is correlated to intolerance, we can hardly expect further progress in the oral diabetes therapy from new blood sugar decreasing guanidine derivatives.

Further substances proved as oral anti-diabetic drugs

A. Salicylate and salicylate derivatives

Salicylate and other benzoic acid derivatives have been used for several decades in rheumatism therapy. There are numerous experimental and clinical publications on this drug. In this review, only the blood sugar decreasing properties of salicylate and some derivatives will be discussed. We refer to the following authors in respect to the other properties, especially to the toxicology— HANZLIK (1927), GROSS and GREENBERG (1948) (more than 4000 literary references) also SMITH (1953).

The hypoglycaemic action of salicylic acid in diabetes mellitus has been known for a considerable time (EBSTEIN 1876, BARTELS 1878, GREENHOW 1880, NICOLAIER 1893, WILLIAMSON 1901). Improvement of the following symptoms has been described: glucosuria with connected polyuria, metabolic status (weight increase, improvement in the general condition). The conditions for an effect to take place was a sufficiently long therapy (several days to weeks) and a relatively high dosage. Already before the introduction of insulin, the application of salicylates in diabetes therapy was discontinued. The reason for this could have been the frequently appearing side-effects and the ineffectiveness of this drug in severe forms of diabetes.

I. Experimental investigations

a) Blood sugar decrease in the animal

Salicylate produced no hypoglycaemia in normal experimental animals. The blood sugar of dogs was even elevated (BARBOUR and HERMANN), also of rats (SMITH 1955; SÖLING, JARRE and SCHMIDT) and of mice (SPROULL). Only SMITH, MEADE and BORNSTEIN found no change in the blood sugar at all in healthy rats receiving salicylate. In alloxan diabetic rats, salicylate (100 mg/rat) effected a definite blood sugar decrease (SMITH, MEADE and BORNSTEIN; BORNSTEIN; MEADE and SMITH; SÖLING, JARRE and SCHMIDT). The same was described for the diabetes occurring after partial pancreatectomy in the rat (INGLE and MEEKS). Also in adrenalectomised, cortisone substituted rats, aspirin led to a blood sugar decrease (INGLE; SMITH 1954). This findings suggests that the supra-renals play an important part in the absent blood sugar decrease of the normal animal.

After the positive experience with adrenal cortical steroids in rheumatism therapy, it was believed that salicylates and steroids had the same mechanism of action. Recent investigations have meanwhile shown that the individual effect of each substance is very different, but that salicylate and salicylate derivatives do in fact lead to an increased liberation of adrenal cortical steroids (BLANCHARD; HETZEL; HETZEL and HINE, LÖWENTHAL and JAQUES; VAN CAUWENBERGE); their effect can partly overshadow that of salicylate. By this, the fact that salicylate does not depress the blood sugar in the non-diabetic rat unless not only the adrenal medulla, but also the adrenal cortex has been extirpated, is explained (SMITH 1955). As in hypophysectomised animals there is no ascorbic acid depletion in the adrenals usually observed after salicylate administration (BLANCHARD; VAN CAUWEN BERGE; CRONHEIM and KING), it is believed that salicylate acts via an increased ACTH liberation on the adrenal cortex.

b) Investigations on the mechanism of the blood sugar decrease

1. Investigations in vitro

Glucose uptake. MANCHESTER, RANDLE and SMITH found on incubating the isolated rat diaphragm in a carbonate-bicarbonate buffer, an increased glucose uptake under salicylate action (5×10^{-3} m). This effect is unspecific as under these conditions d-xylose uptake is also increased. Recently SEGAR, BLAIR and WEINBERG did not find, in a carbonate-bicarbonate buffer, an effect of salicylate (1.9×10^{-3} m) on the glucose uptake by the diaphragm of normal or alloxan diabetic rats. The same was found on incubating in a phosphate buffer (JEFFREY and SMITH).

Oxygen consumption. The O_2 consumption of tissue slices is increased by salicylate (1×10^{-3} m) (BRODY). Hereby glycolysis is increased while the *P/O* quotient is decreased (BRODY). This corresponds to the findings of SEGAR, BLAIR and WEINBERG. These authors found an increased formation of $^{14}CO_2$ from ^{14}C-labelled glucose, pyruvate and palmitate in the muscle, less in the epididymal adipose tissue of the rat. Salicylate had no detectable effect on glucose oxidation in the liver. The rate of the $^{14}CO_2$ formation from $^{14}C_1$-respectively $^{14}C_6$-labelled glucose remained unchanged by salicylate.

Amino acid incorporation. The incorporation of amino acids in protein by the isolated rat diaphragm is inhibited by salicylate (5×10^{-3} m) (MANCHESTER, RANDLE and SMITH).

Effect on single enzymes. KAPLAN described an inhibiting action of salicylate on the dehydrogenase of the tri-carbonic acid cycle. Here inhibition of α-keto-glutarate dehydrogenase and of succino dehydrogenase stands in the foreground. Inhibition is abolished by the addition of Mg^{++} ions. BRODY could not reproduce this finding. The activity of muscle phosphorylase is diminished. However the remaining activity is sufficient for performing increased glycogenolysis under the influence of salicylate (SEGAL, BLAIR and WEINBERG). MITIDIERI and AFFONSO described an increase of the xanthine-dehydrogenase activity in the blood on simultaneous decrease in the liver. Here there is obviously an unspecific effect in the sense of an enzyme release from the damaged liver cells; this can be explained by the high dosage (500 mg salicylate per rat i.p.).

2. Experiments in vivo

Liver and muscle glycogen. In normal rats, salicylate (100 mg per animal s.c.) leads to a definite reduction in liver glycogen, attaining its maximum after 4—7 hrs (LUTWAK-MANN; SMITH 1954; SMITH, MEADE and BORNSTEIN). After 24 hrs, the liver glycogen content is higher than in the controls (LUTWAK-MANN; SMITH 1954). Also muscle glycogen is decreased (WINTERS and MORILL). The elevation of the liver glycogen content instigated by glucocorticoids can be inhibited by salicylate (WINTERS and MORILL). There is also no increase in the liver glycogen following glucose loading if salicylate is administered (EDELMANN, BOGNER and STEELE). Liver glycogen augmentation caused by stilboestrol is also inhibited by salicylate (BARNETTI and TEAGUE). However, the liver glycogen content in alloxanised rats is not significantly changed by salicylate (SMITH, MEADE and BORNSTEIN).

O_2-consumption. Salicylate causes an increased O_2 consumption in experimental animals (ANDREWS; SINGER; HSIEH and CHIU; D. E. HALL et al.; ROWE et al.; WALTNER et al.). This increase is only partly due to stimulation of the respiratory centre (HSIEH and CHIU; TENNEY and MILLER). Increased respiration is accompanied by augmented glycolysis (SMITH and JEFFREY; STOWERS, CONSTABLE and HUNTER).

Gluconeogenesis. Hardly anything has been published of the effect of salicylate on gluconeogenesis. Only WINTERS and MORILL described a slight increase in nitrogen excretion following salicylate application.

3. Uncoupling of oxidative phosphorylation

As mentioned above BRODY proved that salicylates uncouple oxidation from phosphorylation (see also KIRPEKAR and LEWIS). The different organs obviously display varying sensitivity. Thus the O_2 consumption of the kidney is not increased even on relatively high salicylate concentrations. Investigations with rat brain tissue, indicate that besides the uncoupling, other mechanisms are implicated in increasing the O_2 consumption (PATEL and HEIN).

The uncoupling effect of the salicylates can in the first place be made responsible for a blood sugar decrease in the animal experiment. This assumption is supported by the following results:

1. Other uncoupling reagents are also capable of lowering the blood sugar (e.g. 2,4-dinitrophenol s. p. 147). Increased glucose uptake through the isolated rat diaphragm was observed for 2,4-dinitrophenol (RANDLE and SMITH) and also for thyroxine (COSMA). Other effects of the salicylates also correspond to those of uncoupling substances (e.g. increased potassium output from the isolated rat diaphragm, lowering of the blood cholesterol level).

2. Only those benzoic acid derivatives have a blood-sugar lowering and a glycogenolytic effect that also cause increased O_2-consumption (e.g. salicylate and aspirin), while others, also anti-rheumatically active derivatives (e.g. salicylamide or gentisinic acid) have no increasing, but rather a decreasing effect on the O_2-consumption (ANDREWS 1958, 1960). Uncoupling leads to an increased accumulation of anorganic phosphate and ADP (adenosine di-phosphate). By this the Pasteur effect, said to be caused mainly by a deficiency of anorganic phosphate, is abolished. The uncoupling of oxidation and phosphorylation causes an increase in glucose utilization by increasing aerobic glycolysis. The energy gained is relatively slight. Augmented glucose by the means of increased *aerobic* glycolysis, is introduced into the tri-carbonic acid cycle. The energy is lost for the greater part in the form of heat, as it cannot be transformed to the phosphate bond, rich in energy, owing to the uncoupling. The uncoupling salicylate effect is also responsible for the decrease in the blood cholesterol level (WREIGHT and LOEB; s. also the review of LOOMIS and LIPMAN).

II. Investigations with salicylates and salicylate derivatives in man

a) The effect of salicylates and salicylate derivatives on the metabolism of non-diabetics

According to most investigators salicylate leads to a *blood sugar rise* in non-diabetics (SCHADT and PURNELL; CHARTERS; MORRIS and GRAHAM). HECHT and GOLDNER however correctly indicated that in these cases there are more or less severe salicylate intoxications. HECHT even found among 90 cases of salicylate poisoning a blood sugar rise only three time. After acute i.v. salicylic acid loading DIBENEDETTO DELL'AQUILA et al. saw an elevation of the blood glucose; COCHRAN, WATSON and REID described the appearance of hyperglycaemia in rheumatics during salicylate treatment. On the other hand HECHT and GOLDNER found in 13 non-diabetics receiving 4.8 g of aspirin orally, daily for 1—3 weeks, in 12 cases a decrease in the blood sugar (in 8 cases the decrease was significant, averaging 23 mg-%). The *glucose tolerance curve* was definitely lowered in 7 from 10 patients receiving the same premedication with aspirin. However, the *insulin sensitivity* remained unchanged in 2 of the examined patients.

Not only in the animal experiment but also on application in man, salicylates can have effects very similar to those caused by the *adrenal-cortical* steroids (s. review by HAILMAN also HETZEL, WILLIAMS and LANDER). This is not an effect peculiar to the salicylates, but an increased corticoid production effected by the release of ACTH (CRONHEIM and HYDER). The picture of acute salicylate poisoning is determined by this "stress" effect of the salicylates, thus the hyperglycaemia often described for salicylate intoxication can also be understood.

Salicylate and aspirin also effect an increased O_2 *consumption* in man (BARBOUR and DEVENIS; COCHRAN 1954 and 1956; BALOGH et al.; WALTNER; TANOS and Kelemen; Rowe; Hetzel, Charnock and Lander; Alexander and Johnson). Cochran (1954) described a reduction in the respiratory quotient.

Blood cholesterol is decreased by salicylates (Hetzel, Charnock and Lander).

b) The effect in diabetes mellitus

The high salicylate, respectively aspirin doses necessary for treating diabetics *recommend the estimation of the plasma level* of these drugs. The estimation is generally carried out with the method of Trinder, less frequently with that of Loberg.

If during the treatment of diabetes, glucosuria is determined by reduction methods, salicylate degradation products can cause increased reduction and therefore simulate elevated glucosuria (Reid 1959).

1. Clinical experience

The publications from the past decades of the previous century have already been referred to (comp. p. 141 f.). Recently Reid et al. also Hecht and Goldner reported of the treatment of diabetics with salicylate. Following experience was made:

Similar as in alloxan diabetes, salicylate, respectively aspirin, effect a definite blood sugar decrease in diabetics. Reid Macdougall and Andrews saw in all of 7 patients with diabetes of varying severity, recession of glucosuria and a decrease in the fasting blood sugar. Goldner and Hecht also attained a significant blood sugar decrease in 9 from 12 diabetics receiving aspirin. Ketonuria can also recede through aspirin treatment (Reid, Macdougall and Andrews; Reid 1959). Hecht and Goldner saw a normal hyperglycaemic reaction in the glucagon tolerance test (0.1 mg glucagon i.v.) in 4 patients.

According to Reid (1959) the response to salicylates is independent of the height of the insulin dose required previously. By treating with aspirin, respectively salicylate, insulin can be reduced (Reid, 1959; Hecht and Goldner). In cases of severe diabetes the blood sugar is sometimes not influenced, however the amount of insulin can be reduced. In single cases it was possible to reduce this by more than 40 U (maximally 72 U) (Reid 1959). Insulin and aspirin seem to have an additive effect, when measured by the decrease in the blood sugar (Hecht and Goldner). Also the combination of tolbutamide (D 860) and aspirin leads to an increased blood sugar effect (Hecht and Goldner). In the case of brittle diabetes with a high insulin requirement, the metabolic state is said to be improved by aspirin, and the danger of hypoglycaemia is reduced (Reid 1959).

Dosage. The dose necessary for lowering the blood sugar is relatively high. Reid, Macdougall and Andrews gave their patients between 1 and 1.6 g aspirin in the space of 4 hrs. Hecht and Goldner administered similar doses (minimum dose 4.8 g aspirin per day). The plasma aspirin level necessary for a blood sugar decreasing effect, lies between 30 and 50 mg-% (Reid, Macdougall and Andrews; Reid 1959). The responsiveness of the individual patients varies at the same plasma level. In the single case however, effectiveness and plasma level are proportional.

The effect of salicylate treatment only appears after some time (5—7 days). On the other hand the effect lasts some time on discontinuing therapy (Reid 1959; Macdougall and Andrews; Hecht and Goldner).

2. Side-effects

Hecht and Goldner observed side-effects only twice, among 13 patients (stomach complaints), they disappeared after discontinuation of the therapy.

REID (1959) however, describes strong symptoms of intolerance. In about 50% of the patients examined by REID, persistent nausea occured followed by vomiting in 2 cases. In both cases the plasma level was very high (52 mg-%). The complaints vanished on reducing the dose.

Besides these unspecific symptoms of intolerance, other signs, characteristic for salicylate intoxication, appear: in almost all patients the hearing ability deteriorates, accompanied by tinnitus in single cases (REID, MACDOUGALL and ANDREWS; REID 1959). The complaints disappear after discontinuing aspirin treatment or reducing the dose.

Symptoms of severe salicylate poisoning (disturbed consciousness, respiratory alkalosis resulting in metabolic acidosis, s. the review of CANN and VERHULST) do not appear within the recommended dose range. However in the case of severe gastro-intestinal symptoms, a decreased food intake with carbohydrate deprivation can result which is followed by starvation acidosis (REID 1959). Toxic organ damage, especially damage of the bone marrow function does not occur, according to the experience made in the rheumatism therapy, even after long-term application of therapeutic doses. Hypoglycaemia was not observed with salicylate treatment alone.

3. Practical value of the salicylates in the diabetes therapy

The doses necessary for lowering the blood sugar correspond to those applied in the animal experiments. Increased O_2 consumption is also seen in the treated diabetics (REID, MACDOUGALL and ANDREWS). This indicates that the uncoupling effect of the salicylates plays a large role in the blood sugar decrease. The fact that the blood sugar lowering effect of the salicylates is much stronger than that of 2,4-dinitrophenol at the same elevated O_2 consumption, indicates the cooperation of another mechanism (REID 1958). Whether stimulation of insulin secretion plays a part here has not been investigated.

According to experience to date, the practical value of salicylate therapy in diabetes mellitus is slight. First, the necessary doses are very high and therefore cause side-effects relatively often. Secondly, the actual improvement in metabolism is not great when compared to that of the other orally applicable anti-diabetic drugs. Finally a theoretical reason against salicylate treatment is the fact that it is not known to what extent the blood sugar decrease is due to an uncoupling effect. If this effect plays an important part in the blood sugar decrease then salicylate therapy has not much sense. The reduction in the blood glucose would be the expression of increased glucose metabolism, but not however of increased glucose utilization, as the energy freed on degradation in the organism is, for the greater part lost.

B. Other benzoic acid derivatives

I. p-amino benzoic acid (PABA)

ALSTRÖM (1951) described a rise in the blood sugar in rats receiving a diet poor in PABA. The liver glycogen content was lowered. This aberrancy is normalised by adding 200 γ PABA/100 g of food.

Adding 20 mg/100 g food also leads to hyperglycaemia, which is remarkable (ALSTRÖM 1957). Despite the fact that these investigations say nothing of a blood sugar lowering effect, PABA is already, combined with ascorbic acid and sodium salicylate as an oral anti-diabetic drug, on the market (Pascon®). The effectiveness of this combination is apparently due to a real salicylate effect (NILSSON). In the animal experiment no increased O_2 consumption after PABA can be proved (ANDREWS).

II. p-aminosalicylic acid (PAS)

LANGERON, MICHAUX, DESTOMBES and PAUL saw a blood sugar lowering effect during the treatment of tubercular diabetics with high PAS doses. No further details are given. PAS does not lead to increased O_2 consumption in the animal experiment (ANDREWS).

C. 2,4-dinitrophenol (DNP)

The uncoupling effect of DNP has already been mentioned (comp. p. 144). DNP effects increased glucose uptake in the isolated rat diaphragm (RANDLE and SMITH; FORBATH and CLARKE). The increased permeability through DNP is unspecific, as the uptake of other sugars is also elevated (RANDLE and SMITH; FORBATH and CLARKE). On the whole the effects of 2,4-dinitrophenol in vitro resemble those of salicylate (SEGAL, BLAIR and WEINBERG).

REID (1959) investigated the effect of DNP on the blood sugar of 8 female maturity-onset diabetics. He administered daily 100—300 mg. DNP orally for 14 days, continuously controlling the plasma DNP level (using PARKER's method for determination). The plasma level was between 3.5 and 5.0 mg-%. 5 patients displayed a slight to definite decrease in the fasting blood sugar after 7 days. The decrease augmented during the following 8 days. In the patient with the mildest diabetes, moderate hyperglycaemia appeared. In the other cases, glucosuria was reduced by DNP, but disappeared only in one case. The oral glucose tolerance test showed a slight flattening in the blood sugar curve. In the remaining patients the glucose tolerance remained unchanged. Patients receiving DNP showed a clear increase in the basal metabolic rate proportional to the plasma DNP level.

There were no side-effects or symptoms of intolerance. Six of the patients were subsequently changed over to salicylate; a much more extensive blood sugar decrease was then seen.

DNP cannot be used as an anti-diabetic drug, already on the grounds of its small blood sugar lowering effect.

D. Mesoxalic acid

KOBAYASHI, OHASHI and TAKEUCHI reported in 1951 the blood sugar decreasing effect of this drug. The earlier investigations of JACOBS (1937) on non-diabetic rabbits however, showed no blood sugar effectiveness; he gives no details as to the amount applied.

$$OH\diagdown \diagup COOH$$
$$C$$
$$OH\diagup \diagdown COOH$$

mesoxalic acid

I. Experimental investigations

a) Toxicity

No toxic symptoms could be found in rats, acutely or chronically receiving high doses of mesoxalic acid (KOBAYASHI, OHASHI et al.). The authors could not definitely state a minimum toxic dose. Growth was not influenced in young rats and rabbits chronically receiving high doses of mesoxalate. No organ damaging action was found by KOBAYASHI, OHASHI, TAKEUCHI and IKEDA for mesoxalate. No histological damage was seen in the liver, kidney or pancreas in rats and rabbits treated for 15 months, with mesoxalic acid.

10*

b) Mechanism of action

The investigations on the mechanism of action of mesoxalic acid showed similar results to those found with the sulphonylureas; therefore this drug is closely connected to the sulphonylureas in this respect.

Kobayashi et al. found already in 1951 that the salts of mesoxalic acid had the following effect: parenterally and orally administered they lowered the blood sugar in normal and alloxanised rabbits and dogs, while having no effect in totally pancreatectomised dogs. The infusion of sodium-mesoxalate solution (of 4—0.8%, 1 ml/min) in the common hepatic artery (thus before the origin of the pancreatico-duodenal artery) led to a definite blood sugar decrease in the dog, and on higher concentrations causing death in the state of hypoglycaemic shock. If an infusion of equal concentration was made via the portal vein, there was no hypoglycaemia. A slight blood sugar decrease was only observed on infusing more than 1.3 ml/min of a 4% solution. Infusing concentrations over 4% into the jugular vein resulted in death during hypoglycaemic shock. When infusing malonate, succinate and other intermediate substances into the common hepatic artery, the blood sugar remained unchanged. These experiments seem to confirm the assumption of Kobayashi and Ohashi (1955) namely that mesoxalic acid affects the blood sugar by stimulating the β-cells in the pancreas. This conception was corroberated by the findings of Kobayashi, Ohashi, Takeuchi and Ikeda. They saw in rats and also rabbits receiving calcium oxalate for several months (rabbits 50—200 mg/kg, rats 50—500 mg/kg) hypertrophy and regeneration of islets, and relative and absolute augmentation of the β-cells. Correspondingly, the plasma and pancreatic insulin content increases in the dog receiving mesoxalate (Kobayashi). Mesoxalic acid causes increased liver glycogen synthesis in healthy and diabetic rats; both with and without previous glucose doses (Takeda, Nakano and Wakabayashi).

II. Clinical investigations

Takeda et al. also Kobayashi (1957) investigated the effect of mesoxalic acid in about 100 diabetics. According to their findings, mesoxalate only has an effect in older diabetics without ketosis tendency. This correlates with the assumption of a similar mechanism of action as that of the sulphonylureas. In such cases the urine sugar excretion can recede or disappear. While Takeda saw a less impressive effect on the fasting blood sugar, Kobayashi (1957) described a definite blood sugar decrease, an increased glucose tolerance and improvement in the subjective complaints. Complete change-over is only successful, even on correct selection of the patients, in a small number of cases, according to present reports. Mostly insulin in varying amounts must also be given.

Complications have not been seen to date even in treatment lasting almost 1 year. Mesoxalate alone is said to cause no hypoglycaemia in diabetics (Kobayashi 1957).

Dosage. The daily mesoxalate doses lie between 0.3 and 2 g per os. Symptoms of intolerance have not been reported, even on higher doses.

Calcium oxalate has been on the Japanese market as "Mesoxan®" (Shionogi and Co.) for 2 years.

Kobayashi and his group of workers are the only ones who have investigated this drug. Publications from other research workers are still to be expected.

E. Antihistamines and sympathicolytica

There are only very few publications on the blood sugar lowering action of these substances. However, there are facts that speak for their effect on the blood sugar having the same, or at least a very similar mechanism of action.

The compounds to be considered can be divided into three groups.
1. Secalealkaloides
2. Sympatheticolytic imidazole derivatives
3. Antihistamines.

I. Secalealkaloides

It has already been mentioned in the discussion on the guanidine derivatives that the hyperglycaemia seen in experimental animals receiving guanidine (comp. p. 95) galegine (comp. p. 108) and synthalin (comp. p. 108) can be suppressed by ergotamine.

Ergotamine can inhibit the glycogenolytic properties, in the liver, of the increased epinephrine secretion stimulated by the above cited drugs.

Dehydrated secalealkaloides (e.g. Hydergin, KRONEBERG and STOEPEL), have the same effect. Not only can the blood sugar rise caused by epinephrine be inhibited or reduced by secalealkaloides, but also—with corresponding dosage—a certain blood sugar decrease can be achieved.

SHERIF, RAZZAK and HASSABALLAH saw, in 3 healthy control subjects receiving 5 γ/kg Hydergin s.c., a slight blood sugar decrease of 27% (mean value) after 90 mins. The blood sugar decrease through Hydergin (5 γ/kg s.c.) was clearer in 3 diabetics: here the mean blood sugar decrease was 38% after 90 mins, and regained its original level after 3—4 hrs.

HARVEY, WANG and NICKERSON had shown that the metabolic effect of the ergotalkaloides was independent from their ability for influencing other epinephrine effects (e.g. the effect on the smooth muscle or on the circulatory system). Thus e.g. ergonovine suppresses the epinephrine hyperglycaemia in experimental animals (3.5 mg/kg) and has no effect on all other epinephrine properties.

II. Sympatheticolytic imidazole derivatives

SHERIF, RAZZAK and HASSABALLAH investigated the effect of *tolazolin* (Priscol ®) and *phentolamine* (Regitin ®) on the blood sugar.

Tolazoline (3 mg/kg s.c.) lowered the blood sugar 40% in rabbits. Phentolamine (3 mg/kg s.c.) only caused a weak blood sugar decrease in some animals and in others hyperglycaemia.

The inhibition of the epinephrine hyperglycaemia in rabbits through tolazoline or phentolamine is definitely weaker than through Hydergin.

In man however, both drugs suppressed the epinephrine hyperglycaemia. In healthy controls both drugs caused a decrease in the fasting blood sugar (of 38% respectively 37% after 90 mins). The blood sugar values regained their original level after 3—4 hrs.

The blood sugar decreasing effect was also greater than that of Hydergin in diabetic patients. Tolazoline lowered the blood sugar 46%, phentolamine 40% (mean values). This correlates with the experiences FRIEB also CARVALHO made with tolazolin.

III. Antihistamines

GENAZZINI et al. (1951) also GOLDNER and JAUREGUI (1954) reported of the blood sugar lowering effect of antihistamine. Antazoline (Antistin ®) and pyrilamine (Neo-Antergan ®) were found to be effective. Also pyribenzamine seems to have certain blood sugar lowering effect (ZWANG and JACUBEIT).

JAUREGUI and GOLDNER (1954 b) investigated the metabolic effect of Antistin in the isolated perfused liver of the frog. At a concentration of 5 mg-% in the perfusing fluid, Antistin suppressed glycogenolysis stimulated by epinephrine and histamine. Spontaneous glycogenolysis was also inhibited by Antistin.

Healthy controls show a blood sugar decrease between 20 and 27% after i.v. injection of 150 mg. Antistin (GOLDNER and JAUREGUI 1954a). *Orally* administered

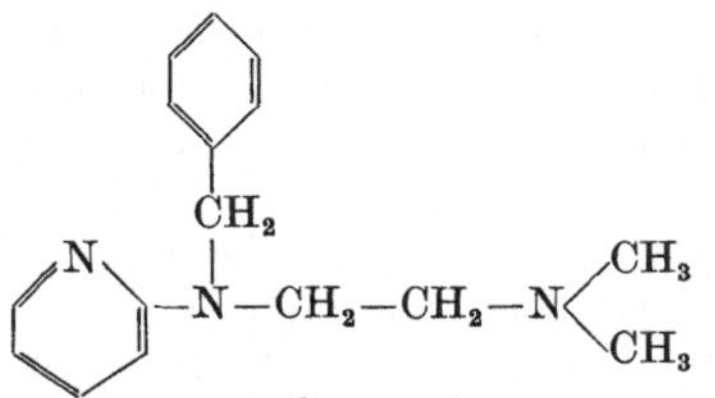

pyribenzamine

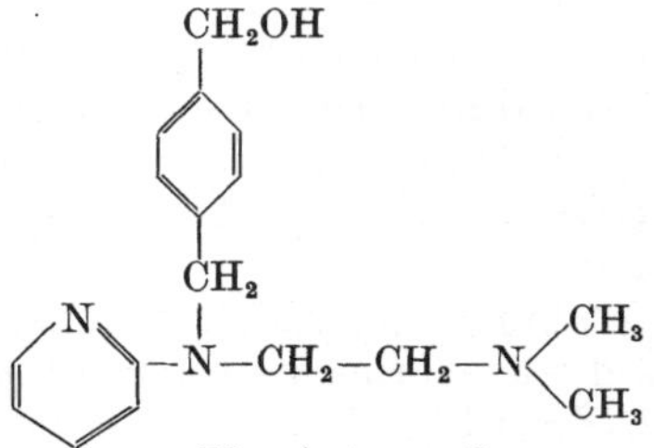

Neo-Antergan®

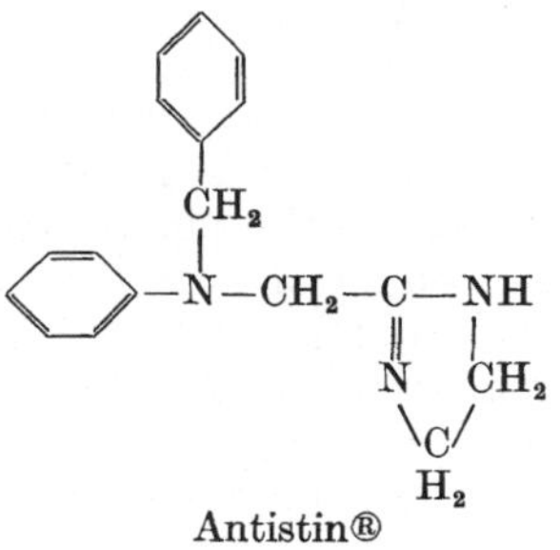

Antistin®

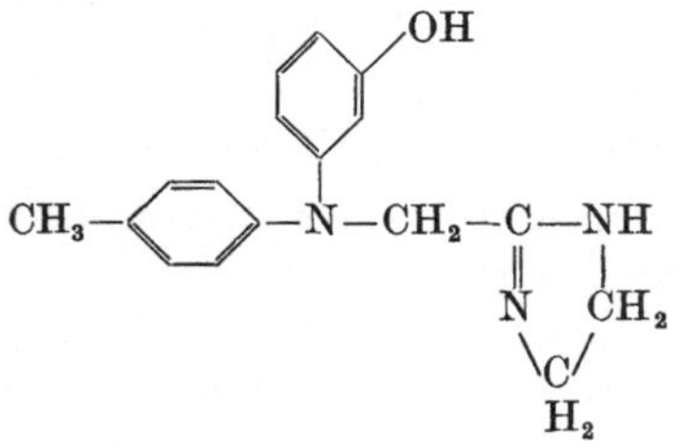

Regitin®

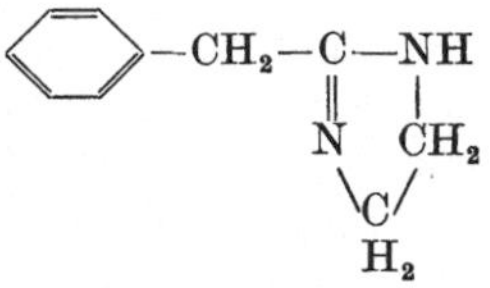

Priscol®

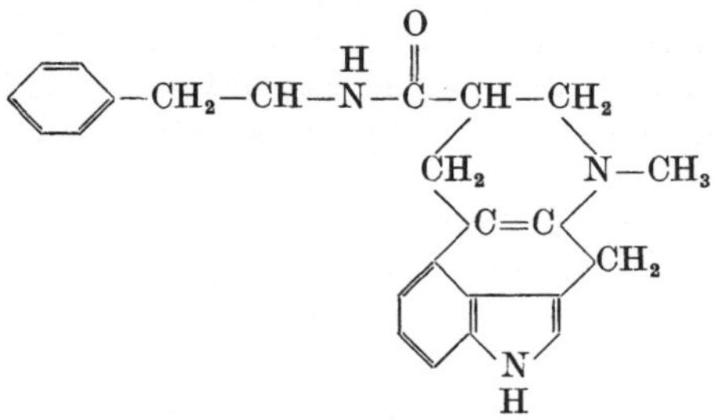

ergotamine

doses up to 600 mg. Antistin do not affect the blood sugar. In diabetics whose insulin dose was reduced to half that necessary for optimal control, Antistin prevented the blood sugar rise in some cases with doses of at least 600 mg/day. However maximally only 20 U insulin could be reduced for a longer time (GOLDNER and JAUREGUI). 2 patients with mild diabetes not requiring insulin previously, could be controlled by 600 mg/day Antistin. Withheld experiments objectivated the effectiveness of Antistin. In diabetics who were optimally controlled before and during the experiment by diet or insulin, only a weak blood sugar decrease, within physiological limits, could be achieved by 600 mg Antistin per day (GOLD-NER and JAUREGUI).

IV. Mechanism of action

Exact experimental investigations are limited to the work done by JAUREGUI and GOLDNER. Thus one has to answer the question on the mode of action partly theoretically. All 3 groups of drugs have the following common properties: they inhibit the glycogenolytic epinephrine effect, show structural similarities as they all have an ethylamine group (comp. Tab. 8) and only have a weak blood sugar decreasing effect in the healthy organism; however a more definite blood sugar lowering effect in the diabetic.

The inhibition of the epinephrine instigated hyperglycaemia and the anti-glycogenolytic effect (JAUREGUI and GOLDNER) speak for direct intervention of the named drugs in the process of glycogenolysis. The interference with the epinephrine effect refers to an inhibition of phosphorylase activation or of phosphorylase itself in the liver. No proof was found for the assumption of ZWANG and JACUBEIT that insulin secretion is stimulated. The drugs are effective in the isolated organs in the depancreatised animal (JAUREGUI, cited from GOLDNER and JAUREGUI).

The above mentioned drugs are as yet of no practical value in the diabetes therapy.

Blood sugar lowering substances without clinical significance

A. Hypoglycin A and B

The hypoglycins deserve only theoretical interest as the mechanism of action, known for the greater part; forbids their use in the treatment of diabetics.

The hypoglycins are blood sugar active substances that are found in the seeds and meat of the unripe fruit of *Blighia sapida*. The ripe fruit of the tree, known in Jamaica as "acee" or "akie", and in Africa as "ishin" is eaten in Jamaica, Central America and Florida. The unripe fruit can cause the typical "vomiting sickness" often ending fatally. The clinical picture is characterised by a severe hypoglycaemia accompanied by glycogen depletion and fat augmentation in the liver (HILL 1953, JELIFFE and STUART 1954).

I. Structure of the hypoglycins

The structure of hypoglycin A was simultaneously elucidated by VON HOLT and LEPPLA (1958a and b) also WILKINSON (1958) and DE ROPP et al. It is a β-(methylene-cyclopropyl)-α-amino-propionic acid.

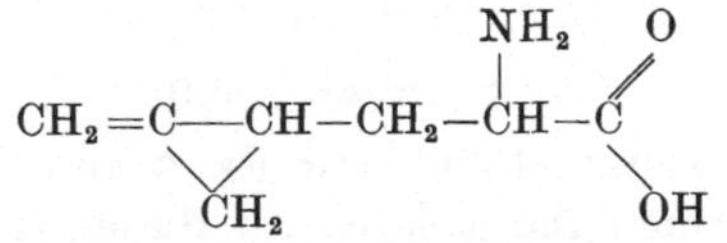

$$CH_2=C-CH-CH_2-CH-C \overset{NH_2 \quad O}{\underset{CH_2 \qquad\qquad OH}{}}$$

β-(methylene-cyclopropyl)-α-aminopropionic acid (hypoglycin A)

The structure was acertained by synthesis (CARBON et al.). Further investigations on the structure have been published by ELLINGTON et al. and ANDERSON et al.

Hypoglycin B is a dipeptide from hypoglycin A and glutarate (v. HOLT, LEPPLA, KRÖNER and v. HOLT 1956, v. HOLT and LEPPLA 1959). While N-acetyl derivatives of the hypoglycin A are similarly blood sugar effective (100 mg/kg rat), dehydration of the double bond of the molecule results in the loss of effect (DE ROPP et al.).

II. Experimental investigations

a) Toxicity and the blood sugar lowering

CHEN, ANDERSON et al. (1957) also HASSALL investigated the toxicity of the hypoglycins. In the animal experiment hypoglycin A and also hypoglycin B were highly toxic. The effectiveness of hypoglycin A is much greater.

In mice (100—160 mg/kg i.v. or s.c.), rats (75—100 mg/kg i.v. or orally), monkeys (20—40 mg/kg i.v.) hypoglycin A and also hypoglycin B in higher doses lead to marked hypoglycaemia. The animals mostly die during the hypoglycaemic shock. In cats (5—40 mg/kg i.v.), dogs (30 mg/kg i.v.) and pigeons (25—100 mg/kg i.v.) no hypoglycaemia could be found. These animals also died. In contrast to the other animals, vomiting is a regular symptom of intoxication in cats, dogs, and pigeons.

A blood sugar decrease is also seen in alloxan diabetic rats given hypoglycin A in the acute experiment (CHEN, ANDERSON et al. 1957). It is remarkable that these animals die after the same hypoglycin doses without recession of glucosuria (CHEN, ANDERSON et al. 1957). In contrast to this L. v. HOLT and C. v. HOLT were able to reduce glucosuria in alloxan diabetic rats orally receiving 40 mg/day hypoglycin A, for a longer period.

In 2 pancreatectomised dogs, hypoglycin A (15 mg/kg i.v.) once led to a slight blood sugar decrease, while the blood sugar of the other animal remained unchanged (CHEN, ANDERSON et al. 1957). Adrenalectomised mice showed increased sensitivity towards the blood sugar decreasing effect (CHEN, ANDERSON et al., 1957). The blood sugar decrease caused by hypoglycin depends on the dose given (FENG and PATRICK). Animals who were in fasting condition before poisoning reacted much more strongly (FENG and PATRICK; HASSALL, REYLE and FENG).

The hypoglycin poisoning can only temporarily be improved by glucose doses, according to corresponding results of many authors.

Histological investigations of the hypoglycin poisoned animals show a strong *reduction in liver glycogen* accompanied by a definite *fatty liver degeneration* (PATRICK 1954, CHEN, ANDERSON, McLOWEN and HARRIS). The picture corresponds to that found in man by HILL also JELIFF and STUART. The reduction in liver glycogen commences several hours before the blood sugar decreases (PATRICK).

There are controversial results from the histological investigations on the *islets* of the *pancreas*. LEPPLA and v. HOLT also CHEN, ANDERSON et al. (1957) saw no damage. However FENG, on applying 150—300 mg/kg hypoglycin A (lethal dose) to guinea-pigs and rats, saw massive α-cell-damage. FENG did not believe the α-cell changes to be responsible for the blood sugar decrease (comp. also p. 118).

b) Mechanism of action

1. Investigations in vitro

Neither v. HOLT and LEPPLA (1956), nor FENG and PATRICK could find increased glucose uptake through the isolated rat diaphragm, under the influence of hypoglycin A (to 200 mg-% in the incubation medium). However the glycogen synthesis was inhibited or prevented, in the rat diaphragm and in liver slices, while the respiratory quotient was simultaneously increased (DE ROPP, v. METER et al.; BELL et al.). Besides this, inhibition of oxidative phosphorylation in isolated liver mitochondria is described (DE ROPP et al.). In contrast to this FENG and PATRICK found no change in the O_2 consumption, in the respiratory quotient or in the glycogen synthesis of liver slices (rat).

2. Investigations in vivo

Hypoglycin causes an increase of lipid concentration (DE ROPP et al.) and of the urea concentration (HASSALL, REYLE and FENG) in the blood. Lactate and pyruvate levels remain unchanged under these conditions (FENG and PATRICK). While the blood sugar rise on loading with glucose is reduced through insulin, hypoglycin treated animals show a much stronger blood sugar rise than the controls (FENG and PATRICK, CHEN, ANDERSON et al., BELL et al.).

After loading with U-^{14}C glucose, BELL saw an elevation in the liver lipid content, accompanied by an increase of blood lipid concentration. The liver lipids contained ^{14}C activity. The $^{14}CO_2$ formation remained unchanged, while after injection of ^{14}C acetate the $^{14}CO_2$ portion in the totally expired CO_2 showed a significant reduction (BELL et al.). v. HOLT and BENEDICT saw under hypoglycin A (40 mg/kg orally) after a dose of U^{14}C-glucose, an increased $^{14}CO_2$ output in relation to the total CO_2 output, when compared to controls; this indicates increased glucose oxidation. The oxidation of ^{14}C labelled capronate was not inhibited by hypoglycin A (40 mg/kg orally) while that of ^{14}C labelled palmitate was.

L. v. HOLT and C. v. HOLT have shown that the effect of the hypoglycins causing a decrease in the blood sugar and fatty liver degeneration, can be inhibited by lactoflavin administration.

The experimental findings indicate a primary disturbance in the fat metabolism as causing the hypoglycin hypoglycaemia (HILL 1953, BELL et al.; LEPPLA and v. HOLT; C. v. HOLT and L. v. HOLT; v. HOLT and BENEDICT), and can be summarised thus: β-methylene-cyclopropyl-α-amino-propionic acid (hypoglycin A) is desaminised in the organism (liver ?) to a non-physiological fatty acid (v. HOLT unpublished, cited from v. HOLT and BENEDICT). This non-physiological fatty acid competitively inhibits an enzyme of the fatty acid degradation. Here probably inhibition of the ethylene reductase occurs (acyldehydrogenase) (v. HOLT and BENEDICT). For this speaks 1. The protective effect of riboflavin [ethylene reductase has at least one co-enzyme, containing FAD (flavin adenine dinucleotide)]. 2. The fact that the fatty acid synthesis does not seem to be disturbed (comp. the findings of BELL et al., also the histological findings). If one of the 3 other enzymes implicated in the fatty acid degradation (crotonase, β-hydroxy-acyl-dehydrogenase, thiolase) were inhibited, then degradation and synthesis would have been disturbed in the same way, for these enzymes catalyse oxidation and reduction respectively, the apposition and splitting off of acetate, in the same manner. However the ethylene reductase only catalyses oxidation of the fatty acids while the corresponding reduction stage is catalysed by Lynen's "reducing enzyme of the fatty acid cycle".

According to the findings of v. HOLT and BENEDICT, only the oxidation of long chain fatty acids in inhibited, as the capronate oxidation is unchanged by hypoglycin. The fats in the organism and those contained in the diet, mostly have fatty acids with long chains. The inhibition of the fatty acid degradation leads to compensatory increase of glucose oxidation. As the amount of glucose available is very limited, glycogenolysis and increased gluconeogenesis occur, from protein. The decrease in blood sugar commences as soon as these reserves are exhausted. Thus this mechanism shows the unsuitability of the hypoglycins in the diabetes therapy.

B. Mono-iodo-acetic acid and iodo-acetamide

HULTQUIST (1958) found in rats given 50 mg/kg mono-iodo-acetamide or 30 mg per kg. iodo-acetamide (s.c.), a definite blood sugar decrease.

$$CH_2J \cdot C \begin{smallmatrix} O \\ OH \end{smallmatrix} \qquad CH_2J \cdot C \begin{smallmatrix} O \\ NH_2 \end{smallmatrix}$$

Mono-iodo-acetic acid   Mono-iodo-acetamide

HULTQUIST saw signs of increased activity of the β-cells on histologically examining the pancreas, while the α-cells displayed only slight, rapidly disappearing disturbances. Therefore he interpreted that the brief blood sugar decrease caused by the named drugs was due to stimulation of the insulin secretion. There are no further investigations.

C. Tris (hydroxy-methyl)-amino-methane (TRIS-buffer)

TARALL and BENNET observed a definite blood sugar decrease in healthy dogs and in healthy humans after i.v. infusion of Tris solution.

$$NH_2 - C \begin{smallmatrix} CH_2OH \\ CH_2OH \\ CH_2OH \end{smallmatrix}$$

Tris-(hydroxy-methyl-) aminomethane

The blood sugar lowering effect was proportional to the dose. If the dose was high enough (0.3 m Tris solution in 0.03 m NaCl and 0.005 m KCl, 0.7—1.0 ml per kg/min) dogs suffered from severe hypoglycaemic shock. The decrease in the blood sugar was accompanied by a reduction in blood anorganic phosphate and an increased blood p_H value, plasma CO_2 content, incontinence and excretion of sodium, chlorine, and potassium. Tris had no effect *in vitro*.

TARALL and BENNET therefore discuss a stimulation of insulin secretion. This is supported by the reduction in blood phosphate. No results were gained from investigating the blood potassium, as potassium was induced by the infusion. Further investigations must be awaited.

D. Less important blood sugar decreasing drugs and insufficiently investigated preparations

In conclusion, some other blood sugar decreasing substances are mentioned that cannot be fully discussed in this review. These are substances whose blood sugar effectiveness is only slight or is doubted. α-liponic acid belongs to this series (PAGLIARO 1956a and b, SCHIROSA and PAGLIARO; SCHIROSA and FURITANO, CUTOLO and REDUZZI, BRUSA and SERAFINI), also nicotinic acid (GURIAN and ADLERSBERG; UNGER), nicotin (BERRY) and phenylbutazon (comp. the review by ZÜRN).

Regarding the blood sugar lowering properties of substances of herbal origin, that have not been defined chemically, we recommend the review of PETERS (1957).

References

AARSETH, S., u. H. WILLUMSEN: Pancytopeni og agranulocytose efter carbutamid ved diabetes. Nord. Med. 1958, 564—565.

ACHELIS, J. D.: Vom Wirkungsmechanismus der oralen Antidiabetica. Diabetes mellitus. 3. Kongreß der internat. Diabetes Federation. Düsseldorf 1958, S. 286—292. Stuttgart: Georg Thieme 1959.

— u. K. HARDEBECK: Über eine neue blutzuckersenkende Substanz. Dtsch. med. Wschr. 1955, 1452—1455.

ADAM, A.: Über Insulinersatz durch Synthalin. Med. Klin. 1927, 1218.

ADAMI, E., V. LARDARUCCIO e C. CARDANI: Azione ipoglicemizzante di alcune N-alchil-(aril-solfonil) uree. Minerva med. (Torino) 49, 1466—1468 (1958).

ADLER, A.: Über die Nebenwirkungen des Synthalins und ihre Beseitigung. Klin. Wschr. 1927, 493.

AIMAN, R. and N. CHAUDRAY: Mechanism of action of oral anti-diabetic drugs. Brit. J. Pharmacol. 14, 377—379 (1959).

AIMAN, R., and R. D. KULKARNI: The effect of human plasma on the glucose uptake of the rat diaphragma before and after administration of carbutamide. Brit. J. Pharmacol. 12, 475—478 (1957).

ALEXANDER, W. D., and K. W. M. JOHNSON: A comparison of the effects of acetylsalicylic acid and d, l-Triid othyronine in patients with myxoedema. Clin. Sci. 15, 593—601 (1956).

ALLES, G. A.: The comparative physiological action of some derivatives of guanidine. J. Pharmacol. exp. Ther. 28, 251—276 (1926).

ALSTRÖM, I.: In verkan av sulfanilamid och dess antagonist Para-amino benzoesyra på den djuriska organismen huvudsakligen med hänsyn till kolhydratom-sättningen. Diss. suppl. till Scand. vet. tidskrift 4 (1948).

— Effect of para-aminobenzoic acid on the blood sugar level and the liver glycogen content of white rats. Acta med. scand. 157, 327 (1957).

ALWALL, N.: Steigerung des Citratstoffwechsels in vitro durch Salicylsäure. Acta med. scand. 102, 390—395 (1939).

ANDERSON, E., and J. A. LONG: The effect of hyperglycemia on insulin secretion as determined with the isolated rat pancreas in a perfusion apparatus. Endocrinology 40, 92 (1947).

ANDERSON, G. E., A. J. PERFETTO, CH. M. TERMINE and R. R. MONACO: Hypoglycemic action of orinase. Effect on output of glucose by liver. Proc. Soc. exp. Biol. (N. Y.) 92, 340—345 (1956).

ANDERSON, H. V., J. L. JOHNSON, J. W. NELSON, E. C. OLSON, M. E. SPEETER and J. J. VAVRA: Chem. and Ind. 1958, 330. Zit. nach v. HOLT und LEPPLA (1959).

ANDERSON, R. C., H. M. WORTH and P. N. HARRIS: Toxicological studies on carbutamide. Diabetes 6, 2—7 (1957).

ANDREU-KERN, F., H. D. SÖLING u. W. CREUTZFELDT: Untersuchungen über die Wirkung einer Kombination von DBI mit Insulin bzw. Tolbutamid auf den Kohlenhydratstoffwechsel des Meerschweinchens. (In Vorbereitung.)

ANDREWS, M. M.: The relative potencies of some substituted salicylic acids as metabolic stimulants in the intact rat. Brit. J. Pharmacol. 13, 419—423 (1958).

— The glycogenolytic activity of some substituted salicylic acids. Biochem. J. 75, 298—303 (1960).

ANGELI, G.: Il trattamento orale del diabete mellito con la N_1-p-toluil-sulfonil-N_2-n-butil-carbamide (D 860). Minerva med. (Torino) 48, 2772—2785 (1957).

— e B. ALBERINI: Un nuovo farmaco ad azione ipolgicemizzante nella terapia orale del diabete mellito: la 1-cicloesil-3-p-tolil-solfonilurea (K 386). Minerva med. (Torino) 48, 360 (1957).

ANTILA, V., A. N. KUUSISTO u. G. HÄRTEL: Über die Wirkung des peroralen Antidiabeticums N-[4-Methyl-benzolsulfonyl]-N'butylharnstoff und Serumcholesterin der Ratte. Ann. Med. exp. Fenn. 35, 272—276 (1957).

APEL, S.: Klinische Erfahrungen beim Diabetes mellitus des Fleischfressers Berl. Münch. tierärztl. Wschr. 72, 295—314 (1959).

APPEL, W.: Körperbaustudien an Diabetikern. Dtsch. Arch. klin. Med. 198, 172—181 (1951).

ARNDT, H. J., E. MÜLLER u. E. SCHEMANN: Experimentelle Beiträge zur Frage der Synthalin-wirkung. Klin. Wschr. 1927, 2283—2287.

ASHMORE, J., G. F. CAHILL, A EARLE and S. ZOTTU: Studies on the disposition of blood glucose. Diabetes 7, 1—8 (1958).

— — and A. B. HASTINGS: Inhibition of glucose-6-phosphatase by hypoglycemic sulfonylureas. Metabolism 5, 774—777 (1956).

— A. B. HASTINGS, F. B. NESBETT and A. E. RENOLD: Studies on carbohydrate metabolism in rat liver slices. IV. Hormonal factors influencing glucose-6-phosphatase. J. biol. Chem. 218, 77 (1956).

ASHWORTH, M. A., and R. E. HAIST: Some effects of BZ 55 on the growth of the islets of Langerhans. Canad. med. Ass. J. 74, 975—976 (1956).

Azérad, E.: Essai de traitement du diabète sucré de l'adulte par des hypoglycémiants de synthèse de la série des sulfamido-thiodiazols (2254 et 2261 RP). Bull. Soc. méd. Hôp. Paris Sér. 4, 72, 424—435 (1956).
— et J. Lubetzki: Traitement du diabète par le N-N-diméthyl diguanid (LA 6023). Presse méd. 1959, 765.
Baer, J., u. L. Blum: Über die Einwirkung chemischer Substanzen auf die Zuckerausscheidung und die Acidose. Naunyn-Schmiedebergs Arch. exp. Path. Pharmak. 63, 1—33 (1911).
Baier, H.: Über die Wirkung von Sulfonylharnstoffen auf die Fruktoseverwertung bei Diabetes. Klin. Wschr. 1959, 399—401.
Baird, C. W., and J. Bornstein: Plasma-Insulin and Insulin resistance. Lancet 1957I, 1111—1113.
Baird, J. D.: The new oral hypoglycemic agents. Nutrition 12, 3—7 (1958).
— and L. J. P. Duncan: The interpretation of the intravenous glucose tolerance test. Clin. Sci. 16, 147—153 (1957).
— — An analysis of the hypoglycaemic response to tolbutamide. Scot. med. J. 2, 341—350(1957).
Baird, R. W., and J. G. Hull: Cholestatic jaundice from tolbutamide. Ann. intern. Med. 53, 194—196 (1960).
Balogh, L., Sz. Donhoffer, Gy. Mestyán, T. Pap u. I. Tóth: Über die Wirkung der Natriumsalze der Benzoe- und Salicylsäure, ihrer p-Aminoverbindungen und des Salicylamids auf den Sauerstoffverbrauch und die Körpertemperatur der Ratte. Naunyn-Schmiedebergs Arch. exp. Path. Pharmak. 214, 299—307 (1952).
Bänder, A.: Die Wirkung von N-(4-Methyl-benzolsulfonyl)-N'-butylharnstoff auf das Nebennierenmark. Arzneimittel-Forsch. 8, 459—462 (1958).
— Histologische Untersuchungen nach Gaben des oralen Antidiabeticums Rastinon. Med. u. Chem. VI, 119—133 (1958).
— Pharmacological studies of the sulfonylureas. Ann. N. Y. Acad. Sci. 82, 508—512 (1959).
— Zum Wirkungsmechanismus blutzuckersenkender Sulfonylharnstoffe D 860 und BZ 55. Dtsch. med. Wschr. 1959, 996—1002.
— A. Häussler u. J. Scholz: Ergänzende pharmakologische Untersuchungen über Rastinon. Dtsch. med. Wschr. 1957, 1557—1564.
— u. J. Scholz: Spezielle pharmakologische Untersuchungen mit D 860. Dtsch. med. Wschr. 1956, 889—891.
Barbour, H. G., and N. M. Devenis: Acetyl salicylic acid and heat regulation in normal individuals. J. Pharmacol. exp. Ther. 13, 499—500 (1919).
— and J. B. Herrmann: The relation of the dextrose and water contents of the blood to antipyretic drug action. J. Pharmacol. exp. Ther. 18, 165—183 (1921).
Barger, G., and F. D. White: The constitution of Galegin. Biochem. J. 17, 827 (1923).
Barnett, G. O., and R. S. Teague: The antagonism of salicylate to diathylstilboesterol upon liver glycogen in the rat. Endocrinology 63, 205—211 (1958).
La Barre, J., et J. Reuse: A propos de l'action hypoglycémiante de certains dérivés sulfamidés. Arch. néerl. Physiol. 28, 475—480 (1947).
Barros Barreto, H. P., and L. Recant: Tolbutamide studies in prediabetes. Ann. N. Y. Acad. Sci. 82, 560—569 (1959).
Bartelheimer, H.: Extrainsuläre hormonale Regulatoren im diabetischen Stoffwechsel. Ergebn. inn. Med. Kinderheilk. 59, 595—752 (1940).
— Letal verlaufende Encephalomyelitis post- oder propter BZ 55-Therapie eines Diabetes? Ärztl. Wschr. 1957, 283.
— u. H. Maring: Der Einfluß eines hypoglykämisierenden Sulfonamidderivates (BZ 55) auf die Insulinwirksamkeit bei Diabetikern. Klin. Wschr. 1956, 1011—1016.
Bartels: Über die therapeutische Verwertung der Salicylsäure und ihres Natronsalzes in der inneren Medizin. Dtsch. med. Wschr. 1878, 435—437.
Barth, H., u. M. Kleinsorge: Pharmakologische und klinische Untersuchungen mit Sulfanilylharnstoffen. Schriftenreihe d. Z. ges. inn. Med. Heft 11, 124—139 (1959).
Bastenie, P. A., J. R. M. Franckson, R. de Meutter, J. C. Demanet and V. Conard: Metabolic effects of carbutamide in selected diabetics. Lancet 1957I, 504—507.
Bastiani, G. de, e L. Granata: Effetti del pretrattamento con il preparato sulfamidico 2254 RP sulla insorgenza e sul decorso del diabete da allossana nel coniglio. Arch. ital. Sci. farmacol. 1, 3—8 (1957).
Batts, A. A.: Effect of hypophysectomy and growth hormone administration upon the Golgi-apparatus in the islets of Langerhans. Endocrinology 64, 610—614 (1959).
Bayliss, R. I. S., and A. W. Steinbeck: Salicylates and the plasma level of adrenal steroids. Lancet 1954I, 1010.
Bayreuther, H.: Über die Verwendungsmöglichkeit und den Wirkungsmechanismus blutzuckersenkender Sulfonamidderivate bei der Insulin-Schock-Behandlung in der Psychiatrie. Arch. Psychiat. Nervenkr. 195, 435—445 (1957).

BAYREUTHER, H.: u. N. SPECHT: Über die Brauchbarkeit blutzuckersenkender Sulfonamidabkömmlinge für die Insulin-Schockbehandlung in der Psychiatrie. Arch. Psychiat. Nervenkr. **195**, 132—139 (1956).

BEARN, A. G., B. H. BILLING and SH. SHERLOCK: Response of the liver to insulin; hepatic vein catheterization studies in man. Ciba Foundation Colloquia on Endocrinology. Vol. VI: Hormonal factors in carbohydrate metabolism. London **1953**, 250—260.

BEASER, S. B.: The use fo orinase in diabetes. Metabolism **5**, 933—939 (1956).

— Further experience with the use of sulfonylureas in diabetes. Ann. N. Y. Acad. Sci. **71**, 264—267 (1957).

— Therapy of diabetes mellitus with combinations of drugs given orally. New Engl. J. Med. **259**, 1207—1210 (1958).

— The correlation between oral dosage, blood levels and clinical and metabolic activity of chlorpropamide in the treatment of diabetes mellitus. Ann. N. Y. Acad. Sci. **74**, 701—708 (1959).

BEBER, B. A., and M. BEBER: The effect of tolbutamide (Orinase) on the liver. Amer. J. Med. Sci. **238**, 433—442 (1959).

BECKER, W. H., E. BUDDECKE u. H. MÜLLER: Blutzuckerwirkung von Nadisan (BZ 55) beim pankreasresezierten Hund. Klin. Wschr. **1956**, 920.

BELL, P. H., E. C. DE RENZO and K. W. MCKERNS: Biological activities of hypogycin A. Abstr. IV. Int. Conf. Biochem. Wien 1958, 9/15 (S. 104).

BELLENS, R., et V. CONARD: Influence d'une dose et de doses répétées d'un sulfamide hypoglycémiant sur des épreuves d'hyperglycémie successives. Ann. Endocr. (Paris) **19**, 1197—1205 (1958).

— R. DEMEUTTER et V. CONARD: Influence d'une dose unique de BZ 55 sur l'assimilation glucidique et la sensibilité à l'insuline du rat normal. C. R. Soc. Biol. (Paris) **150**, 1630—1633 (1956).

— A. H. OOMS, J. R. FRANCKSON, V. CONARD et P. A. BASTENIE: Influence d'une dose unique d'un sulfamide hypoglycémiant sur l'assimilation glucidique du chien. C. R. Soc. Biol. (Paris) **152**, 1403—1404 (1958).

BENCOSME, S. A., S. MARIZ and J. FREI: Further studies on the relationship of glucagon to the alpha cell of the pancreas. Can. J. Biochem. **35**, 1197—1203 (1957).

— — — Changes in dogs devoid of A cells. Endocrinology **61**, 1—11 (1957).

BENDTFELDT, E., O. ERNST, R. FLÜGGE u. H. OTTO: Das Verhalten der Darmflora unter der oralen Diabetestherapie mit BZ 55 und D 860. Medizinische **1957**, 634—637.

— u. H. OTTO: Schwere hypoglykämische Reaktion im Verlauf der peroralen Diabetesbehandlung mit BZ 55. Münch. med. Wschr. **1956**, 1136—1137.

BERGEN, S. S., J. G. HILTON and W. S. NORTON: Effect of phenethylbiguanide on adrenal function and responsiveness as measured by ACTH-test. Proc. Soc. exp. Biol. (N. Y.) **98**, 625 (1958).

— and W. S. NORTON: Clinical and metabolic effects of phenethylbiguanide. Diabetes **9**, 183—185 (1960).

BERGENSTAL, D. M., H. A. LUBS, L. F. HALLMAN and J. A. SCHRICKER: Effects of tolbutamide on the diabetes of acromegaly and on the bloodsugar in patients with altered endocrine states. Ann. N. Y. Acad. Sci. **71**, 215—232 (1957).

BERINGER, A.: Zur Beeinflussung des Stoffwechsels durch Insulin und die blutzuckersenkenden Sulfonamide. Wien. med. Wschr. **107**, 972 (1957).

— Zur Behandlung der Zuckerkrankheit mit Biguaniden. Wien. med. Wschr. **1958**, 880—882.

— Unterschiede in der Insulin- und der Sulfonamidwirkung zwischen Mensch und Versuchstier. Wien. med. Wschr. **109**, 245—246 (1959).

— Experimentelle und klinische Untersuchungen beim menschlichen Diabetes mit Biguaniden. In BERTRAM und MICHAEL: Internationales Biguanid-Symposium, S. 49—55. Stuttgart: G. Thieme 1960.

— u. F. HELMER: Zit. nach A. BERINGER, K. HUPKA, K. MÖSSBACHER, K. MOSER u. R. WENGER. Wien. med. Wschr. **108**, 639—643 (1958).

— u. D. HOFMANN-CREDNER: Über eine Affinität der Leber zum Zucker. Wien. med. Wschr. **1957**, 94—96.

— K. HUPKA, K. MÖSSLACHER, K. MOSER u. R. WENGER: Zur Beeinflussung des menschlichen Diabetes mit Insulin, blutzuckersenkenden Sulfonamiden sowie den Biguaniden. Wien. med. Wschr. **1958**, 639—643 (1958).

— u. E. KEIBL: Untersuchungen mit den blutzuckersenkenden Sulfonamiden beim Menschen und beim Versuchstier. Wien. med. Wschr. **106**, 792—798 (1956).

— u. A. LINDNER: Zur Frage des Wirkungsmechanismus blutzuckersenkender Sulfonamide. Wien. klin. Wschr. **68**, 316 (1956).

— u. M. PANTLITSCHKO: Experimentelle Untersuchungen mit neuen blutzuckersenkenden Substanzen. Wien. med. Wschr. **108**, 481—483 (1958).

— u. H. THALER: Zur oralen Diabetesbehandlung. Medizinische **1959**, 41—43.

BERRY, M. G.: Tobacco hypoglycemia. Ann. intern. Med. 50, 1149—1157 (1959).

BERSON, S. A., and R. S. YALOW: Some remarks on the mechanism of action of the sulfonyl-ureas. Diabetes 6, 274—277 (1957).

— — Recent studies on insulin-binding antibodies. Ann. N. Y. Acad. Sci. 82, 338—344 (1959).

— — S. WEISENFELD, M. G. GOLDNER and B. M. VOLK: The effect of sulfonylureas on the rates of metabolic degradation of insulin-I^{131} and glucagon-I^{131} in vivo and in vitro. Diabetes 6, 54—60 (1957).

BERTHET, J., E. W. SUTHERLAND and M. H. MAKMAN: Observations on the action of certain sulfonylurea derivatives. Metabolism 5, 768—773 (1956).

BERTRAM, F.: Die periphere Steuerung der Blutzuckerreaktion auf Gifte. Naunyn-Schmiede-bergs Arch. exp. Path. Pharmak. 126, 267 (1927).

— Zum Wirkungsmechanismus des Synthalins. Dtsch. Arch. klin. Med. 158, 76 (1928).

— Die Behandlung des Diabetes mellitus mit kleinen Dosen von Guanidinderivaten. Med. Klin. 1928, 1229.

— Die Zuckerkrankheit. 1. Aufl. Leipzig 1934; 4. Aufl. Stuttgart 1953.

— Ergebnisse einer dreijährigen oralen Therapie des Diabetes mellitus. Arzneimittel-Forsch. 8, 427—430 (1958).

— Indikationen und Ergebnisse der oralen Diabetesbehandlung. IV. Dtsch. med. Wschr. 1958, 1260—1261.

— Die Klinik der oralen Therapie des Diabetes mellitus. Diabetes mellitus. III. Congress of International Diabetes Federation, Juli 1958. Stuttgart: Georg Thieme 1959.

— E. BENDTFELDT u. H. OTTO: Über ein wirksames perorales Antidiabeticum (BZ 55). Dtsch. med. Wschr. 1955, 1455—1460.

— — — Indikationen und Erfolge der peroralen Behandlung des Diabetes mellitus mit einem Sulfonylharnstoffderivat. Dtsch. med. Wschr. 1956, 274.

— — — Derzeitiger Stand der oralen Diabetesbehandlung. Schweiz. med. Wschr. 87, 25—30 (1957).

— u. J. KUNTZE: Aktuelle Diabetesfragen, Symposion in Hamburg. Stuttgart: Georg Thieme 1957.

BEST, C. H., R. E. HAIST and J. H. RIDOUT: Diet and the insulin content of the pancreas. J. Physiol. (Lond.) 97, 107—119 (1939).

BIERMAN, E. L., T. N. ROBERTS and V. P. DOLE: Effect of tolbutamide (orinase) on plasma non-esterfied fatty acids. Proc. Soc. exp. Biol. (N. Y.) 95, 437—439 (1957).

BILHAN, N.: Über einen besonderen Fall von Synergie von Insulin und D 860. Diabetes mel-litus. 3. Kongreß der internat. Diabet. Federation. Düsseldorf 1958. S. 468—470. Stutt-gart: Georg Thieme 1959.

BIRÓ, L., K. WEISZ, T. BÁNYÁSZ u. H. FRIED: Die Wirkung des Invenols auf die Zucker-resorption aus dem Dünndarm. Klin. Wschr. 1959, 768—769.

BISCHOFF, F., M. SAHYUN and M. L. LONG: Guanidine structure and hypoglycemia. J. biol. Chem. 81, 325 (1928).

BLANCHARD, K. C., E. H. DEARBORN, T. H. WARREN and E. K. MARSHALL: Stimulation of anterior pituitary by certain cinchoninic acid derivatives. Bull. Johns Hopk. Hosp. 86, 83 (1950).

BLATHERWICK, N. R., M. SAHYUN and E. HILL: Some effects of synthalin on metabolism. J. biol. Chem. 75, 671 (1927).

BLECHER, O.: Diabetes und Tuberkulose. Erfahrungen aus einer Lungenheilstätte. Z. Tuberk. 111, 57—63 (1958).

BLÖCH, J., and A. LENHARDT: Advantages and disadvantages in shifting patients from tolbut-amide to chlorpropamide. Ann. N. Y. Acad. Sci. 74, 954—961 (1959).

— — Vorläufiger Bericht über die Erfahrungen mit W 32 und W 37 an 71 diabetischen Patienten. In BERTRAM und MICHAEL: Internationales Biguanid-Symposium, S. 149—152. Stuttgart: G. Thieme 1960.

BÖCK, J., A. LINDNER u. H. OBENAUS: Untersuchungen über die Wirkung von Insulin und-blutzuckersenkenden Sulfonylharnstoffverbindungen auf den Glukosegehalt des Kammer-wassers. Wien. klin. Wschr. 70, 644—648 (1958).

— J. STEPANIK u. T. TERES: Tonographische Untersuchungen über die Wirkung von N_2-(p-Aminobenzolsulfonyl)-N_2-butylharnstoff auf den Kammerwasserhaushalt des Menschen. Wien. klin. Wschr. 71, 952—953 (1959).

BODO, R., and H. P. MARKS: The relation of synthalin to carbohydrate metabolism. J. Physiol. 65, 83 (1928).

BODO, R. C. DE, A. ALTSZULER, A. DUNN, R. STEELE, D. T. ARMSTRONG and J. S. BISHOP: Effects of exogenous and endogenous insulin on glucose utilization and production. Ann. N. Y. Acad. Sci. 82, 431—449 (1959).

— R. STEELE, N. ALTSZULER, A. DUNN, D. T. ARMSTRONG and J. S. BISHOP: Further studies on the mechanism of action of insulin. Metabolism 8, 520—530 (1959).

BOECKH: Diskussionsbemerkung in BERTRAM und MICHAEL: Internationales Biguanid-Sym-posium, S. 167. Stuttgart: G. Thieme 1960.

BÖHLE, E., E. F. PFEIFFER, K. SCHÖFFLING u. H. STEIGERWALD: Das Verhalten der Blutlipide unter D 860. Dtsch. med. Wschr. 1956, 838.
BOIS, C. DE, W. J. DEFAU et J. HOET: Sur le mécanisme d'action d'un dérive polymethyle de la guanidine. C. R. Soc. Biol. (Paris) 97, 1420 (1927).
BOL, M., H. D. SÖLING u. W. CREUTZFELDT: Wirkung von Guanidinderivaten auf die Glucoseabsorption des isolierten Dünndarms von Ratten in vivo. To be published.
BOLINGER, R. E., and H. J. GRADY: Effect of aryl sulfonylurea on the plasma disappearance of labeled insulin in diabetics. Amer. J. med. Sci. 233, 182—184 (1957).
— W. P. MCKEE and J. W. DAVIS: Comparative effects of DBI and insulin on glucose uptake of rat diaphragm. Metabolism 9, 30 (1960).
— P. WALLACE, W. P. MCKEE and J. W. DAVIS: Interaction effects of DBI, insulin and epinephrine on the isolated rat diaphragm. Symposium on "A new Oral Hypoglycemic Agent, Phenformin (DBI)". Houston (Texas) 1959.
BOLLER, R., u. E. KÖCK: Zur peroralen Diabetestherapie. Wien. med. Wschr. 107, 351—355 (1957).
BONHÔTE, D.: Aspects du mode d'action de certaines substances sulfamidées hypoglycémiantes révélés chez l'homme normal et diabétique par leur effet sur des surcharges intraveineuses de fructose. Schweiz. med. Wschr. 87, 1318—1321 (1957).
BORNSTEIN, J.: Insulin-reversible inhibition of glucose utilization by serum lipoprotein fractions. J. biol. Chem. 205, 513 (1953).
— Inhibition of alanine transaminase by the hypoglycaemic sulphonylurea derivatives. Nature (Lond.) 179, 534—535 (1957).
— u. R. D. LAWRENCE: Plasma-insulin in human diabetes mellitus. Brit. med. J. 1951, 4747, 1541—1544.
— B. W. MEADE and M. J. H. SMITH: Salicylates and carbohydrate metabolism. Nature (Lond.) 169, 115—116 (1952).
— and C. R. PARK: Inhibition of glucose uptake by serum lipoprotein fractions. J. biol. Chem. 205, 503 (1953).
BOSHELL, B. R., G. R. ZAHND and A. E. RENOLD: An effect of tolbutamide on ketogenesis, in vivo and in vitro. Metabolism 9, 21—29 (1960).
BÖTTCHER, K.: Wirkung des N-(4-Methylbenzolsulfonyl-)-N'butylcarbamids (D 860) auf den Alloxandiabetes des Kaninchens. Inaug.-Diss. Freiburg 1957.
BOULET, P., J. MIROUZE et Y. SCHMOUKER: Intérêt de l'association arylsulfamide-biguanide dans le traitement du diabète sucré. Presse méd. 1960. 2123—2126.
BOULIN, R.: Essais de traitment du diabète sucré par le BZ 55. Presse méd. 64, 643 (1956).
BOVET. D., et P. DUBOST: Activité hypoglycemiante des amino-benzène-sulfamido-alkylthiodiazols. Rapports entre la constitution chimique et l'activité pharmaco-dynamique. C. R. Soc. Biol. (Paris) 138, 764 (1944).
BRADLEY, R. F.: Note of oral blood sugar lowering agents in the management of diabetes. Current trends in research and clinical management of diabetes. Ann. N. Y. Acad. Sci. 82, 513—530 (1959).
BRATTON, C., and E. K. MARSHALL JR.: A new coupling component for sulfanilamide determination. J. biol. Chem. 128, 537—550 (1939).
BRAUCH, F.: Tuberkulose und Diabetes. Ärztl. Wschr. 12, 929—936 (1957).
BRAUN, T., B. MOSINGER and V. KUJALOWÁ: A contribution on the mode of action of D 860. Experientia (Basel) 15, 190—191 (1959).
BRAVERMAN, A. E., N.-W. DREY and S. SHERRY: Experience with orinase in the management of adult diabetes. Metabolism 5, 911—918 (1956).
BREDNOW, W., u. D. JORKE: Klinische Erfahrungen in der Diabetesbehandlung mit hypoglykämisierenden Sulfonamidkörpern. Münch. med. Wschr. 1957, 101—105.
BRENEMAN, J. C.: Clinical use of tolbutamide (orinase) in office and home care of diabetes. J. Amer. med. Ass. 164, 627—633 (1957).
BRESSLER, R., and F. L. ENGEL: Some metabolic actions of orinase. Proc. Soc. exp. Biol. (N. Y.) 95, 738—741 (1957).
BROD, R. C.: Blood dyscrasias associated with tolbutamide therapy. J. Amer. med. Ass. 171, 296—297 (1959).
BRODY, T. M.: Action of sodium salicylate and related compounds on tissue metabolism in vitro. J. Pharmacol. exp. Ther. 117, 39—51 (1956).
BROGLIE, M., G. VOSS, E. G. BERG u. O. RÜHLING: Vorläufige Erfahrungen bei der peroralen Behandlung des Diabetes mit dem Sulfonamid „Nadisan". Medizinische 1956, 656—659.
BROWN, J., and D. H. SOLOMON: Effects of tulbutamide and carbutamide on thyroid function. Metabolism 5, 813—829 (1956).
— — Mechanism of antithyroid effects of a sulfonylurea in the rat. Endocrinology 63, 473—480 (1958).

BROWN, G., J. ZOIDIS and M. SPRING: Hepatic damage during chlorpropamide therapy. J. Amer. med. Ass. 170, 2085—2088 (1959).

BRUSA, P., e L. SERAFINI: L'acido tioctico. Richerche sul suo effetto ipoglicemizzante nel bambino sano. Minerva pediat. (Torino) 10, 932—937 (1958).

BULGARELLI, R.: Prime ricerche sulla curva glicemica da BZ 55 nel morbo di Gierke, confronta con la curva glicemica da BZ 55 in bambini sani e in bambini diabetici. Minerva paediat. (Torino) 40, 1177—1182 (1956).

BURCKHARDT, W., u. K. u. M. SCHWARZ-SPECK: Photoallergische Ekzeme durch Nadisan. Schweiz. med. Wschr. 87, 954 (1957).

BÜRGER, M., u. H. KOHL: Über kristallinisches Insulin. VI. Über die Einwirkung kristallinischen Insulins auf den Glykogengehalt der Leber. Naunyn-Schmiedebergs Arch. exp. Path. Pharmak. 178, 269—281 (1935).

BUTTERFIELD, J., I. K. FRY and E. HOLLING: Effects of insulin, tolbutamide and phenethyldiguanide on peripheral glucose uptake in man. Diabetes 7, 449—454 (1958).

BUTTERFIELD, W. J. H., J. L. CAMP, C. HARDWICK and H. E. HOLLING: Clinical studies on the hypoglycemic action of the sulfonylureas. Lancet 1957 I, 753—756.

— and R. H. S. THOMPSON: The effect of dimercaprol (BAL) on blood sugar and pyruvate levels in diabetes mellitus. Clin. Sci. 16, 679 (1957).

BÜTTNER, H.: Diskussionsbemerkung. Verh. dtsch. Ges. inn. Med. 64, 297 (1958).

— u. F. PORTWICH: Wirkung des N-(4-Methyl-benzolsulfonyl)-N'-butylharnstoffs (D 860) auf den Stoffwechsel des Äthanols. Naunyn-Schmiedebergs Arch. exp. Path. Pharmak. 238, 45 (1960).

CABARROU, A., H. V. CAINO, F. SCHAPOSNIK, L. PIANZOLA and N. O. BIANCHI: Liver biopsies in diabetics treated with sulfonamides. Diabetes mellitus. 3. Kongreß der internationalen Diab. Feder. Düsseldorf 1958, S. 436—439. Stuttgart: Georg Thieme 1959.

CAHILL, G. F., A. B. HAISTINGS and J. ASHMORE: Effects of substituted sulfonylureas on rat diaphragm and liver tissue. Diabetes 6, 26—27 (1957).

CAMERINI-DAVALOS, R., A. MARBLE and H. F. ROOT: Clinical experience with orinase. Metabolism 5, 904—910 (1956).

— — P. WHITE, M. BELMONTE and L. SARGEANT: Effect of sulfonylurea compounds in diabetic children. New Engl. J. Med. 256, 817—822 (1957).

— — ROOT, H. F., and A. MARBLE: Clinical experience with carbutamide (BZ 55) Diabetes 6, 74—77 (1957).

CAMPBELL, G. D. (Durban): Persönliche Mitteilung (1960).

— Chlorpropamide in the natal indian. Med. Proc. S. Africa 5, 559—563 (1959).

CAMPBELL, J., and V. LAZIDINS: The action of BZ 55 in dogs. II. Obersvations on the pancreatized and metahypophyseal diabetic dogs. Canad. med. Ass. J. 74, 962—965 (1956).

CAMPENHOUT, E. VAN: Effets du BZ 55 sur le pancréas endocrine du cobaye. C. R. Soc. Biol. (Paris) 151, 1438—1440.

CANAL, N., S. GARATTINI e L. TESSARI: Un nuova ippoglicemizzante: la N_1-sulfanilil-N_2-n-butilcarbamide. II. Sul mecanismo d'azione periferico dei nuovi ipoglicemizzanti. Clin. ter. 11, 472—476 (1956).

CANARY, J. J., R. STOFFER, DE WITT E. DE LAWTER and J. M. MOSS: The response of tolbutamide-treated patients to the stress of surgery. Med. Ann. D. C. 28, 614—670 (1959).

CANN, H. M., and H. L. VERHULST: The salicylate problem with special reference to methyl salicylate. J. Pediat. 53, 271—276 (1958).

CARBON, J. A., W. B. MARTIN and L. R. SWETT: Synthesis of α-Amino-methylene cyclopropane-propionic acid. (Hypoglycin A). J. Amer. chem. Soc. 80, 1002 (1958).

CAREN, R., and L. CORBO: The potentiation of exogenous insulin by tolbutamide in depancreatized dogs. J. clin. Invest. 36, 1546—1550 (1957).

CARLOZZI, M., D. G. LEZZONI and L. SILVER: Blood levels of chlorpropamide in normal men following chronic administration. Ann. N. Y. Acad. Sci. 74, 788—793 (1959).

CARVALHO, J. M.: Vasodilatation and glycemia. Portugal. méd. 26, 486 (1942).

CATTANEO, R.: Chetonemia, piruvicemia e lattacidemia in diabetici trattati con sulfabutilurea. Arch. Stud. Fisiopat. Ricambio 21, 351—352 (1957).

CAUWENBERGE, H. VAN: Relation of salicylate action to pituitary gland. Observations in rat. Lancet 1951 II, 374—375.

CERLETTI, P., and C. GREGOLIN: The effect of sulfonylureas on the respiratory quotient in diabetic and normal animals. Clin. chim. Acta 4, 579—582 (1959).

CHARTERS, A. D.: A case of aspirin poisening. Brit. med. J. 1944, 10—11 (1).

CHEN, K. K., and R. C. ANDERSON: The toxicity and general pharmacology of N_1-parachlorophenyl-N_5-isopropyl-biguanide. J. Pharmacol. exp. Ther. 91, 157 (1947).

— — M. C. McCOWEN and P. N. HARRIS: Pharmacologic action of hypoglycin A and B. J. Pharmacol. exp. Ther. 121, 272—285 (1957).

CHEN, K. K., R. C. ANLERSON and N. MAZE: Hypoglycemic action of sulfanilamido-cyclo-propylthiadiazole in rabbits and its reversal by alloxan. Proc. Soc. exp. Biol. (N. Y.) **63**, 483 (1946).

CHERNICK, S. S., I. L. CHAIKOFF and S. ABRAHAM: Localization of initial block in glucose metabolism in diabetic liver slices. J. biol. Chem. **193**, 793 (1951).

CHRISTOFFEL, P.: Dauerdosierung und Verschiedenwertigkeit oraler Antidiabetika sowie Insulinbedarf nach deren erfolgloser Verwendung. Medizinische **1959**, 414—417.

CHRISTOPHE, J., R. BELLENS et W. GEPTS: Etude expérimentale d'un sulfamide hypoglycémiant. II. Action du R. P. 2254 sur la glycémie du rat normal et du rat diabétique. Ann. Endocr. (Paris) **16**, 956—961 (1956).

— — — Etude expérimentale de l'action du BZ 55 sur le rat normal ou alloxanisé. II. Action sur la glycémie. Ann. Endocr. (Paris) **17**, 291—298 (1956).

— et V. CONARD: Effets d'un traitement aigu et prolongé au BZ 55 chez le chien normal. Ann. Endocr. (Paris) **18**, 1046—1056 (1957).

— and J. MAYER: Effects of chronic treatment with carbutamide on distribution and biosynthesis of fatty acids and cholesterol in obese-hyperglycemic mice. Ann. J. Physiol. **196**, 603—606 (1959).

— — Effects of acute and chronic treatment with carbutamide (BZ 55) on obese-hyperglycemic mice and their lean littermates. Endocrinology **64**, 664—670 (1959).

CLARK, G. A.: Interrelation of parathyroids, suprarenals and pancreas. J. Physiol. **58**, 294 (1923/24).

CLARKE, D. W., M. DAVIDSON, E. SCHÖNBAUM and H. SENMAN: Some in vitro studies with BZ 55. Canad. med. Ass. J. **74**, 966—968 (1956).

— and N. FORBATH: Some studies on the mode of action of DBI. Metabolism 8, 553 (1959).

— — The effects of Phenformin on the isolated rat diaphragm. Diabetes **9**, 167—169 (1960).

— and H. SENMAN: Fourteen-day administration of carbutamide, tolbutamide and cortisone. Effects on metabolism of rat liver and diaphragm. Diabetes **7**, 283—287 (1958).

COATES, J. R., and J. J. ROBBINS: Severe hypoglycemic shock due to chlorpropamide. J. Amer. med. Ass. **170**, 941—943 (1959).

COCHRAN, J. B.: The respiratory effects of salicylate. Brit. med. J. **2**, 964 (1952).

— R. D. WATSON and J. REID: Mild Cushing's syndrome due to aspirin. Brit. med. J. **1950**, 1411—1413 (2).

COHEN, J. L., and A. D. COHEN: Pustular acne, staphyloderma and its treatment with tolbutamide. Canad. med. Ass. J. **80**, 629—632 (1959).

COLWELL, A. R., and J. A. COLWELL: Pancreatic action of the sulfonylureas. J. Lab. clin. Med. **53**, 376—395 (1959).

COLWELL, A. R. jr., J. A. COLWELL and A. R. COLWELL: Intrapancreatic perfusion of the antidiabetic sulfonylureas. Metabolism **5**, 749—756 (1956).

— — and A. R. COLWELL SR.: Perfusion studies with sulfonylureas in dogs. Ann. N. Y. Acad. Sci. **71**, 125—130 (1957).

COMSA, J.: Influence of in vitro added thyroxin upon the glucose uptake of the rat diaphragm. Experientia (Basel) **XIII**, 499 (1957).

CONARD, V.: Mesure de l'assimilisation du glucose. Acta méd. belg. éd. Bruxelles 1955.

— J. CHRISTOPHE, R. BELLENS, J. C. DEMANET et P. A. BASTENIE: Modifications métaboliques induites chez le rat normal par des traitements chroniques à la cortisone et au BZ 55. Acta endocr. **25**, 303—311 (1957).

CONSTAM, G. R.: Sulfonylurea compounds in the treatment of diabetes. Northw. Med. (Seattle) **1957**, 1155—1156.

— D. BONHÔTE, H. FELLMANN, A. HELLER, A. LABHART, O. SPÜHLER u. V. WENGER: Über blutzuckersenkende Sulfonamide. Schweiz. med. Wschr. **86**, 699—705 (1956).

CORI, C. F., and G. T. CORI: The influence of insulin and epinephrine on glycogen formation in the liver. J. biol. Chem. **85**, 275 (1929).

— — Die Kohlehydratbilanz an der hungernden Ratte nach Insulin- und Adrenalininjektion. Biochem. Z. **206**, 39—55 (1929).

COX, R. W., E. D. HENLEY, E. B. FERGUS and R. H. WILLIAMS: Sulfonylureas and diabetes mellitus. I. Clinical evaluation. Diabetes **5**, 358—365 (1956).

— — and R. H. WILLIAMS: Sulfonylureas and diabetes mellitus. II. Preliminary studies of the mechanism of action. Diabetes **5**, 366—371 (1956).

CRAIG, J. W., W. R. DRUCKER, M. MILLER, H. WOODWARD and V. MOLZAHN: A comparison of the influence of tolbutamide and small doses of insulin on the splanchnic output and peripheral uptake of glucose in man. Ann. N. Y. Acad. Sci. **74**, 537—547 (1959).

— M. MILLER, F. D. MILLS and N. NICKERSON: A comparison of the acute hypoglycemic potencies of tolbutamide and chlorpropamide. Ann. N. Y. Acad. Sci. **74**, 618—620 (1959).

— — H. WOODWARD JR., and E. MERIK: Influence of Phenethylbiguanide on lactic, pyruvic and citric acids in diabetic patients. Diabetes **9**, 186—193 (1960).

CREUTZFELDT, W.: Pankreasbefunde bei Diabetikern nach Behandlung mit D 860. Dtsch. med. Wschr. **1956**, 841—844.
— Alpha cell cytotoxins. Diabetes **6**, 135—145 (1957).
— Die pathologische Morphologie der Langerhans'schen Inseln im Experiment, besonders beim experimentellen Diabetes. Verh. dtsch. Ges. Path. **42**, 85—106 (1959).
— A-Zellveränderungen nach Synthalin und DBI und die Bedeutung des Glucagons für den Wirkungsmechanismus der Guanidinderivate. Mod. Probl. Pädiat. IV, 306—317 (1959).
— Morphologische Befunde an der Leber von Diabetikern nach langfristiger Sulfonylharnstoff-behandlung und an verschiedenen Organen nach Synthalin und DBI-Vergiftung beim Tier. Diabetes mellitus. 3. Kongreß der internat. Diab. Feder. Düsseldorf 1958, S. 267—274. Stuttgart: Georg Thieme 1959.
— Klinische Beziehungen zwischen Diabetes mellitus und Leber. Acta hepatol. (Hamburg) **6**, 156—177 (1959).
— F. ANDREU-KERN and R. DISCHER: Correlation of plasma levels of oral antidiabetic agents with blood sugar responses. Ann. N. Y. Acad. Sci. **82**, 537—546 (1959).
— u. K. BÖTTCHER: Die Wirkung des D 860 auf den Alloxandiabetes des Kaninchens. Dtsch. med. Wschr. **1956**, 896—899.
— L. DETERING u. O. WELTE: Das B-Zellsystem von normalen und hypophysektomierten Ratten sowie von Kaninchen unter D 860 und diabetogenen Hormonen. Dtsch. med. Wschr. **1957**, 1564—1568.
— u. DEUTICKE u. H. D. SÖLING: lPotenzierung der Wirkung von exogenem Insulin durch N-(4-Methylbenzolsulfonyl)-N-butycarbamid und N_1, n-Butylbiguanid. Klin. Wschr. **1961**, in press.
— u. H. FINTER: Blutzucker und histologische Veränderungen nach D 860 bei normalen Kaninchen. Dtsch. med. Wschr. **1956**, 892—896.
— — Unpublished investigations 1959.
— u. G. GEGINAT: Glukosetoleranz und Inselregeneration bei teilpankreatektomierten Ratten unter ACTH und langfristiger Behandlung mit N-(4-Methylbenzolsulfonyl) N'-butyl-harnstoff. Arzneimittel-Forsch. **8**, 464—469 (1958).
— F. KÜMMERLE u. E. KERN: Beobachtungen an vier Patienten mit totaler Duodenopankrea-tektomie wegen eines Karzinoms des Pankreas. Dtsch. med. Wschr. **1959**, 541—549.
— u. H. J. LEHMANN: Verhalten der alkalischen Phosphatase in den A-Zellen der Ratte nach D 860. Dtsch. med. Wschr. **1956**, 900.
— u. A. MOENCH: Vergleichende Untersuchungen mit den blutzuckersenkenden Guanidin-derivaten Synthalin B und Phenylätayldiguanid (DBI). (Ein Beitrag zur Frage der sog. A-Zellgifte). Endokrinologie **36**, 167 (1958).
— u. ST. SCHLAGINTWEIT: Kasuistischer Beitrag zur Wirkung der Sulfonylharnstoffe bei einigen Sonderformen der Zuckerkrankheit. Dtsch. med. Wschr. **1957**, 1539—1541.
— et H. SÜTTERLE: Recherches expérimentales sur le méchanisme d'action des sulfonamides hypoglycémiants. Ann. Endocr. (Paris) **18**, 184 (1957).
— — Vergleichende Untersuchungen über das Verhalten des Leber- und Diaphragma-Glykogens der Ratte unter Insulin und D 860. Dtsch. med. Wschr. **1957**, 1574—1576.
— u. E. TECKLENBORG: Synthalinhypoglykämie, A-Zellen und Glucagon. Klin. Wschr. **1955**, 43—44.
— — Experimentelle Untersuchungen zur Funktion der A-Zellen der Pankreasinseln und zur Glucagonwirkung. Naunyn-Schmiedebergs Arch. exp. Path. Pharmak. **227**, 23—61(1955).
CRONHEIM, G., and N. HYDER: Effect of salicylic acid on adrenal pituitary system. III. Studies on mechanism of this effect. Proc. Soc. exp. Biol. (N. Y.) **86**, 409—413 (1954).
— J. S. KING JR., and N. HYDER: Effect of salicylic acid and similar compounds on the adrenal-pituitary system. Proc. Soc. exp. Biol. (N. Y.) **80**, 51—55 (1952).
CROWLEY, M. F., F. W. WOLFF and A. BLOOM: Tolbutamide in diabetes. Some clinical and biochemical studies. Brit. med. J. **1957** II, 327—331.
CUGADDA, E., A. MANOLINI, R. LISPENEA: Variazoni dell'effetto insulinico del plasma in soggetti sani e diabitici trattati con carbutamide e tolbutamide. Minerva med. (Torino) **49**, 1500 (1958).
CUTOLO, E., e F. REDUZZI: L'acido tioctico inibisce l'insorgere del diabete da allossana nel ratto. Boll. Soc. ital. Biol. sper. **31**, 1532 (1955).
CZYZYK, A.: Der Einfluß von BZ 55 auf den Verlauf des Alloxandiabetes bei Kaninchen und auf den Glukagongehalt des Hundepankreas. Arzneimittel-Forsch. **6**, 700—701 (1956).
— u. G. MOHNIKE: Über die Beeinflussung der Alkoholtoleranz durch blutzuckersenkende Harnstoffderivate. Dtsch. med. Wschr. **1957**, 1585—1586.
DALE, H. H., G. GRAHAM, R. D. LAWRENCE and P. J. CAMMIDGE: Proc. roy. Soc. Med. **21**, 21 (1958).
DANOWSKI, T. S., M. H. KUNKEL, F. M. MATEER and F. A. WEIGAND: Lessened insulin hypo-phosphatemia following N-sulfanilyl-N'-butylurea (BZ 55 or carbutamide). Proc. Soc. exp. Biol. (N. Y.) **94**, 325—327 (1957).

DAVID: Synthalin und Leberschädigung. Dtsch. med. Wschr. **1928**, 473.

DAVIS, J. C.: Hydropic degeneration of the alpha-cells of the pancreatic islets produced by synthalin A. J. Path. Bact. **64**, 575—584 (1952).

DAVIS, T. W., R. B. KERR and A. BOGOCH: Experience with glipasol (R. F. 2259) — an antidiabetic sulfonamide drug. Canad. med. Ass. J. **81**, 101—107 (1959).

DE LAWTER, DE WITT, E., J. M. MOSS, S. TYROLER and J. J. CANARY: Secondary failure of response to tolbutamide therapy. J. Amer. med. Ass. **171**, 1786—1792 (1959).

DEUIL, R.: Le traitement du diabète par les hypoglycémiants oraux (sulfamides et biguanidines). Rev. Prat. **1959**, 2985—2992.

DEUTICKE, U., u. W. CREUTZFELDT: Wirkung von Sulfonylharnstoffen und Guanidinderivaten auf den Blutzucker und die Insulinempfindlichkeit der eviscerierten, nephrektomierten Ratte. Klin. Wschr. **1961** (in press).

DIBENEDETTO DELL'AQUILA, M., e D. ANGARANO: Azione del salicilato di sodio sul ricambio glicidico nell'uomo normale e diabetico. Folia endocr. (Pisa) **7**, 5—18 (1954).

DIENGOTT, D., and I. A. MIRSKY: Relation to quantity of sulfonylurea by mouth to the hypoglycemic response in normal human subjects. J. Pharmacol. exp. Ther. **118**, 168—173 (1956).

DITSCHUNEIT, H., E. F. PFEIFFER u. H. G. ROSSENBECK: Über die Bestimmung von Insulin im Blute am epididymalen Fettanhang der Ratte mit Hilfe markierter Glucose. III. Die Wirkung von Sulfonylharnstoffen und Biguanid (DBI) auf den Kohlenhydratstoffwechsel des isolierten Rattenfettgewebes und Rattenzwerchfells. Klin. Wschr. **1961**, 71—76.

DOBSON, H. L.: Diskussionsbemerkung. Conference on insulin and the oral hypoglycemic agents. (Indianapolis, Febr. 1959). Metabolism 8, 558 (1959).

— H. GUILAK, R. E. CARTER, H. MONTGOMERY and J. A. GREENE: The use of chlorpropamide in brittle and poorly controlled diabetes mellitus. Ann. N. Y. Acad. Sci. **74**, 940—952 (1959).

— — J. SCOGIN and R. E. CARTER: Clinical comparison of metahexamide with other oral hypoglycemic agents. Metabolism 8, 659—666 (1959).

DOLGER, H.: Clinical experience with orinase. Metabolism **5**, 946—952 (1956).

— Experience with the tolbutamide treatment of five hundred cases of diabetes on an ambulatory basis. Ann. N. Y. Acad. Sci. **71**, 275—279 (1957).

— An assessment of oral antidiabetic therapy. Ann. N. Y. Acad. Sci. **82**, 531—536 (1959).

— Combination of DBI with tolbutamide in diabetic therapy. Symposium on "A New Hypoglycemic Agent, Phenformin (DBI)". Houston (Texas) 1959.

DOMANOWSKY, K., W. LIMBACH, W. PRESSER u. F. J. ZAPP: Über die Nebenwirkungen der oralen Diabetestherapie mit besonderer Berücksichtigung eines Falles von schwerster allergischer Polyneuritis. Med. Klin. **1958**, 459.

DONE, A. K., R. S. ELY and V. C. KELLEY: Response of plasma 17-hydroxycorticosteroids to salicylate administration in normal human subjects. Metabolism 4, 129 (1955).

DORFMÜLLER, TH.: Untersuchung des Urins auf Eiweiß bei Verabreichung von D 860, einem neuen peroralen Antidiabeticum ohne antibakterielle Wirkung auf Koli. Ärztl. Lab. **2**, 264 (1956).

— Nachweis und Isolierung des Ausscheidungsproduktes von D 860. Dtsch. med. Wschr. **1956**, 888.

DOTEVALL, G.: Secondary resistance in oral treatment of diabetes. Acta med. scand. **161**, 251—256 (1958).

DOWNIE, E., J. BORNSTEIN and H. BREIDAHL: Preliminary clinical and experimental studies with chlorpropamide in diabetes mellitus. Ann. N. Y. Acad. Sci. **74**, 810—816 (1959).

— — B. HUDSON and K. TAYLOR: The role of sulphonylurea derivatives in the management of diabetes mellitus — a preliminary report. Med. J. Aust. **1956** I, 1072.

DREY, N. W., M. KARL, B. L. TAUSSIG, R. RUBIN, R. A. JOSHI and H. T. BLUMENTHAL: Preliminary observations on liver histochemistry and histopathology in diabetic patients receiving sulfonylurea euglycemic agents. Metabolism 8, 676—682 (1959).

DRILL, V. A.: Pharmacology in medicine. McGraw-Hill Book Co. Inc. 1958.

DULIN, W. E., and R. L. JOHNSTON: Studies concerning the role of the liver in the hypoglycemic response of animals to tolbutamide. Ann. N. Y. Acad. Sci. **71**, 177—191 (1957).

— and W. L. MILLER: Role of the pituitary in the response of rats to tolbutamide. Diabetes 8, 199—204 (1959).

— E. H. MORLEY and J. E. NEZAMIS: Role of adrenal in response to orinase. Proc. Soc. exp. Biol. (N. Y.) **93**, 132—136 (1956).

— Effects of long-term tolbutamide therapy on severety of diabetes in partially depancreatized rats. Metabolism **9**, 884—889 (1960).

DUMMER, G. M.: Die orale Diabetesbehandlung in der Chirurgie. Chirurg **28**, 7 (1957).

DUNCAN, L. J. P., and J. D. BAIRD: Oral insulin substitutes. Scot. med. J. **2**, 171—182 (1957).

— — and D. M. DUNLOP: A clinical trial of BZ 55. Brit. med. J. **1956** II, 433—439.

— J. D. N. NABARRO, W. G. OAKLEY and F. W. WOLFF: A warning note. Brit. med. J. **1956**, 454.

164 References

DUNLOP, D. M., J. D. BAIRD and L. J. P. DUNCAN: The antidiabetic sulphonamides. J. Endocrin. 15, 45—48 (1957).
DUNN, D. F., B. FRIEDMANN, A. R. MAAS, G. A. REICHARD and S. WEINHOUSE: Effects of insulin on blood glucose entry and removal rates in normal dogs. J. biol. Chem. 225, 225 (1957).
DUVE, CH. DE: The hepatic action of insulin. Ciba Foundation, Colloquia on Endocrinology. Vol. 9, Internal Secretions of the pancreas. London 1956, p. 203—222.
EBSTEIN, W.: Zur Therapie des Diabetes mellitus, insbesondere über die Anwendung des Salicyl-sauren Natron bei demselben. Berl. klin. Wschr. 13, 337—340 (1876).
EDELMANN, A., R. L. BOGNER and R. STEELE: Anethole, sodium salicylate and glycogen deposition in adrenalectomized fasted rat. Fed. Proc. 13, 39—40 (1954).
EDLEN, A., T. HERMANSSON u. S. STRANDQUIST: Oral Diabetesbehandling. Nord. Med. 58, 1658—1662 (1957).
EGELI, E. S., u. H. ALP: Die Glukose-6-Phosphatase-Aktivität der Leber bei normalen Menschen und Diabetikern. Z. klin. Med. 155, 191—194 (1958).
EGER, W., u. A. REINCKE: Sulfonamidderivate als nekrotrope Leberschutzstoffe. Arzneimittel-Forsch. 9, 363—365 (1959).
EHRHARDT, G.: Über neue peroral wirksame blutzuckersenkende Substanzen. Naturwissenschaften 43, 93 (1956).
EICKSTEDT, K. W. V.: Die Beeinflussung experimentell erzeugter Lebernekrosen durch blutzuckersenkende Sulfonylharnstoffverbindungen. Arzneimittel-Forsch. 8, 454—459 (1958).
EISMAYER, G.: Zur Synthalinbehandlung des Diabetes mellitus. Klin. Wschr. 1932, 860.
ELLENBERG, M.: Diabetic neuropathy precipitated by diabetic control with tolbutamide. J. Amer. med. Ass. 169, 1755—1757 (1959).
ELLINGTON, E. V., C. H. HASSALL and J. R. PLIMMER: Constitution of hypoglycin A. Chem. and Ind. 1958, 339—340.
ELRICK, H., and R. PURNELL: The response of kidney, liver and peripheral tissues to tolbutamide and insulin. Ann. N. Y. Acad. Sci. 71, 38—45 (1957).
ESMANN, V., K. LUNDBAEK and P. H. MADSEN: Clinical and laboratory effects of chlorpropamide, a new oral antidiabetic compound. Acta med. scand. 164, 73—79 (1959).
ESKUCHEN: Synthalinbehandlung des Diabetes. Klin. Wschr. 1928, 238 (Sitzungsbericht).
FABRYKANT, M.: Favorable effects of supplemental orinase in insulin-treated labile diabetes. Metabolism 6, 509—517 (1957).
— Use of orinase as a basic adjuvant in management of insulin-dependent diabetes. Metabolism 7, 213—221 (1958).
— and B. I. ASHE: Combined insulin-tolbutamide therapy in the management of insulin-dependent diabetes. Ann. N. Y. Acad. Sci. 82, 585—589 (1959).
FAJANS, ST. S., and J. W. CONN: An intravenous tolbutamide test as an adjunct in the diagnosis of functioning pancreatic islet cell adenomas. J. Lab. clin. Med. 54, 811—812 (1959).
— — Tolbutamide-induced amelioration of diabetes of young people with restoration of normal carbohydrate tolerance in some. Ann. Meet. Am. Diab. Ass. Atlantic City 1959.
— — Tolbutamide-induced improvement in carbohydrate tolerance of young people with mild diabetes mellitus. Diabetes 9, 83—88 (1960).
— L. H. LOUIS, H. S. SELTZER, R. D. GITTLER, A. R. HENNES, B. L. WAJCHENBERG, I. P. ACKERMANN and J. W. CONN: Metabolic effects of arylsulfonylurea compounds in normal men and in diabetic subjects. Metabolism 5, 820—839 (1956).
— J. A. MOORHOUSE, H. DOORENBOS, H. L. LAWRENCE and J. W. CONN: Metabolic effects of phenethylbiguanide in normal subjects and in diabetic patients. Diabetes 9, 194—201 (1960).
— — — L. H. LOUIS and J. W. CONN: Metabolic effects of phenethyl formamidinyliminourea in normal subjects and in diabetic patients. Clin. Res. 4, 252 (1958).
FALTA, W., u. F. HÖGLER: Die Zuckerkrankheit. 4. Aufl. Halle 1953.
FEENEY, G. C., P. CARLÓ and P. K. SMITH: Action of salicylates and related compounds on carbohydrate metabolism and on adrenal ascorbic acid and cholesterol concentrations. J. Pharmacol. exp. Ther. 114, 299—305 (1955).
FELLER, J., u. H. J. KÜPPER: Über einen Fall von schwerster allergischer Reaktion bei der peroralen Behandlung des Diabetes mellitus mit einem Sulfonylharnstoffderivat. (N_1-sulfanilyl-N_2-n-butylcarbamid). Medizinische 1956, 1641—1645.
FENG, P. C.: Effect of hypoglycin A on the alpha cells of the pancreas. Nature (Lond.) 180, 855—856 (1957).
— and S. J. PATRICK: Studies of the action of hypoglycin A, an hypoglycaemic substance. Brit. J. Pharmacol. 13, 125—130 (1958).
FERNER, H., and W. RUNGE: Synthalin A as selective mitotic poison acting on alpha-cells of the islets of Langerhans. Science 122, 420 (1955).
— — Morphologische Untersuchungen über die Wirkung des N_1-Sulfanilyl-N_2-n-butyl-carbamid auf die Inselzellen von Kaninchen und Ratten. Arzneimittel-Forsch. 6, 256—260 (1956).

FERNER, H., and W. RUNGE: Die Langerhans'schen Inseln von Diabetikern nach Behandlung mit dem oralen Antidiabeticum BZ 55. Dtsch. med. Wschr. 1956, 331—333.

FERRET, P., et J. IZARD: Un nouveau cas de diabète infantile sensible aux sulfamides hypoglycémiants. Presse méd. 67, 417 (1959).

FIELD. J. B., and D. D. FEDERMAN: Sudden death in a diabetic subject during treatment with BZ 55. Diabetes 6, 67 (1957).

— — Effects of carbutamide in the diabetes associated with acromegaly. Diabetes 6, 70—72 (1957).

— and M. L. WOODSON: Effect of oral hypoglycemic drug (carbutamide) on glycogen deposition by isolated rat diaphragm. Proc. Soc. exp. Biol. (N. Y.) 93, 534—536 (1956).

FISHGOLD, J. T., J. FIELD and V. E. HALL: Effect of sodium salicylate and acetylsalicylate on metabolism of rat brain and liver in vitro. Amer. J. Physiol. 164, 727 (1951).

FISTER, V., D. BAIĆ u. L. RABADJIJA: Verhinderung von Alloxandiabetes bei Ratten mittels BZ 55, D 860 und Sulfathiazole. Diabetes mellitus. 3. Kongreß der internat. Diab. Feder. Düsseldorf 1958, S. 352—354. Stuttgart: Georg Thieme 1959.

FOÀ, P. P., G. GALANSINO, G. D.'Amico and D. KANAMAISHI: Comparison of some metabolic effects of insulin, chlorpropamide and other hypoglycemic substances. Ann. N. Y. Acad. Sci. 74, 570—574 (1959).

— H. R. WEINSTEIN and J. A. SMITH: Secretion of insulin and of a hyperglycemic substance studied by means of pancreatic-femoral cross circulation experiments. Amer. J. Physiol. 157, 197 (1949).

FODDEN, J. H.: Experiments with chemicals noxious to the pancreatic alpha cells. Amer. J. clin. Path. 23, 1002—1011 (1953).

— and W. O. READ: The activity of extracted pancreatic hyperglycemic-glycogenolytic factor after cobaltous chloride and synthalin A. Endocrinology 54, 303 (1954).

FORBATH, N., and D. W. CLARKE: The effect of phenethylbiguanide upon the metabolism of the isolated rat diaphragm. Canad. J. Biochem. 37, 881 (1959).

FORIST, A. A.: Determination of metahexamide in human plasma. Ann. N. Y. Acad. Sci. 82, 496—501 (1959).

— W. L. MILLER, J. KRAKE and W. A. STRUCK: Determination of plasma levels of tolbutamide. Proc. Soc. exp. Biol. (N. Y.) 96, 180—183 (1957).

FORNEY, R. B., and H. R. HULPIEU: Lack of effect of carbutamide (BZ 55) on the metabolism of alcohol. Diabetes 6, 28—30 (1957).

FORSHAM, P. H.: Summary of the monograph "Current trends in research and clinical management of diabetes". Ann. N. Y. Acad. Sci. 82, 640—643 (1959).

— G. J. MAGID and D. E. DOROSIN: A clinical comparison of chlorpropamide and tolbutamide. Ann. N. Y. Acad. Sci. 74, 672—682 (1959).

FRAENKEL. K. A., u. K. SCHULZ: Kritische Betrachtungen zur Wirkungsweise des oralen Antidiabetikums Nadisan. Dtsch. med. J. 7, 209 (1956).

FRAENKEL-CONRAT, H. L., V. V. HERRING, M. E. SIMPSON and H. M. EVANS: Effect of purified pituitary preparations on the insulin content of the rat's pancreas. Amer. J. Physiol. 135, 404—410 (1942).

FRANCISCIS, P. DE, N. RUSSO, L. BERNINI e B. CAMPANELLI: Osservazioni sul compartomento glucidico dei cani diabetici trattati con i nuovi farmaci ipoglicemizzanti. Minerva med. (Torino) 49, 1504 (1958).

FRANK, E.: Synthalin. Med. Klin. 1928, 1218.

— M. NOTHMANN u. A. WAGNER: Über synthetisch dargestellte Körper mit insulinartiger Wirkung auf den normalen und den diabetischen Organismus. Klin. Wschr. 1926, 2100—2107.

— — — Über die experimentelle und klinische Wirkung des Synthalins B. Klin. Wschr. 1928, 1996—2000.

— — — Über die Guanidinhypoglykämie. Naunyn-Schmiedebergs Arch. exp. Path. Pharmak. 115, 55—63 (1926).

— — — Die Synthalinbehandlung des Diabetes mellitus. Dtsch. med. Wschr. 1926, Nr. 49/50.

— R. STERN u. M. NOTHMANN: Die Guanidin- und Dimethylguanidin-Toxikose des Säugetiers und ihre physiopathologische Bedeutung. Z. ges. exp. Med. 24, 341 (1921).

FRANKE, H., u. J. FUCHS: Ein neues antidiabetisches Prinzip. Dtsch. med. Wschr. 1955, 1449—1452.

FRASER, R., M. HARRISON, G. JOPLIN, G. STUART, J. VALLANCE-OWEN and F. WOLFF: The type of diabetic patient responding to oral sulphonamides. Diabetes mellitus. 3. Kongreß internat. Diab. Feder. 1958. Stuttgart 1959, 408—409.

FRAWLEY, TH. F., ST. SEGAL, M. M. CAMUS and J. FOLEY: A concept of the mechanism of sulfonylurea-induced hypoglycemia based on studies of glucose and pentose disposition in man. Ann. N. A. Acad. Sci. 71, 81—96 (1957).

FRAWLEY, TH. F., TH. F. SHELLEY, J. W. RUNYAN, E. J. MARGULIES and J. J. CINCOTTI: Further studies on the significant role of the liver in sulfonylurea hypoglycemia. Ann. N. Y. Acad. Sci. **82**, 460—478 (1959).

FREDERICQ, E.: The association of insulin molecular units in aqueous solutions. Arch. Biochem. **65**, 218 (1956).

FREINKEL, N., and S. H. INGBAR: The effects of the arylsulfonylureas on the respiratory activity and glucose metabolism of isolated rabbit kidney cortex. Endocrinology **64**, 1002—1009 (1959).

FREY, V.: Wird durch Carbutamid (Nadisan)-Behandlung die Kapillarbrüchigkeit von Zuckerkranken gesteigert? Schweiz. med. Wschr. **1959**, 933—934.

FRIEB, J.: Functional effects of priscol on various organs. (A comparison with nicotinic acid). Cas. Lék. Ces. **81**, 570—574 (1942).

FRIEDLANDER, E. O.: Use of tolbutamide in insulin-resistant diabetes. New Engl. J. Med. **257**, 11—14 (1957).

— and M. D. BRYANT: Idiopathic insulin-resistant diabetes mellitus. Amer. J. Med. **26**, 139—145 (1959).

FRIEDLICH, T. L., M. A. ASHWORTH, R. D. HAWKINS and R. E. HAIST: An effect of BZ 55 on the rate of absorption of glucose from the gastrointestinal tract. Canad. med. Ass. J. **74**, 973—974 (1956).

FRIEDMAN, M. B., and A. MARBLE: Island hyperplasia in partially depancreatized rat. Endocrinology **29**, 577 (1941).

FRITZ, I. B., J. V. MORTON, M. WEINSTEIN and R. LEVINE: Studies on the mechanism of action of the sulfonylureas. Metabolism **5**, 744—748 (1956).

— M. WEINSTEIN, J. V. MORTON and R. LEVINE: The effects of carbutamide (BZ 55) on blood sugar levels of depancreaticed dogs given insulin. Endocrinology **60**, 76—79 (1957).

FROST, I.: Carbutamide in treatment of schizophrenia. Brit. med. J. **1958 I**, 381—383.

FRY, I. K., and P. H. WRIGHT: The action of hypoglycemic sulphonylureas on carbohydrate metabolism in the fasted rat. Brit. J. Pharmacol. **12**, 350—355 (1957).

FUCHS, K. H., W. MICHEL u. H. K. FOERDER: Klinische Erfahrungen mit dem Sulfonylharnstoff BZ 55. Medizinische **1957**, 1290—1296.

FÜHNER, H.: Die Guanidingruppe. Handbuch der experimentellen Pharmakologie. Bd. I, S. 684—701. Berlin: Springer-Verlag 1923.

FULMER, H. S., A. H. DUBE and CH. W. LLOYD: Clinical experience with orinase. Metabolism **5**, 940—946 (1956).

FURTHMÜLLER, W., P. KÜHNE, F. MARTINI u. G. STÖTTER: Das Verhalten des Eiweißhaushaltes unter Rastinoneinwirkung. Dtsch. med. Wschr. **1957**, 1531—1533.

GABBE: Über die Wirkung des Synthalins auf den Gasstoffwechsel. Sitzungsbericht. Münch. med. Wschr. **1927**, 438.

GALANSINO, G., G. D'AMICO, D. KANAMEISHI and P. P. FOÀ: Mode of action of insulin, carbutamide and tolbutamide. Proc. Soc. exp. Biol. (N. Y.) **99**, 447—451 (1958).

— D. KANAMEISHI, F. G. BERLINGER and P. P. FOÀ: Comparison of the mode of action o. insulin and metahexamide. Metabolism **8**, 587—592 (1959).

GAMBASSI, G., e A. PIRELLI: Sul problema del mecanismo d'azione delle sulfoniluree ipoglicemizzanti. Arch. Pat. clin. med. **34**, 161—242 (1957).

GARATTINI, S., R. PAOLETTI and L. TESSARI: Influence of N_1-sulfonilyl-N_2-n-butyl-carbamide on glucose-V-C^{14} metabolism in the isolated rat diaphragm. Arzneimittel-Forsch. **8**, 477—479 (1958).

GARBERS, H.: Zur Frage des Wirkungsmechanismus der oralen Diabetestherapie mit BZ 55 und D 860 an Hand eines Falles von Diabetes mellitus beim Hund. Dtsch. tierärztl. Wschr. **64**, 104—105 (1957).

GELFAND, M. L.: Gastrointestinal bleeding during tolbutamide therapy. J. Amer. med. Ass. **171**, 258—260 (1959).

GENAZZINI, E., T. JAVICOLI e L. DONATELLI: Variazoni glicemiche da istamina e neoantergan. Boll. Soc. ital. Biol. sper. **27**, 787—788 (1951).

GEORGE, R., and L. E. WAY: The hypothalamus as an intermediary for pituitary-adrenal activation by aspirin. J. Pharmacol. exp. Ther. **119**, 310 (1957).

GEORGII, A., H. MEHNERT, R. PROSIEGEL, H. KASTEIN u. G. STOCK: Tierexperimentelle Leberbefunde nach langfristigen Sulfonylharnstoffgaben (D 860) und gleichzeitiger Leberschädigung mit Thioacetamid. Z. ges. exp. Med. **131**, 181—190 (1959).

— Tierexperimentelle Befunde zur Organtoxizität der Biguanide. In BERTRAM und MICHAEL: Internationales Biguanid-Symposium, S. 44—49. Stuttgart: G. Thieme 1960.

GEPTS, W.: Contribution à l'étude morphologique des îlots de Langerhans au cours du diabètes Les éditions «Acta Medica belgica», Bruxelles 1957.

GEPTS, W: Etude histologique de l'effet des sulfamides hypoglycémiants sur les îlots de Langerhans du rat. Ann. Endocr. (Paris) **18**, 204—217 (1957).

GEPS, W.: Die histopathologischen Veränderungen der Langerhansschen Inseln und ihre Bedeutung in der Frage der Pathogenese des menschlichen Diabetes. Endokrinologie **36**, 185—211 (1958).
— Histopathologie des îlots de Langerhans après traitement oral du diabète. Diabète **1958**, 215—222.
— J. CHRISTOPHE et R. BELLENS: Etude expérimentale d'un sulfamide hypoglycémiant. I. Modifications morphologiques provoquées chez le rat normal et le rat diabétique par le R. P. 2254. Ann. Endocr. (Paris) **16**, 946—955 (1956).
— — — Etude expérimentale du BZ 55 sur le rat normal ou alloxanisé. Modifications morphologiques et en particulier pancréatiques. Ann. Endocr. (Paris) **17**, 278—290 (1956).
— — and J. MAYER: Pancreatic islets in mice with the obesehyperglycemic syndrome. Lack of effect of carbutamide. Diabetes **9**, 63—69 (1960).
GERSCHENFELD, H. M., et A. J. SOLARI: Action d'un sulfamide hypoglycémiant sur les mitoses. C. R. Soc. Biol. **151**, 1017—1018 (1957).
— — Antimitotic action of tolbutamide. Lancet **1957** II, 544—545.
GERSTENBERG, E., A. HASSELBLATT u. G. SCHMIDT: Wirkung hoher Dosen des oralen Antidiabeticum D 860 („Artosin", „Rastinon") auf neuromotorische Funktionen, besonders des Rückenmarkes. Naunyn-Schmiedebergs Arch. exp. Path. Pharmak. **231**, 407—418 (1957).
GESSNER, O.: Über Synthalin. 1. Mitteilung: Die Beeinflussung der Metamorphose unter Schilddrüsenwirkung stehender Amphibien-Larven durch Synthalin. Naunyn-Schmiedebergs Arch. exp. Path. Pharmak. **127**, 223 (1928).
GHANEM, M. H., and M. N. MIKHAIL: The role of oral arylsulfonurea compounds in the managemant of diabetes mellitus. Alexandria med. J. **1957**, 383—409.
GIALRONI-GRASSI, G., C. GRASSI e F. VERGANI: Tests di tolleranza glucidica in corso di trattamento con sulfoniluree: modeficazioni dei tassi ematici di glucosio, fosforo, acido piruvico e acido lattico. G. ital. Tuberc. **11**, 3—7 (1957).
GITTLER, R. D., G. ZUCKER, R. EISENGER and N. STOLLER: Amelioration of diabetes mellitus by an insulinoma. New Engl. J. Med. **258**, 932—935 (1958).
GOETZ, F. C., and R. G. EGDAHL: Direct demonstration of insulin release from the pancreas by tolbutamide. Fed. Proc. **17**, 55 (1958).
— A. S. GILBERTSEN and V. JOSEPHSON: Acute effects of orinase on peripheral glucose utilization. Metabolism **5**, 788—800 (1956).
GOLD, A.: The treatment of diabetes mellitus with oral tolbutamide. Canad. J. Biochem. **35**, 953—960 (1957).
GOLDNER, M. G.: Historical review of oral substitutes for insulin. Diabetes **6**, 259—262 (1957).
— Diskussionsbemerkung. Symposium on the hypoglycemic agents. Metabolism **8**, 557 (1959).
— and R. H. JAUREGUI: Hypoglycemic action of an antihistaminic. A clinical evaluation. Amer. J. Dis. Child. **21**, 160—163 (1954).
— — Effect of histamine, epinephrine and antihistamine (antistine) on glucose turnover in the isolated liver. Proc. Soc. exp. Biol. (N. Y.) **85**, 347—349 (1954).
— SH. WEISENFELD u. G. HUGHES: Glukagon und die blutzuckersenkenden Sulfonylharnstoffe. Arzneimittel-Forsch. **8**, 432—435 (1958).
GONNARD, P., et J. DALLION: Etude expérimentale sur le BZ 55. Presse méd. **65**, 777—780 (1957).
— A. PELOU et C. NGUYEN PHILIPPON: Action de la carbutamide (BZ 55) sur l'adrénalinogénèse. Bull. Soc. Chim. biol. (Paris) **41**, 127—132 (1959).
GOOD, T. A., A. K. DONE, R. S. ELY and V. C. KELLEY: Effects of salicylate on plasma 17-hydroxy-corticosteroids in hypophysectomized and adrenalectomized guinea pigs. Metabolism **6**, 346 (1957).
GOOR, D. C., en J. TH. R. SCHREUDER: Polyneuritis na gebruick van nadisan. Ned. Ti. Geneesk. **101**, 402—403 (1957).
GORDON, R. S. jr., and A. CHERKES: Unesterified fatty acid in human blood plasma. J. clin. Invest. **35**, 206 (1956).
GORDON, M. F., J. F. BUSE and F. D. W. LUKENS: Hypoglycemic sulfonylureas in various types of experimental diabetes. Diabetes **6**, 7—12 (1957).
GORMAN, C. K., and J. A. WEAVER: Interrelations of tolbutamide and glucagon. Lancet **1959** II, 21—22.
GOURLEY, D. R. H.: Relation between structure of sulfonylurea compounds and their effect on frog muscle metabolism. Proc. Soc. exp. Biol. (N. Y.) **99**, 69—71 (1958).
— and R. H. DODD: In vitro effects of carbutamide on isolated frog muscle. Amer. J. Physiol. **192**, 471—475 (1958).
GRAFE, E., u. F. MEYTHALER: Beitrag zur Kenntnis der Regulation der Insulinproduktion. I. Der Traubenzucker als Hormon für die Insulinabgabe. Naunyn-Schmiedebergs Arch. exp. Path. Pharmak. **125**, 181—192 (1927).
GRANDE, F., and C. MARTÍNEZ: The effect of chlorpropamide on alloxan diabetes in mice. Ann. N. Y. Acad. Sci. **74**, 817—819 (1959).

GRANVILLE-GROSSMAN, K. L., S. CRAWFURD, M. F. CROWLEY and A. BLOOM: Further experience with oral therapy in diabetes. Brit. med. J. 1959 II, 841—847.

GREENHOUSE, B.: Clinical experience with chlorpropamide. Ann. N. Y. Acad. Sci. 74, 643—655 (1959).

GREENHOW, E. H.: Med. Times 1, 597 (1880); zit. nach GROSS, M., and L. A. GREENBERG.

GREIF, ST.: Erfahrungen mit der oralen Diabetesbehandlung. Wien. med. Wschr. 108, 318—322 (1958).

GRODSKY, G. M., and C. T. PENG: Insulin measured by immuno-chemical assay: effect of tolbutamide. Proc. Soc. exp. Biol. (N. Y.) 101, 100—103 (1959).

GROEN, J., H. VAN DER GELD, R. E. BOLINGER and A. F. WILLEBRANDS: The anti-insulin effect of epinephrine. Its significance for the determination of serum insulin by the rat diaphragm method. Diabetes 7, 272 (1958).

GROSS, M., and L. A. GREENBERG: The salicylates. New Haven/Con. Hillhouse Press: (1948).

GUGLIELMI, G., e ZUCCONI: Fissazione et eliminazione negli organi della carbutamide marcata con S^{35}. Minerva med. (Torino) 49, 1509—1511 (1958).

GURIAN, H., and D. ADLERSBERG: The effect of large doses of nicotinic acid on circulating lipids and carbohydrate tolerance. Amer. J. med. Sci. 237, 12—22 (1959).

GUSEK, W., u. J. KRACHT: Elektronenmikroskopische Untersuchungen über Inselwachstum und acinoinsuläre Transformation. Frankfurt. Z. Path. 70, 98—106 (1959).

— — Elektronenmikroskopische Befunde an der aktivierten Insel. Vortrag Dtsch. Ges. Endokrinol. April 1959.

GUTMAN, A., H. ZIFFER, and J. L. GABRILOVE: Effect of orinase (1-butyl-3-para-toluene sulfonylurea) on adrenal response to corticotropin. J. Mt. Sinai Hosp. 24, 516—518 (1957).

GUTSCHE, H.: Beeinflussung des Staub-Traugott-Effektes bei Biguanidbehandlung. In BERTRAM und MICHAEL: Internationales Biguanid-Symposium. S. 102—110. Stuttgart: G. Thieme 1960.

GYÖRGY, P., u. H. VOLLMER: Beeinflussung der Guanidinvergiftung durch Säurezufuhr. Naunyn-Schmiedebergs Arch. exp. Path. Pharmak. 95, 200—205 (1925).

HAACK, E.: Sulfanilyl- und Sulfonylcarbaminosäure-Derivate und ihre blutzuckersenkende Wirkung. Arzneimittel-Forsch. 8, 444—448 (1958).

HADLEY, W. B., A. KHACHADURIAN and A. MARBLE: Studies with chlorpropamide in diabetic patients. Ann. N. Y. Acad. Sci. 74, 621—624 (1959).

HÄGGBLOM, G.: Diabetes mellitus med dermatitis herpetiformis behandlad med carbutamide. Nord. Med. 59, 365 (1958).

HAILMAN, H. F.: ACTH and cortisone versus salicylates. J. clin. Endocr. 12, 454 (1952).

HAIST, R. E.: The pituitary and the insulin content of pancreas. J. Physiol. (Lond.) 98, 419—423 (1940).

— Factors affecting the insulin content of the pancreas. Physiol. Rev. 24, 409—444 (1944).

— Islet cell function. Ann. N. Y. Acad. Sci. 82, 266—286 (1959).

HALL, D. E., E. G. TOMICH, and E. A. WOOLETT: Metabolic effect of salicylate. Brit. med. J. 1954 II, 99.

HALL, G. H., M. F. CROWLEY and A. BLOOM: Oral treatment of diabetes. Brit. med. J. 2, 71 (1958).

HALLER, H.: Klinische Untersuchungen zur peroralen Diabetestherapie mit einem Sulfonylharnstoffderivat. Z. Ges. inn. Med. 12, 150—158 (1957).

— u. S. E. STRAUZENBERG: Ein Beitrag zur Beurteilung der Testverfahren für die Indikationsstellung der Behandlung des Diabetes mellitus mit Sulfonylharnstoffen. Dtsch. Gesundh.-Wes. 13, 1715—1719 (1958).

HAMFF, L. H., H. A. FERRIS, E. C. EVANS and H. W. WHITEMAN: The effects of tolbutamide and chlorpropamide on patients exhibiting jaundice as a result of previous chlorpropamide therapy. Ann. N. Y. Acad. Sci. 74, 820—829 (1959).

HAMWI, G. J., TH. G. SKILLMAN, L. R. FREEDY and L. A. ALEXANDER: Metabolic studies with metahexamide. Metabolism 8, 631—643 (1959).

— — F. A. KRUGER, W. H. ROUSH and L. R. FREEDY: Comparative pharmacology and clinical responses to metahexamide. Ann. N. Y. Acad. Sci. 82, 547—559 (1959).

HANDLER, P.: The effects of various inhibitors of carbohydrate metabolism in vivo. J. biol. Chem. 161, 53 (1945).

HANUSCH, A., u. D. JORKE: Sulfonamidblutspiegelbestimmungen bei Diabetikern. Ärztl. Forsch. 11 I, 451—457 (1957).

HÄRTEL, G.: Über die Bedeutung der Schilddrüse für das Auftreten von erhöhten Serumcholesterinwerten bei Ratten nach Fütterung von N_1-Sulfanilyl-N_2-n-butylcarbamid (BZ 55). Acta endocr. (Kbh.) 29, 267—272 (1958).

— u. V. ANTILA: Die Wirkung von N_1-sulfanilyl-N_2-n-butylcarbamid auf Serumcholesterin und Gesamtlipoide der Ratte. Arzneimittel-Forsch. 6, 701—703 (1956).

HARVEY, S. C., C. Y. WANG and M. NICKERSON: Blockade of epinephrine induced hyperglycemia. J. Pharmacol. exp. Ther. **104**, 363—376 (1952).

HASSALL, C. H., K. REYLE and P. FENG: Hypoglycin A, B: Biologically active polypeptides from blighia sapida. Nature (Lond.) **173**, 356 (1954).

— — Hypoglycin A and B, two biologically active polypeptides from Blighia sapida. Biochem. J. **60**, 334—339 (1955).

HASSELBLATT, A., u. G. BASTIAN: Vergleichende Untersuchungen über die krampferregende Wirkung von Insulin und N_1-(4-Methyl-benzolsulfonyl)-N_2-butyl-harnstoff an der Maus unter normalen und nach einer Behandlung mit Thyroxin verminderten Stoffwechselverhältnissen. Arzneimittel-Forsch. **8**, 590—594 (1958).

— u. W. BLUDAU: Dosisabhängigkeit von Serumkonzentration und Blutzuckerwirkung des N-4-Methylbenzolsulfonyl-N-butylharnstoff (D 860) bei intravenösen Dauerinfusionen. Klin. Wschr. **1958**, 157—163.

— u. G. HAUN: Die Insulinaktivität in Pfortader- und Venenblut des Kaninchens unter Insulin-, Rastinon- und Glucoseinfusionen. Z. ges. exp. Med. **133**, 163—176 (1960).

— — Die Bedeutung der sympathischen Innervation der Leber für die hemmende Wirkung von Chlorpromazin (Megaphen) und Veronal auf die Rastinonhypoglykämie. Klin. Wschr. **1960**, 1108—1112.

— u. R. SCHUSTER: Wirkung von Megaphen und Veronal auf die Rastinonhypoglykämie. Klin. Wschr. **1958**, 814—819.

HÄUSSLER, A.: Die Bestimmung von N_1-sulfanilyl-N_2-n-butylcarbamid im Serum, im Harn und im Kot. Arzneimittel-Forsch. **6**, 393—394 (1956).

HAWKINS, R. D., and R. E. HAIST: The effect of BZ 55 (carbutamide) on the glucose-6-phosphatase activity in the livers of intact and alloxanized female rats. Canad. J. Biochem. **35**, 215—218 (1957).

— M. A. ASHWORTH and E. E. HAIST: The effect of BZ 55 on glucose-6-phosphatase activity. Canad. med. Ass. J. **74**, 972—973 (1956).

HAZELWOOD, R. L.: The peripheral action of tolbutamide in domestic fowl. Endocrinology **63**, 611—618 (1958).

HECHT, A.: Unpublished data; zit. nach HECHT u. GOLDNER. Metabolism 8, 418—428 (1959).

— and G. GOLDNER: Reappraisal of the hypoglycemic action of acetylsalicylate. Metabolism 8, 418—428 (1959).

HEINEMANN, A., M. WEINSTEIN and R. LEVINE: Clinical experience with carbutamide and tolbutamide. Metabolism **5**, 972—977 (1956).

HEINIVAARA, O.: Studies on the effect of BZ 55 and D 860 on the pancreatic islet cells of rat. Ann. Med. intern. Fenn. **45**, 63—66 (1956).

HEINSEN, H. A.: Über die sogenannten „Spätversager" der peroralen Diabetestherapie. Endokrinologie **36**, 229—236 (1958).

— G. DEHN u. H. HAGEN: Klinische Untersuchungen an Zuckerkranken mit P 607 (Chlorpropamid), einem neuen peroralen Antidiabeticum. Med. Klin. **53**, 1685—1688 (1958).

— u. H. HAGEN: Kritisches zur peroralen Diabetestherapie. Med. Klin. **1956**, 1217—1221.

HENNES, A. R., B. L. WAJCHENBERGER, ST. S. FAJANS and J. W. CONN: Comparative effects of insulin and orinase on blood levels of pyruvate and alphaketoglutarate in normal subjects. Metabolism **6**, 63—69 (1959).

HENNING, N., H. KINZLMEIER, G. ZEITLER, I. NEUGEBAUER u. G. KOUTSOURIS: Über die Wirkung von BZ 55 und D 860 auf die Azidität und Motilität des Magens. Gastroenterologia (Basel) **87**, 65 (1957).

HENRY, W. L., J. H. KIM and A. S. HALL: Factors determining the liver glycogenating action of orinase. Amer. J Physiol. **192**, 514—516 (1958).

HERNANDEZ, D. M., R. R. CANDELA y J. L. R. CANDELA: Acción "in vitro" del DBI sobre el consumo de oxígeno y glucosa del cerebro y diafragma aislado de rata. Rev. ibér. Endocr. **25**, 39 (1958).

HESSE, E., u. G. TAUBMANN: Die Wirkung des Biguanids und seiner Derivate auf den Zuckerstoffwechsel. Naunyn-Schmiedebergs Arch. exp. Path. Pharmak. **142**, 290 (1929).

HESSE, L.: Experimentelle Untersuchungen über die Wirkung von Cortison, Prednisolon, N-[4-Methyl-benzolsulfonyl]-N′-butylharnstoff (D 860) und 5-(O-Tolyl-sulfonamido)-3-methyl-1,2,4-thiodiazol (Bayer 3282) auf die chronische CCl_4-Vergiftung der Ratte. Dissertation. Freiburg i. Br. 1960.

HETZEL, B. S., J. S. CHARNOCK and H. LANDER: Metabolic effects of salicylate in Man. Metabolism 8, 205—213 (1959).

— and D. C. HINE: The effect of salicylates on the pituitary and suprarenal glands Lancet **1951 II**, 94.

— R. WILLIAMS and H. LANDER: Early metabolic effects of triidothyronine and hydrocortisone in Man. Austr. Ann. Med. **6**, 218 (1957).

HILL, K. R.: Hypoglycemia and fatty metamorphosis of the liver in the vomiting sickness of Jamaica. J. Path. Bact. **66**, 334—335 (1953).

HIRSCH-KAUFFMANN, H., u. A. WAGNER: Zur Frage der Milchsäure-Produktion bei Synthalingebrauch. Klin. Wschr. **1928**, 1866.

HIRSCH-Mamroth, P., u. G. PERLMANN: Das synthetische Guanidinderivat Synthalin in der ambulanten Praxis. Dtsch. med. Wschr. **1927**, Nr. 3.

HOEPKER, W.: Insulinbedarfsminimum und Sulfonylharnstoffbehandlung des Diabetes mellitus. Klin. Wschr. **1957**, 668—672.

HOFSTETTER, J. R., et CL. RAMEL: L'application des sulfonyl-urées au traitement du diabète sucré. Schweiz. med. Wschr. **88**, 821—827 (1958).

HOLLUNGER, G.: Guanidines and oxidative phosphorylation. Acta Pharmacol. (Kbh.) **11**, Sup. 1, 7 (1955).

HOLT, C. v., u. I. BENEDICT: Biochemie des Hypoglycins A. II. Der Einfluß des Hypoglycins auf die Oxydation von Glucose und Fettsäuren. Biochem. Z. **331**, 430—435 (1959).

— u. H. FERNER: Morphologie der A-Zellbildung und der Entinselung des Pankreas. Z. Zellforsch. **42**, 305—330 (1955).

— et L. v. HOLT: Pancréas endocrine et antidiabétiques par voie orale. Ann. Endocr. (Paris) **18**, 171—173 (1957).

— — Der Einbau von V-C^{14}-Glukose in Leber- und Muskelglykogen unter Einwirkung von Aminobenzolsulfonylbutylharnstoff. Biochem. Z. **330**, 108—112 (1958).

— — Der Einfluß von Aminobenzolsulfonylbutylharnstoff auf die Glukoseabgabe der Leber und Glukoseaufnahme der Körperperipherie. Biochem. Z. **330**, 378—384 (1958).

— — Über die Wirkung von Arylsulfonylharnstoffen auf den Kohlehydratstoffwechsel. Endokrinologie **36**, 158—167 (1958).

— — J. KRACHT, B. KRÖNER and J. KÜHNAU: Carbutamide and plasma insulin activity. Science **125**, 735—736 (1957).

— — u. B. KRÖNER: Das Verhalten des Blutzuckers und des Leberglykogens adrenalektomierter Ratten bei isolierter Zerstörung der A-Zellen des Pankreas. Dtsch. med. Wschr. **80**, 648—649 (1955).

— — — Über die Wirkung von N_1-sulfanilyl-N_2-n-butylcarbamid auf den Kohlenhydratstoffwechsel. Naturwissenschaften **43**, 162 (1956).

— — — u. J. KÜHNAU: Chemische Ausschaltung der A-Zellen der Langerhansschen Inseln. Naturwissenschaften **41**, 166 (1954).

— — — — Chemische Ausschaltung der A-Zellen der Langerhansschen Inseln. Naunyn-Schmiedebergs Arch. exp. Path. Pharmak. **224**, 66—77 (1955).

— — — — Über die Wirkung der chemischen Ausschaltung der A-Zellen der Langerhansschen Inseln auf den Alloxandiabetes. Naunyn-Schmiedebergs Arch. exp. Path. Pharmak. **224**, 78—94 (1955).

— — — — Ciba foundation. Colloquia on Endocrinology **9**, 14—26 (1956).

— J. KRACHT, B. KRÖNER u. L. v. HOLT: Wirkung von N_1-Sulfanilyl-N_2-n-butylcarbamid auf Kohlenhydratstoffwechsel und endokrines System. Schweiz. med. Wschr. **86**, 1123 (1956).

— u. W. LEPPLA: Die Konstitution von Hypoglycin A. Angew. Chem. **70**, 25 (1958).

— — Die Konstitution von Hypoglycin A und B. Z. physiol. Chem. **313**, 276—290 (1958).

— — B. KRÖNER u. L. v. HOLT: Zur chemischen Kennzeichnung der Hypoglycine. Naturwissenschaften **43**, 279 (1956).

HOLT, L. v., u. C. v. HOLT: Biochemie des Hypoglycins A. I. Die Wirkung des Riboflavins auf den Hypoglycineffekt. Biochem. Z. **331**, 422—429 (1959).

— I. NOLTE u. C. v. HOLT: Wirkung der portalen Infusion von Insulin auf den Einbau von U-^{14}C-Glukose in Leber- und Muskelglykogen. Endokrinologie **37**, 36—42 (1959).

HORNUNG, ST.: Synthalin und Leberschädigung. Klin. Wschr. **1928**, 69.

HOUSSAY, B. A., et R. H. MIGLIORINI: Renforcement de l'action de l'insuline par les sulfamides hypoglycémiants. C. R. Soc. Biol. (Paris) **150**, 1620—1621 (1956).

— and J. C. PENHOS: Action of the hypoglycemic sulfonyl compounds in hypophysectomized, adrenalectomized and depancreatized animals. Metabolism **5**, 727—732 (1956).

— — N. TEODOSIO, J. BOWKETT and J. APELBAUM: Action of the hypoglycemic sulfonyl compounds in hypophysectomized, adrenalectomized and depancreatized animals. Ann. N. Y. Acad. Sci. **71**, 12—24 (1957).

— — E. URGOITI, N. TEODOSIO, J. APELBAUM and J. BOWKETT: The role of insulin in the action of the hypoglycemic sulfonyl compounds. Ann. N. Y. Acad. Sci. **71**, 25—34 (1957).

HSIEH, A. C. C., and C. C. CHIU: The effects of sodium salicylate on the oxygen consumption of the rat. Brit. J. Pharmacol. **14**, 219—221 (1959).

HUCKABEE, W. E.: Relationships of pyruvate and lactate during anaerobic metabolism. I. Effects of infusion of pyruvate or glucose and of hyperventilation. J. clin. Invest. **37**, 244 (1958).

HULTQUIST, G. T.: Hypoglycemic effect of monoiodoacetic acid and iodoacetamide in rats. Nature (Lond.) 182, 318—319 (1958).

HULTQUIST, G., G. NATHORST-WINDAHL och L. JOHANSSON: Några synpunkter på mekanismen för den antidiabetiska verkan av sulfonamidurinämnepreparat. Nord. Med. 58, 1873 (1957).

HUMBEL, R., M. STAUB u. E. R. FROESCH: Der Einfluß von Insulin und oralen Antidiabetica auf die Glukoseaufnahme und den Gasaustausch von isoliertem Fettgewebe. Schweiz. med. Wschr. 89, 381—382 (1959).

HUMBEL, R. E., K. VÖLLM, E. R. FROESCH u. A. LABHART: Insulinaktivität im Blut der V. hepatica und V. portae nach i. v. Carbutamid beim Menschen. Schweiz. med. Wschr. 89, 1217 (1959).

HUNT, J. A., W. OAKLEY and R. D. LAWRENCE: Clinical trial of the new oral hypoglycemic agent BZ 55. Brit. med. J. 1956, 4990, 445—448.

HURWITZ, D., and A. C. McCUISTION: Tolbutamide. A double-blind study of its effect in diabetes. New Engl. J. Med. 257, 931—933 (1957).

HUUASAKO, H.: Einfluß des Synthalins auf den Kohlehydratstoffwechsel des Kaninchens. Mitt. med. Akad. Kioto 28, 1107 (1940).

ILLIG, H.: Unterschiede zwischen Rastinon und Invenol bei der ambulanten Behandlung des Diabetes mellitus. Münch. med. Wschr. 1958, 117—119.

— TH. V. UEXKÜLL u. H. H. WAGNER: Nil nocere! Zur Frage der Leberschäden bei oraler Diabetestherapie. Münch. med. Wschr. 1959, 2121—2123.

INGLE, D. J.: Discussion. Recent Progr. Hormone Res. 7, 462 (1952).

— D. F. BEARY and A. PURMALIS: The effect of aspirin upon the glucosuria of partially depancreatized rats in the presence and absence of the adrenal glands. Endocrinology 52, 403—406 (1953).

— and R. C. MEEKS: Suppression of glycosuria during administration of large doses of aspirin to force-fed partially depancreatectomized rats. Amer. J. Physiol. 171, 600—603 (1952).

IRSKENS, K. J.: Über Erfahrungen mit der peroralen Diabetesbehandlung bei tuberkulösen Zuckerkranken. Ärztl. Wschr. 13, 346—348 (1958).

IZZO, J. L.: Metabolic effects of continued administration of sulfonylurea derivatives in selected diabetic subjects: interrelations with glucagon. Ann. N. Y. Acad. Sci. 74, 582—602 (1959).

JACKSON, W. P. U., and J. B. HERMAN: Agranulocytosis caused by BZ 55. Brit. med. J. 1956 II, 607.

— G. C. LINDER, S. SAUNDERS, R. HOFFENBERG, J. B. HERMAN, M. J. BAILEY, I. GRAYCE and R. WEINBERG: A clinical trial of D 860 (Rastinon) in diabetes. S. Afr. med. J. 31, 146—152 (1957).

JACOBI, J., u. K. BRÜLL: Über unsere Erfahrungen mit der Synthalintherapie des Diabetes mellitus. Med. Klin. 1927, 1017.

— u. M. KAMMRATH: Klinische Erfahrungen mit peroraler Diabetestherapie. Ärztl. Wschr. 11, 301—305 (1956).

JACOBS, G., G. REICHARD, E. H. GOODMAN, B. FRIEDMANN and S. WEINHOUSE: Action of insulin and tolbutamide on blood glucose entry and removal. Diabetes 7, 358—364 (1958).

JACONO, G., A. BRANCACCIO, B. D'ALESSANDRO e R. DE LUCA: Sul trattamento orale del diabete mellito con il 1-cicloesil-2-p-tolil-sulfanilurea (K 386). Minerva med. (Torino) 48, 3691—3697 (1957).

JANBON, M., J. CHAPTAL, A. VEDEL et J. SCHAAP: Accidents hypoglycémiques graves par un sulfamido-thiodiazol (le V. K. 57 ou 2254 R. P.). Communications. Soc. Sci. méd. biol. Montpellier 1942, 222—250; Montpellier méd. 1942, 441.

— P. LAZERGES et J. H. METROPOLITANSKI: Etude du métabolisme du sulfaisopropylthiodiazol chez le sujet sain et en cours de traitement comportement de la glycémie. Communications. Soc. Sci. méd. biol. Montpellier 1942, 212—221; Montpellier méd. 1942, 489.

JANES, R. G., H. A. ALERT and N. D. PAUL: Influence of glucose and tolbutamide in the fasted animal. Diabetes 8, 466—471 (1959).

JANSEN, W. H., u. H. BAUR: Klinische Erfahrungen mit Synthalin nebst Bemerkungen zum Mechanismus der Synthalinwirkung. Münch. med. Wschr. 1927, 441.

JELLIFFE, D. B, and K. L. STUART: Acute toxic hypoglycaemia in the vomiting sickness of Jamaica. Brit. med. J. 1954 I, 75.

JENSEN, S. E., K. LUNDBAEK, B. MÜLLER and O. J. RAFAELSEN: Effect of oral antidiabetic drugs on blood sugar and in organic phosphate curves in oral and intravenous glucose tolerance test. Acta med. scand. 160, 67—74 (1958).

JOHNSON, PH. C., A. R. HENNES, TH. DRISCOLL and K. M. WEST: Metabolic fate of chlorpropamide in man. Ann. N. Y. Acad. Sci. 74, 459—470 (1959).

JOPLIN, G. F., R. FRASER and J. VALLANCE-OWEN: Tolbutamide control of diabetes mellitus, selection of patients and persistence of response. Lancet 1959 I, 582—584.

JORDAN, H.: Veränderungen der Blutzuckerregulation durch den Cholinesterasehemmstoff Neoeserin. 1. Mitteilung. Dtsch. Z. Verdau- u. Stoffwechselkr. 18, 183—189 (1958).

JORES, J., u. J. KRACHT: Wirkung von Sulfonylharnstoffverbindungen auf die Mitosenfrequenz der insulären B-Zellen. Acta Endocrinologica **32**, 243—254 (1959).

JOST, F.: Blood dyscrasias associated with tolbutamide therapy. J. Amer. med. Ass. **169**, 1468—1469 (1959).

JUNKMANN, K.: Über Synthalin. VII. Mitteilung. Naunyn-Schmiedebergs Arch. exp. Path. Pharmak. **122**, 184 (1927).

KABELITZ, G., u. W. KAPPEL: Sulfonylharnstoffderivate in der Behandlung der Psoriasis vulgaris. Dtsch. med. Wschr. **1958**, 1167.

KÁCL, K., J. PROKES, F. VOREL u. E. AMCHOVÁ-PRAZÁKOVÁ: Bemerkungen zur Biochemie der blutzuckersenkenden Substanzen. Naturwissenschaften **43**, 401 (1956).

KAEDING, A.: Störungen der Leukopoese nach oraler Diabetesbehandlung. Dtsch. Gesundh.-Wes. **14**, 345—348 (1959).

KAHN, M., and V. PEREZ: Jaundice associated with administration of iproniazid: report of nine cases. Amer. J. Med. **25**, 898—916 (1958).

KÁLDOR, A., and G. POGÁTSA: The mode of action of oral antidiabetic compounds. Lancet **1959 I**, 386.

— — Inhibition of glycogenolysis with tolbutamide in liver slices. Lancet **1959 II**, 291.

— — and G. SZINAY: The effect of tolbutamide on toxic liver injury. Diabetes **9**, 126—128 (1960).

KAPLAN, E. H., J. KENNEDY and J. DAVIS: Effects of salicylate and other benzoates on oxidative Enzymes of the tricarbocylic acid cycle in rat tissue homogenate. Arch. Biochem. **51**, 47—61 (1954).

KAPLAN, N., and L. L. MADISON: Effects of endogenous insulinsecretion on the magnitude of hepatic binding of labeled-insulin during a single transhepatic circulation in human subjects. Clin. Res. **7**, 248 (1959).

KARR, W. G., W. P. BELK and O. H. PETTY: The toxicity of synthalin. J. Pharmacol. Ther. **36**, 611 (1929).

KAUFMANN, E.: Chronische Synthalinschäden. Med. Klin. **1928**, 1942.

KAUFMANN-COSLA, O.: and O. VASILCO: Experimentelle Untersuchungen über die Wirkung des Synthalins auf die Oxydation der Zelle. Naunyn-Schmiedebergs Arch. exp. Path. Pharmak. **157**, 154 (1931).

KAUP, H.: Vergleichende Untersuchungen über den Blutzuckerabfall nach intravenöser Gabe von Insulin und N-(4-Methyl-benzolsulfonyl)-N'-butylcarbamid (D 860) bei Lebergesunden und Zirrhotikern. Dissertation. Freiburg i. Br. 1958.

KENNEDY, E. P., and A. L. LEHNINGER: Phosphorus metabolism. Vol. II. Ed. by W. D. MCELROY and B. GLASS. Johns Hopkins Press 1952.

KERP, L., and W. CREUTZFELDT: To be published.

KHACHADURIAN, A. K., and H. S. BADEER: Effect of tolbutamide on glucose utilization by denervated heart-lung preparation. Metabolism **9**, 890—896 (1960).

KIBLER, R. F., and G. GORDON: Effect of tolylsulfonylurea (orinase) on net splanchnic glucose production in man. J. Lab. clin. Med. **48**, 824 (1956).

KINSELL, L. W., G. D. MICHAELS, F. R. BROWN and R. W. FRISKEY: Observations with sulfonylureas in diabetes. Metabolism **5**, 864—867 (1956).

KIRNBERGER, E. J., W. BRAUN, G. STILLE u. V. WOLF: Beziehungen zwischen Leberschutz und Zuckerstoffwechsel. Arzneimittel-Forsch. **8**, 72—76 (1958).

KIRPEKAR, S. M., and J. J. LEWIS: Effects of Reserpine, Chlorpromazine and Sodium Salicylate on the enzymic activity of rat liver. Brit. J. Pzarmacol. Chemotherap. **15**, 175—180 (1960).

KIRTLEY, W. R.: Occurrence of sensitivity and side reactions following carbutamide. Diabetes **6**, 72—73 (1957).

— A. S. RIDOLFO, M. A. ROOT and R. C. ANDERSON: Clinical and pharmacological effects of substance BZ 55 in diabetes. Diabetes **5**, 351—357 (1956).

KLAUS, D., u. W. STRIPECKE: Untersuchungen über die totale und renale Clearance des N_1-Sulfanilyl-N_2-n-butylcarbamide. Z. ges. inn. Med. **12**, 289 (1957).

KLEEBERG, J.: Synthalinbehandlung und ihre Gefahren. Z. klin. Med. **113**, 247—254 (1930).

KLEEFIELD, E. A.: Phenformin (DBI) in management of unstable diabetes in tuberculosis patients. Symposium on "A New Hypoglycemic Agent, Phenformin (DBI)". Houston (Texas) 1959.

KLEIBEL, F., u. J. FRANK: Akute Nierenschädigung bei der oralen Diabetes-Behandlung. Medizinische **1958**, 1147—1148.

KLEINSORGE, H.: Bemerkungen zu den Arbeiten über N_1-sulfanilyl-N_2-n-butylcarbamid als perorales Antidiabeticum. Dtsch. med. Wschr. **1956**, 750—751.

— Blutzuckersenkung durch Sulfonamidverbindungen. Z. ärztl. Fortbild. **50**, 407—411 (1956).

KLIMAS, J. E., and G. W. SEARLE: Effects of tolbutamide on intestinal glucose absorption and blood glucose levels. Proc. Soc. exp. Biol. (N. Y.) **98**, 901—902 (1958).

— — Tolbutamide and the onset of alloxan diabetes in rats. Diabetes **7**, 388—392 (1958).

KLOTZ, H. P., J. AVRIL, L. ISRAËL et GORINS: Premiers résultats du traitement de 15 diabètes par le BZ 55. Bull. Soc. med. Hôp. Paris **72**, 453—455 (1956).

KNAUFF, R. E., ST. J. FAJANS, E. RAMÍREZ and J. W. CONN: Metabolic studies of chlorpropamide in normal men and in diabetic subjects. Ann. N. Y. Acad. Sci. **74**, 603—617 (1959).

— — — — Metabolic half-life times, blood levels, potencies and activity patterns of metahexamide and other sulfonylurea compounds. Metabolism **8**, 606—613 (1959).

KNICK, B.: Zur klinischen Verwendung der oralen Antidiabetica aus der Sulfonylharnstoffreihe. Ärztl. Wschr. **13**, 618—623 (1958).

— u. K. EMRICH: Reversibilität von pathologischem Serum. Labilitätsproben, Elektrophoresediagramm und Leberfunktionstests bei chronischen Lebererkrankungen (chronische Hepatitis, Lebercirrhosen) unter Sulfonylharnstoffgaben (D 860). Klin. Wschr. **1957**, 812—814.

KNICK, B., u. J. RUCKES: Untersuchungen zur Frage der Leberschutzwirkung von Sulfonylharnstoffderivaten. Verh. dtsch. Ges. inn. Med. **65**, 709—712 (1959).

— — u. K. EMRICH: Tierexperimentelle Thioacetamid-Leberschäden unter therapeutischen Sulfonylharnstoffgaben (D 860). Z. exp. Med. **130**, 237—246 (1958).

KNITSCH, K. W.: Beitrag zum Wirkungsmechanismus des blutzuckersenkenden Harnstoffderivates N-(4-Methyl-benzolsulfonyl)-N'-butyl-harnstoff. Hoppe-Seylers Z. physiol. Chem. **309**, 184—189 (1957).

— u. G. MOHNIKE: Über die Wirkung von D 860 auf die Glukose-6-Phosphatase der Leber alloxandiabetischer Ratten. Naturwissenschaften **43**, 474 (1956).

— — Über die Wirkung von N-Sulfanilyl-N'-butylharnstoff auf den Glykogengehalt von Fettgeweben. Naturwissenschaften **45**, 292—293 (1958).

KOBAYASKI, Y.: New antidiabetic agent. On the treatment of diabetes mellitus with calcium mesoxalate (mesoxan). New Drugs and Therapy **1**, 21 (1957).

— and S. OHASHI: Hypoglycemic effect of mesoxalate produced by infusion into the pancreatic circulation in the dog. J. Pharmacol. exp. Ther. **115**, 343—349 (1955).

— — Mechanism of anti-diabetic activity of calcium mesoxalate. Jap. J. Pharmacol. **4**, 103—110 (1955).

— — and S. TAKEUCHI: Effect of salts of meso-oxalic acid on alloxan diabetes mellitus. Jap. J. Pharmacol. **1**, 9—21 (1951).

— — — and Y. IKEDA: Toxicity of mesoxalates and histological observations after continuous administration. Jap. J. Pharmacol. **4**, 111—117 (1955).

KOLAŘÍK, J., u. F. MIKULA: Eine neue therapeutische Anwendung oraler Antidiabetika. Wien. med. Wschr. **109**, 691—692 (1959).

KÖNIG, A.: Wirkungen unterschiedlicher Dosen von N-4-Methylbenzol-sulfonyl-N-butylharnstoff (D 860) und von Insulin auf den Blutzucker des stoffwechselgesunden Kaninchens unter verschiedenen Bedingungen (Vagotomie, Chloralosenarkose). Z. exp. Med. **131**, 131—138 (1959).

KÖNIGSTEIN, R. P., u. H. SUESS: Die Behandlung von tuberkulösen Diabetikern mit dem peroralen Antidiabeticum Invenol (BZ 55) und Rastinon (D 860). Wien. klin. Wschr. **69**, 501 (1957).

KOOPMANN, C.: Erfahrungen mit Biguaniden in der Therapie des Diabetes mellitus. In BERTRAM und MICHAEL: Internationales Biguanid-Symposium, S. 130—133. Stuttgart: G. Thieme 1960.

KORP, W., and PH. M. LE COMPTE: The nature and function of the alpha cells of the pancreas. Diabetes **4**, 347—366 (1955).

KRACHT, J.: In „Aktuelle Diabetesfragen, Symposion in Hamburg am 24. 1. 1957". Bearb. F. BERTRAM u. J. KUNTZE. S. 53. Stuttgart 1957.

— Experimentelle Morphologie des Inselorgans unter BZ 55, D 860 und IPTD. Medizinische **12**, 525 (1959).

— C. v. HOLT u. L. v. HOLT: Morphologische Befunde zur Wirkungsweise oraler Antidiabetica. Endokrinologie **34**, 129—146 (1957).

— B. KRÖNER, L. v. HOLT u. C. v. HOLT: Zunahme von Plasmainsulinaktivität und B-Zellmitosen nach D 860. Naturwissenschaften **44**, 16—17 (1957).

— u. J. G. RAUSCH-STROOMANN: Das Inselzellsystem unter N_1-sulfanilyl-N_2-n-butylcarbamid Naturwissenschaften **43**, 180 (1956).

KRAHL, M. E.: Discussion. Third Lilly Conference on Carbutamide, Sept. 1956. Diabetes **6**, 31 (1957).

KRALL, L. P.: The biguanides: their role in this era of the precise tool. Current trenchs in research and clinical management of diabetes. Ann. N. Y. Acad. Sci. **82**, 603—613 (1959).

— and R. F. BRADLEY: Clinical evaluation of formamidinyliminourea, a new biguanide oral blood sugar lowering compound. Comparison with other hypoglycemic agents. Ann. Int. med. **50**, 586 (1959).

— and R. CAMERINI-DAVALOS: Early clinical evaliation of a new oral non-sulfonylurea hypoglycemic agent. Proc. Soc. exp. Biol. (N. Y.) **95**, 345—347 (1957).

KRALL, L. P. and R. CAMERINI-DAVALOS: Clinical trials with DBI, a new nonsulfonylurea oral hypoglycemic agent. Arch. intern. Med. 102, 25—31 (1958).

KRALL, L. P., P. WHITE and R. F. BRADLEY: Clinical use of the biguanides and their role in stabilizing juvenile-type diabetes. Diabetes 7, 468—477 (1958).

KREBS, E. G., and E. H. FISHER: Zit bei WILLIAMS, TYBERGHEIN, HYDE and NIELSEN. Metabolism 6, 11 (1957).

KRESBACH, H.: Zur Kenntnis der Arzneimittelexantheme durch orale Antidiabetika. Derm. Wschr. 140, 1091—1096 (1959).

KRONEBERG, G., u. K. STOEPEL: Untersuchungen über die Guanidhypoglykämie und die Beeinflussung der Adrenalinwirkung durch β-Phenylacethyl-Biguanid und andere Guanidin-Verbindungen. Arzneimittel-Forsch. 8, 470 (1958).

KRUGER, F., TH. G. SKILLMAN, G. J. HAMWI, R. C. GRUBBS and N. DANFORTH: The mechanism of action of hypoglycemic guanidine derivatives. Diabetes 9, 170—173 (1960).

KUETHER, C. A., M. R. CLARK, E. G. SCOTT, H. M. LEE and C. W. PETTINGA: Lack of effect of carbutamide on activity of rat liver glucose-6-phosphatase. Proc. Soc. exp. Biol. (N. Y.) 93, 215—217 (1956).

KÜHNLEIN, E.: Das Verhalten der diabetischen Stoffwechsellage bei der akuten Hepatitis. Ärztl. Prax. 9, 23, 2—3 (1957).

KUJALOVÁ, V., u. P. FABRY: Der Einfluß von N_1-sulfanilyl-N_2-n-butylharnstoff und N_1-(4-Methylbenzolsulfonyl)-N_2-butylharnstoff auf die Resorption der Glukose aus dem Darm und auf die Motorik des Verdauungstraktes. Arzneimittel-Forsch. 10, 58—60 (1960).

KUNZ, W.: Die Wirkung von N-Sulfanilyl-N-Butyl-Carbamid auf Stoffwechsel und Wachstum von Transplantationstumoren. Naunyn-Schmiedebergs Arch. exp. Path. Pharmak. 232, Pharmak. 232, 350—351 (1957).

KURTZ, M., C. M. HOLTZMAN and E. MEILMAN: Tolbutamide hypoglycemia in acutely depancreatized dogs. J. clin. Invest. 38, 902—906 (1959).

KUUSISTO, A. N., and V. ANTILA: Has the new antidiabetic drug N_1-Sulphanilyl-N_2-n-Butylcarbamide goitrogenic properties? Acta endocr. (Kbh.) 23, 433—436 (1956).

LACY, P. E.: Personal communication.

— and W. ST. HARTROFT: Electron microscopy of the islets of Langerhans. Ann. N. Y. Acad. Sci. 82, 287—301 (1959).

LACHNIT, V., u. A. FERSTL: Klinische Untersuchungen eines blutzuckersenkenden Sulfonamids. Wien. Z. inn. Med. 37, 363—368 (1956).

— u. W. TRETENHAHN: Zur oralen Diabetestherapie. Wien. Z. inn. Med. 38, 123—127 (1957).

— — Serumphosphor bei Dextrosebelastungen vor und nach Gabe von oralen Antidiabetica. Wien. Z. inn. Med. 39, 463—467 (1958).

LAMBERT, S.: Hypoglycémie prolongée après invénol. Rev. méd. Liège 12, 88—89 (1957).

LAMBERT, T. H.: Clinical obersvations with a new oral hypoglycemic agent. Clin. Res. 6, 91 (1958).

LAMPRECHT, W., u. I. TRAUTSCHOLD: Nachweis eines direkten Insulineffektes auf den Kohlenhydratstoffwechsel der Leber. Hoppe-Seylers Z. physiol. Chem. 311, 245—255 (1958).

— — Zum Wirkungsmechanismus des N_1-sulfanilyl-N_2-n-butylcarbamid. Arzneimittel-Forsch. 8, 462—464 (1958).

LANG, ST., and S. SHERRY: Some effects of orinase in the rat. Metabolism 5, 733—738 (1956).

LANGDON, R. G., and D. R. WEAKLEY: The influence of hormonal factors and of diet upon hepatic glucose-6-phosphatase activity. J. biol. Chem. 214, 167 (1955).

LANGERON, L., Q. MICHAUX, A. DESTOMBES et J. PAUL: Action hypoglycémiante du P. A. S. (Note préliminaire). Presse méd. 58, 1037 (1950).

LARDY, H. A., and G. F. MALEY: Metabolic effects of thyroid hormones in vitro. Rec. Progr. Hormone Res. 7, 399 (1954).

LARSSON, Y.: Tolbutamide treatment of juvenile diabetes. Quart. Rev. Pediat. 13, 85 (1958).

LASS, A.: Gefahren der oralen Diabetestherapie während der Schwangerschaft. Geburtsh. u. Fraunheilk. 18, 1167—1171 (1958).

LÁSZLÓ, B., P. BRUCKNER, E. GÖRGEY és B. TÓTH: Acut hepatitises betegek kezelése peroralis antidiabeticummal (Bucarban). Orv. Hetil. 100, 1411—1413 (1959).

LAWRENCE, R. D.: Human and experimental diabetes. Ciba Foundation. Colloquia on Endocrinology. Vol. VI. Hormonal factors in carbohydrate metabolism. p. 243 (London 1953).

— Poisoning by tolbutamide. Brit. med. J. 1959 I, 644.

LAZAROW, A.: Cell types of the islets of Langerhans and the hormones they produce. Diabetes 6, 222—232 (1957).

— and B. TREIBERGS: The effect of long-term administration of tolbutamide to (alloxan)-subdiabetic rats. New Engl. J. Med. 261, 417—423 (1959).

LAZARUS, S. S.: Acid and glucose-6-phosphatase activity of pancreatic B cells after cortisone and sulfonylureas. Proc. Soc. exp. Biol. (N. Y.) 102, 303—306 (1959).

— M. BRADSHAW and B. W. VOLK: Toxic nephrosis in rabbits caused by the hypoglycemic biguanide, phenformin. Diabetes 9, 118—125 (1960).

LAZARUS, S. S., and B. W. VOLK: Functional and morphologic studies on the effect of orinase on the pancreas. Endocrinology **62**, 292—307 (1958).

LEACH, B. E., and J. C. FORBES: Sulfonamide drugs as protective agents against carbon tetrachloride poisoning. Proc. Soc. exp. Biol. (N. Y.) **48**, 361—363 (1941).

LEDERER, J., et R. DE MEYER: Influence de l'ingestion prolongée de BZ 55 à faible dose chez le rat. Ann. Endocr. (Paris) **18**, 252—257 (1957).

LEDUC, E. H., and J. W. WILSON: Injury to liver cells in carbon tetrachloride poisoning. Arch. Path. **65**, 147—157 (1958).

LEE, C. C., R. C. ANDERSON and K. K. CHEN: The effect of carbutamide on tubular glucose transport and glucose tolerance in dogs. Arch. int. pharmacodyn. **113**, 302—312 (1958).

LEE, CH. T., G. L. SCHLESS and G. G. DUNCAN: Clinical experiences with chlorpropamide: a double-blind study. Ann. N. Y. Acad. Sci. **74**, 738—745 (1959).

LEPPLA, W., u. C. V. HOLT: Blutzuckersenkende Peptide aus Blighia Sapida. Vortrag auf der 22. Tagung der Deutschen Pharmakol. Gesellschaft. Naunyn-Schmiedebergs Arch. exp. Path. Pharmak. **228**, 166—167 (1956).

LESTRADET, H., J. BESSE et C. JEZZEQUEL: Etude de l'action des substances hypoglycémiantes sur un groupe de 275 enfants diabétiques. Presse méd. **65**, 553—556 (1957).

LEVIN, M. E., and W. H. DAUGHADAY: Influence of thyroid on adrenocortical function. J. clin. Endocr. **15**, 1499 (1955).

LEVINE, R., M. S. GOLDSTEIN, B. HUDDLESTUN and S. KLEIN: Action of insulin on the "permeability" of cells to tree hexoses, as studied by its effect on the distribution of galactose. Amer. J. Physiol. **163**, 70 (1950).

LEWIS, CH.: Antibacterial properties of orinase in infected mice. Proc. Soc. exp. Biol. (N. Y.) **94**, 772—774 (1957).

LINDEMAN, R. D.: Severe hypoglycemia caused by chlorpropamide. Diabetes **9**, 110—113 (1960).

LINKE, A., K. RIEDERLE u. E. SCHULZ: Vergleichende Untersuchungen über die Wirkung von Sulfonylharnstoff (D 860) und von Insulin auf die Aktivität der Glukose-6-Phosphatase in der Leber von normalen und alloxandiabetischen Ratten. 6. Symposion Dtsch. Ges. Endokrinologie, 1959. Heidelberg: Springer S. 252—258.

LISBOA, P. E., N. CASTEL-BRANCO, M. MACHADO SA'MARQUES, M. J. ARROBAS e M. T. CORTEZ: Primeiros ensaios de terapêutica deambulatória da diabetes pela fenetil-diguanida (DBI). J. Méd. (Pôrto) **39**, 61 (1959).

LOBERG, K.: Eine klinische Methode zur quantitativen Bestimmung von Salicylsäure in Blutserum und Liquor cerebrospinalis. Biochem. Z. **170**, 173—184 (1926).

LOEWENTHAL, J. J., C. ROSS and G. TULLY: Experiences with chlorpropamide, especially in the brittle diabetes. Ann. N. Y. Acad. Sci. **74**, 860—862 (1959).

LOGOTHETOPOULOS, J., and J. M. SALTER: Zit. nach G. A. WRENSHALL (1957).

LOHMANN, D.: Zur Wirkung der peroralen Antidiabetika auf den Eiweißstoffwechsel. Dtsch. Z. Verdau.- u. Stoffwechselkr. **19**, 9—12 (1959).

LOOMIS, W. F., and F. LIPMANN: Reversible Inhibition of the coupling between phosphorylation and Oxidation. J. biol. Chem. **173**, 807—808 (1948).

LOUBATIÈRES, A.: Etude expérimentale chez le chien des accidents nerveux irréversibles consecutifs à l'hypoglycémie prolongée provoquée par le sulfa-isopropyl-thiodiazol. 43e Congrès des méd. alién. neurol. de France. Montpellier 1942; p. 415. Paris: Edit. Masson.

— Analyse du mécanisme de l'action hypoglycémiante du P-Amino-benzène sulfamido thiodiazol (2254 R. P.). C. R. Soc. Biol. (Paris) **138**, 766—767 (1944).

— Rélations entre la structure moléculaire et l'activité hypoglycémiante des amino-benzène-sulfamido-alkylthiodiazols. C. R. Soc. Biol. (Paris) **138**, 830 (1944).

— Physiologie et pharmaco-dynamie de certains dérivés sulfamidés hypoglycémiants. Contribution à l'étude des substances synthétiques à tropisme endocrinien. Thèse Doctorat Sci. naturelles, Montpellier 1946. No. 86. Montpellier: Edit. Causse, Graille et Castelnau 1956.

— Etude physiologique et pharmacodynamique de certains dévirés sulfamidés hypoglycémiants. Arch. int. Physiol. **54**, 174—177 (1946).

— L'utilisation de certaines substances sulfamidées dans le traitement du diabète sucré expérimental. Presse méd. **63**, 1701—1703, 1728—1730 (1955).

— Utilisation de substances sulfamidées dans le traitement du diabète sucré. Thérapie **10**, 907—926 (1955).

— Sulfamides hypoglycémiants et antidiabétiques. Antibiot. et Chemother. (Basel) **4**, 69—114 (1957).

— P. BOUYARD et C. FRUTEAU DE LACLOS: Arguments physiologiques récents en faveur de l'origine intrapancréatique de l'action hypoglycémiante et antidiabétique du p-amino-benzène-sulfamido-isopropyl-thiodiazol. C. R. Soc. Biol. (Paris) **149**, 2187 (1955).

176   References

LOUBATIÈRES A., P. BOUYARD et C. FRUTEAU DE LLGLOS: Etude expérimentale chez le
    diabétique humain du para-aminobenzène-sulfamido-isopropyl-thiodiazol. Sem. Hôp. Paris
    (Ann. Rech. Méd.) 32, 1—6 (1956).
— — — et A. SASSINE: L'hypophyse et les centres diencéphaliques sont ils directement
    impliqués dans l'action hypoglycémiante du para-aminobenzène-sulfamido-isopropyl-
    thiodiazol? C. R. Soc. Biol. (Paris) 150, 770 (1956).
— — — — La «guérison» du diabète sucré méta-alloxanique provoquée chez le chien par les
    sulfamides hypoglycémiants. Conditions expérimentales et caractères. C. R. Soc. Biol.
    (Paris) 151, 2179 (1957).
— — — — et R. ALRIC: Renforcement et prolongation des effets de l'insuline par les sulf-
    amides hypoglycémiants et antidiabétiques. C. R. Soc. Biol. (Paris) 150, 1601—1603 (1956).
— — A. SASSINE et C. FRUTEAU DE LACLOS: Le mécanisme et les conditions du maintien
    de la «guérison» du diabète sucré méta-alloxanique provoquée par les sulfamides hypo-
    glycémiants et antidiabètiques. J. Physiol. (Paris) 50, 383—386 (1958).
LOUIS, L. H., S. S. FAJANS, J. W. CONN, W. A. STRUCK, J. B. WRIGHT and J. L. JOHNSON:
    The structure of a urinary excretion product of 1-butyl-3-p-tolyl-sulfonylurea (orinase).
    J. Amer. chem. Soc. 78, 5701 (1956).
LOUKOPOULOS, L., C. ATHITAKIS u. G. BOUSWAROS: Hypoglykämisches Coma nach Verab-
    reichung von D 860. Münch. med. Wschr. 1957, 1456—1457.
LOEWENTHAL, D., and L. B. JAQUES: A comparative study of the effects of a series of aromatic
    acids on the ascorbic acid content of the adrenal gland. J. Pharmacol. exp. Ther. 107,
    172—177 (1952).
LUBLIN, A.: Der Einfluß des Synthalins auf den respiratorischen Quotienten beim Diabetiker.
    Naunyn-Schmiedebergs Arch. exp. Path. Pharmak. 124, 118 (1927).
LUNDBAEK, K., and K. NIELSEN: A comparative study on the action of three hypoglycemic
    compounds on the bloodsugar and the islet cells of the pancreas in the rat. Acta endocr.
    (Kbh.) 27, 325—338 (1958).
— — and O. J. RAFAELSEN: Mode of action of oral antidiabetic compounds. Lancet 1958 I,
    1036—1039.
LUNDSGAARD, E.: Insulin and glucose uptake by the liver. Acta physiol. scand. 31, 215—220
    (1954).
LUTWAK-MANN, C.: The effect of salicylate and cinchophen on enzymes and metabolic pro-
    gresses. Biochem. J. 36, 706—728 (1942).
LYNEN, F.: In: Conferences et rapports. 3me Congrès Internat. de Biochimie. Bruxelles 1956.
    S. 294. Liège 1956.
MACGREGOR, A. G., and A. R. SOMMER: The antithyroid action of para-aminosalicylic acid.
    Lancet 1954 II, 931—936.
MACH, B., R. A. FIELD and E. B. TAFT: Metahexamide jaundice. New Engl. J. Med. 261,
    438—440 (1959).
MADISON, L. L., B. COMBES, R. H. UNGER and N. KAPLAN: The relationship between the
    mechanism of action of the sulfonylureas and the secretion of insulin into the portal circu-
    lation. Ann. N. Y. Acad. Sci. 74, 548—556 (1959).
— and R. H. UNGER: The physiological significance of the secretion of endogenous insulin
    into the portal circulation. I. Comparison of the effects of glucagon-free insulin administered
    via the portal vein and via a peripheral vein on the magnitude of hypoglycemia and peri-
    pheral glucose utilization. J. clin. Invest. 37, 631—639 (1958).
— — Comparison of the effects of insulin and orinase (tolbutamide) on peripheral glucose
    utilization in the dog. Metabolism 7, 227—239 (1958).
— — Effect of phenformin on peripheral glucose utilization in human diabetic and non-
    diabetic subjects. Diabetes 9, 202—206 (1960).
MAGYAR, I., I. MARTON, Z. MATHE, Z. RÈFI és P. KERTAI: A szájon át ható antidiabeticumok
    hatás-mechanizmusa. Orv. Hetil. 1958, 885—889.
— — — — — Über den Wirkungsmechanismus der peroral wirkenden antidiabetischen
    Mittel. Z. ges. inn. Med. 13, 210—214 (1958).
— K. MEGYESI u. A. PÁLYI: Über die Anwendung von peroral wirksamen antidiabetischen
    Mitteln bei Leberschäden. Z. inn. Med. 12, 1000—1003 (1957).
MAHLER, R., W. C. SHOEMAKER and J. ASHMORE: Hepatic action of insulin. Ann. N. Y. Acad.
    Sci. 82, 452—459 (1959).
MAIER, E.: Todesfall unter peroraler Diabetesbehandlung mit Oranil. Z. ges. inn. Med. 12,
    567 (1957).
MAIER-WEINERTSGRÜN, D.: Guanidinderivate beim Diabetes mellitus (Synthalin, Glukhor-
    ment, Anticoman, Pancresal, Pancresalets). Dtsch. med. Wschr. 1937, 1400—1402.
MAMOU, H.: Myxoedème après traitements par les sulfamidés antidiabétiques. Sem. Hôp.
    Paris 33, 1044—1045 (1957).

MANCHESTER, K. L., P. J. RANDLE and G. H. SMITH: Some effects of sodium salicylate on muscle metabolism. Brit. med. J. 1, 1028 (1958).

MANCINI, R. E., J. C. PENHOS, H. M. GERSCHENFELD et I. IZQUIERDO: Action de l'hypoglycémie par l'insuline ou la tolbutamide sur le testicle du rat. C. R. Soc. Biol. (Paris) 152, 184—188 (1958).

MARBLE, A.: Symposium on "A New Oral Hypoglycemic Agent, Phenformin (DBI)". Diabetes 9, 225—227 (1960).

— and R. CAMERINI-DÁVALOS: Clinical experience with sulfonylurea compounds in diabetes. Ann. N. Y. Acad. Sci. 71, 239—248 (1957).

MARK, R. E.: Vergleichend therapeutische Beurteilung der peroralen Antidiabetika. Wien. med. Wschr. 108, 794—798 (1958).

MÅRTENSSON, J.: Effect of guanidine and synthalin on the citric acid metabolism. Acta med. scand. 125, 82 (1946).

MARTIN, F. I. R., J. R. LEONARDS and M. MILLER: A comparison of the effect of the intraportal and intravenous administration of J^{131}-insulin on peripheral blood glucose and serum radioactivity. Metabolism 8, 472—478 (1959).

MARTINEZ, C.: Effect of barbituric acid on alloxan diabetes in rats and dogs. Amer. J. Physiol. 182, 267—268 (1955).

MASKE, H.: Beobachtungen über das Zink in den Langerhansschen Inseln des Pankreas und seine Beziehungen zur Inselfunktion. Z. Naturforsch. 86, 96—104 (1953)

— Über die Beziehungen zwischen Insulin und Zink in den Langerhansschen Inseln des Pankreas. Experientia (Basel) 11, 122—128 (1955).

— Vorläufige Beobachtungen über das Verhalten des histochemisch nachweisbaren Zinks in den Langerhansschen Inseln von Kaninchen nach i. v. Injektion von D 860. Dtsch. med. Wschr. 1956, 899—900.

— K. MUNK, J. D. H. HCMAN u. R. MATTHIJSEN: Über die Verteilung von Insulin und Zink in verschiedenen Zellbestandteilen der Rieseninseln bei Flundern und Schollen. Z. Naturforsch. 11b, 407—415 (1956).

— B. STAMPFL u. H. GAHN: Untersuchungen zur Verhinderung der diabetogenen Alloxanwirkung durch vorher gegebenes Adrenalin. Z. klin. Med. 152, 68—72 (1953).

— H. WOLFF u. B. STAMPFE: Über die Verhinderung der diabetogenen Alloxanwirkung durch vorhergehende Glucosegaben. Klin. Wschr. 1953, 79—81.

MASSOBRIO, E., e G. BOGLIONE: Terapia antidiabetica per via orale. Minerva med. (Torino) 1956, 273.

McBRYDE, C. M., and B. L. TAUSSIG: Functional changes in liver, heart and muscles, and loss of dextrose tolerance resulting from dinitrophenol. J. Amer. med. Ass. 105, 13 (1935).

McCULLAGH, E. P., and H. W. GOEBERT: Effects of insulin with and without tolbutamide in a pancreatectomized woman. Diabetes 8, 315—316 (1959).

McGAVACK, TH. M.: Diskussionbemerkung. Seventeenth annual meeting of the Amer. Diabet. Assoc. New York City, Juni 1957. Diabetes 7, 91 (1958).

— W. SEEGERS, H. O. HAAR, J. ENZINGER and V. O. ERK: Thyroid function of diabetic patients as influenced by the sulfonylureas. Ann. N. Y. Acad. Sci. 71, 268—274 (1957).

— — H. O. HAAR and V. O. ERK: Some clinical experiences with the aryl sulfonylureas in the management of diabetes mellitus. Metabolism 5, 919—932 (1956).

McKENDRY, J. B. R.: Fatal hypoglycemic coma from the use of tolbutamide (Orinase). Canad. med. Ass. J. 76, 572—573 (1957).

— K. KUWAYTI and P. P. RADO: Clinical experience with DBI (phenformin) in the management of diabetes. Canad. med. Ass. J. 80, 773 (1959).

— — and L. A. SAGLE: Experience with tolbutamide (orinase) in the management of 100 cases of diabetes. Canad. med. Ass. J. 77, 429—438 (1957).

McKENZIE, J. M., P. B. MARSHALL and J. M. STOWERS: BZ 55 in diabetes. Brit. med. J. 1956, 4990, 448—451.

McLAMORE, W. M., G. M. FANELLI, S. Y. P'AN and G. D. LAUBACH: Hypoglycemic sulfonylureas: effect of structure on activity. Ann. N. Y. Acad. Sci. 74, 443—448 (1959).

MEADE, R. C., and H. M. KLITGAARD: Comparison of tolbutamide and insulin pretreatment prior to alloxan induced diabetes. Proc. Soc. exp. Biol. (N. Y.) 102, 410—413 (1959).

MEHNERT, H.: Der Einfluß eines neuen antidiabetisch wirksamen Sulfonamides auf die Darmflora. Klin. Wschr. 1956, 644.

— Über Wirkungsweise und Indikationsbereich oraler Antidiabetika. Dtsch. med. Wschr. 1958, 1273—1279.

— R. CAMERINI-DÁVALOS and A. MARBLE: Results of long-term use of tolbutamide (orinase) in diabetes mellitus. J. Amer. med. Ass. 167, 818—827 (1958).

— u. A. GEORGII: Zur Frage der Lebertoxizität oraler Antidiabetika. Medizinische 1959, 44—47.

MEHNERT, H., u. A. GEORGII: Untersuchungen zur Frage einer kombinierten oralen Diabetestherapie. Verh. dtsch. Ges. inn. Med. 65, 723—726 (1959).
— u. L. P. KRALL: Möglichkeiten und Grenzen der Diabetestherapie mit Biguanidderivaten. Dtsch. med. Wschr. 1960, 577—584.
— u. A. MARBLE: Der Wert des Tabletten-Schnelltests für die Indikationsstellung der Behandlung mit N-(4-Methyl-benzolsulfonyl)-N'-butylharnstoff. Arzneimittel-Forsch. 8, 435—438 (1958).
— u. B. MEHNERT: Zur Frage der Anwendung von BZ 55 oder D 860 als orales Antidiabeticum. Münch. med. Wschr. 1956, 1325—1328.
— u. W. SEITZ: Klinische Erfahrungen mit dem blutzuckersenkenden Biguanid DBI. Münch. med. Wschr. 1958, 1056.
— — Weitere Ergebnisse der Diabetesbehandlung mit blutzuckersenkenden Biguaniden. Münch. med. Wschr. 1958, 1849.
MEIER, H., and G. YERGANIAN: Spontaneous hereditary diabetes mellitus in the chinese hamster (Cricetulus griseus). III. Maintenance of a diabetic hamster colony with the aid of hypoglycemic therapy. Diabetes 10, 19—21 (1961).
MELLANDER, R.: Fall av hypoglykämiskt coma vid invenolbehandling av diabetes mellitus. Svenska Läk.-Tidn. 54, 450—453 (1957).
MELLINGHOFF, C. H.: Orale Diabetestherapie. Med. Klin. 51, 1497—1502 (1956).
MELZER, H., u. B. SACHSSE: Die orale Behandlung des Diabetes mellitus mit D 860 und BZ 55 Ärztl. Wschr. 11, 1058 (1956).
MEUTTER, R. DE, R. BELLENS et V. CONARD: Action d'un traitement prolongé au BZ 55 sur l'assimilation glucidique et la sensibilité à l'insuline du rat normal. C. R. Soc. Biol. (Paris) 150, 1800—1802 (1956).
MEUTTER, R. C. DE, A. K. KHACHADURIAN and A. MARBLE: Immediate effects of intravenous injections of tolbutamide and insulin on blood glucose and amino acids. Proc. Soc. exp. Biol. (N. Y.) 99, 33—35 (1958).
MEYER, R. DE, et M. ISAAC-MATHY: A propos de l'action tératogène d'un sulfamide hypoglycémiant (N-sulfanilil-N'-butylurée-BZ 55). Ann. Endocr. (Paris) 19, 167—172 (1958).
MEYERHOF, O.: Die Energieumwandlungen im Muskel. IV. Mitteilung über die Milchsäurebildung in der zerschnittenen Muskulatur. Pflügers Arch. ges. Physiol. 188, 114 (1921).
MEYER-LEDDIN, H. J.: Über den Wert des akuten Versuches mit dem oralen Antidiabeticum D 860. Med. Klin. 53, 1938—1939 (1958).
MICHEL, W.: Akute Belastungen mit Biguaniden bei Gesunden und Diabetikern. In BERTRAM und MICHAEL: Internationales Biguanid-Symposium, S. 111—116. Stuttgart: G. Thieme 1960.
MIDDLESWORTH, L. VAN, R. F. KLINE and S. W. BRITTON: Carbohydrate regulation under severe anoxic conditions. Amer. J. Physiol. 140, 474—482 (1944).
MILLER, L. L., J. E. SOKAL and E. J. SARCIONE: Effects of glucagon and tolbutamide on glycogen in isolated perfused rat liver. Amer. J. Physiol. 197, 286—288 (1959).
MILLER, M., and J. W. CRAIG: The use of tolbutamide in the management of various types of diabetes mellitus and studies of possible mechanisms of its actions. Metabolism 5, 868—875 (1956).
— — M. S. MACKENZIE, W. R. DRUCKER, M. CAMMARN and H. WOODWARD: Studies of the effect of intravenous tolbutamide on pyruvic and lactic acid concentrations in peripheral venous blood in normal and diabetic subjects and on splanchnic metabolism of fructose and glucose. Ann. N. Y. Acad. Sci. 71, 51—61 (1957).
MILLER, W. L. JR., and W. E. DULIN: Orinase, a new oral hypoglycemic compound. Science 123, 584—585 (1956).
— J. J. KRAKE and M. J. VAN DER BROOK: Studies on the utilization of uniformly labeled C14-glucose by rats given tolbutamide. J. Pharmacol. exp. Ther. 119, 513—521 (1957).
— — — and L. M. REINEKE: Studies on the absorption, mechanism of action and excretion of tolbutamide in the rat. Ann. N. Y. Acad. Sci. 71, 118—124 (1957).
MINOT, A. S.: The mechanism of the hypoglycemia induced by guanidine and carbon tetrachloride poisoning and its relief by calcium modication. J. Pharmacol. exp. Ther. 43, 295 (1931).
— and J. T. CUTLER: Guanidine retention and calcium reserve as antagonistic factors in carbon tetrachloride and chloroform poisoning. J. clin. Invest. 6, 369 (1928).
— — Studies of the response to calcium medication in the hypoglycemic of carbon tetrachloride poisoning. J. Physiol. 93, 674 (1930).
MIRSKY, I. A.: The role of insulinase and insulinase-inhibitors. Metabolism 5, 138—143 (1956).
— Insulinase, insulinase-inhibitors and diabetes mellitus. Recent Progr. Hormone Res. 13, 429 (1956).
— and R. H. BROH-KAHN: The inactivation of insulin by tissue extracts. Arch. Biochem. 20, 1 (1949).

MIRSKY, I. A. and D. DIENGOTT: The hypoglycemic response to insulin in man after sulfonylurea by mouth. J. clin. Endocr. 17, 603—607 (1957).
— — and H. DOLGER: Hypoglycemic action of sulfonylureas in patients with diabetes mellitus. Science 123, 583—584 (1956).
— — — The relation of various variables to the hypoglycemic action of 1-butyl-3-p-Tolylsulfonylurea in patients with diabetes mellitus. Metabolism 5, 875—893 (1956).
— and S. GITELSON: Comparison of the hypoglycemic action of tolbutamide in the fowl and other species. Endocrinology 61, 148—152 (1957).
— — and G. PERISUTTI: Inhibition of the diabetogenic action of somatotropin by tolbutamide. Ann. N. Y. Acad Sci. 74, 499—512 (1959).
— G. PERISUTTI and D. DIENGOTT: The inhibition of insulinase by hypoglycemic sulfonamides. Metabolism 5, 156—161 (1956).
— — and S. GITELSON: The role of insulinase in the hypoglycemic response to sulfonylureas. Ann. N. Y. Acad. Sci. 71, 103—111 (1957).
— — and R. JINKS: Ineffectiveness of sulfonylureas in alloxan diabetic rats. Proc. Soc. exp. Biol. (N. Y.) 91, 475—477 (1956).
MITIDIERI, E., and O. R. AFFONSO: Effect of salicylate on blood and liver xanthine dehydrogenase of Rats. Nature (Lond.) 183, 471—472 (1959).
MIYAKE, H.: Histological studies on the islets of Langerhans in normal rabbits and rats and those treated with sulfonamide derivatives. Endocr. jap. 5, 127—140 (1958).
MOELLER, J.: Die Bedeutung der Nadisan-Clearance und des Glomerulus-Filtrates für die Ansprechbarkeit auf die perorale Diabetesbehandlung. Diabetes mellitus. 3. Kongr. der intern. Diab. Feder. Düsseldorf 1958, S. 364—366. Stuttgart: Georg Thieme 1959.
— u. N. HÜMMER: Blutzuckersenkende Sulfonamide und Nierenfunktion. Verh. dtsch. Ges. inn. Med. 64, 297—299 (1958).
MOHNIKE, G.: Die Beeinflussung des Blutzuckers durch N_1-sulfanilyl-N_2-n-butyl-carbamid und Insulin beim Meta-Alloxan-Diabetes des Kaninchens. Arzneimittel-Forsch. 6, 388 bis 389 (1956).
— Daueranwendung von blutzuckersenkenden Harnstoffderivaten bei stoffwechselgesunden und alloxandiabetischen Hunden. Dtsch. med. Wschr. 1957, 1576—1578.
— u. H. BIBERGEIL: Die Wirkung von BZ 55 und D 860 auf den Blutzucker und den Serumspiegel an Phosphor, Kalium und Natrium von Hunden. Dtsch. med. Wschr. 1956, 900 bis 902.
— — u. A. CZYZYK: Blutzucker, Plasma-Amino-Stickstoff, sowie Phosphor und Kalium im Serum von gesunden und diabetischen Hunden unter akuten Belastungen mit blutzuckersenkenden Harnstoffderivaten. Dtsch. med. Wschr. 1957, 1579—1580.
— A. CZYZYK u. H. BIBERGEIL: Die Veränderungen einiger Blutbestandteile (Dextrose, Plasma-Amino-Stickstoff, Serumphosphor, Serumkalium) bei gesunden Hunden nach peroraler Gabe von blutzuckersenkenden Harnstoff-Derivaten. Arzneimittel-Forsch. 8, 475—477 (1958).
— — u. H. ULRICH: Akute Belastungen zur Frage der Stoffwechselwirkung von N-(4-Methyl-benzol-sulfonyl)-N'butylharnstoff (D 860) bei Gesunden und Diabetikern. Dtsch. med. Wschr. 1957, 1542—1544.
— u. V. HAGEMANN: Die Wirkung verschiedener Dosen von BZ 55 beim Kaninchen. Arzneimittel-Forsch. 6, 389—390 (1956).
— u. W. KNITSCH: Über die Wirkung von D 860 an Leberschnitten. Dtsch. med. Wschr. 1956, 891.
— — Über die Wirkung von D 860 auf die Glucose-6-Phosphatase der Leber. Naturwissensch. 43, 449 (1956).
— K. W. KNITSCH, H. BOSER, G. WERNER u. S. WERNER: Untersuchungen über die Wirkung von N-(4-Methyl-benzolsulfonyl)-N'-butylharnstoff (D 860) an Geweben und Fermenten in vitro. Dtsch. med. Wschr. 1957, 1580—1581.
— u. G. STÖTTER: Klinische Ergebnisse mit D 860. Dtsch. med. Wschr. 1956, 826—835.
— H. ULRICH, H. BIBERGEIL u. A. CZYZYK: Beobachtungen während der Einstellung von Diabetikern auf N-(4-Methyl-benzol-sulfonyl)-N'-butylharnstoff (D 860). Dtsch. med. Wschr. 1957, 1526—1528.
— — u. E. JUTZI: Untersuchungen zur Einstellbarkeit von Diabetikern auf N-(4-Methyl-benzolsulfonyl)-N'-butylharnstoff (D 860). Klin. Wschr. 1957, 845—848.
— — — Kriterien der Einstellbarkeit von Diabetikern auf N-(4-Methyl-benzolsulfonyl)-N'-butylharnstoff (D 860). Dtsch. med. Wschr. 1957, 1514—1515.
— — — Über Dauererfolge der D 860-Therapie. Dtsch. med. Wschr. 1957, 1524—1525.
— u. G. WITTENHAGEN: Über Blutspiegel und Ausscheidung von N-(4-Methyl-benzolsulfonyl)-N'-butylharnstoff (D 860). Dtsch. med. Wschr. 1957, 1556—1557.
— — u. W. LANGENBECK: Über das Ausscheidungsprodukt von N-(4-Methyl-benzolsulfonyl)-N'-butylharnstoff beim Hund. Naturwissenschaften 45, 13 (1958).

MONTENERO, P.: Über einen während Tolbutamidbehandlung aufgetretenen Fall von Myxoedem. Medizinische 1957, 1622—1623.

MOORHOUSE, J. A., S. S. FAJANS and J. W. CONN: The effect of phenethyl-biguanide on pyruvate utilization in man. Clin. Res. 6, 405 (1958).

— and R. M. KARK: Physiologic actions of orinase and their relationship to the types of diabetes in man. Metabolism 5, 847—863 (1956).

— — and D. D. GELLMAN: Effects of tolbutamide and insulin on fructose and glucose metabolism in diabetes mellitus. Ann. N. Y. Acad. Sci. 71, 97—102 (1957).

MORAWITZ, P.: Unsere Erfahrungen mit Synthalin. Münch. med. Wschr. 1927, 571.

MOREAU, R., R. DEUIL, A. SARRAZIN, P. M. DE TRAVERSE et M. MARTINET: Note préliminaire sur le traitement oral du diabète par le D 860. Presse méd. 64, 1261 (1956).

MORGAN, H. E., M. J. HENDERSON, D. M. REGEN and C. R. PARK: Regulation of glucose uptake in heart muscle from normal and alloxan-diabetic rats: The effects of insulin, growth hormone, cortisone and anoxia. Ann. N. Y. Acad. Sci. 82, 387 (1959).

MORGENSTERN, L. L., and E. R. GARRETT: Determination of the half life of metahexamide in normal humans. Ann. N. Y. Acad. Sci. 82, 502—507 (1959).

MORSIANI, M., e S. SERRAVALLI: L'1-Cicloesil-3-p-toluensolfonurea nella terapia del diabete mellito. Arcisped. S. Anna Ferrara 10, 2 (1957).

MORTIMORE, G. E., V. C. DI RAIMONDO and P. H. FORSHAM: Metabolic effects of orinase in diabetes including two cases complicated by other endocrinopathies. Metabolism 5, 840 bis 846 (1956).

— and F. TIETZE: Studies on the mechanism of capture and degradation of Insulin-J^{131} by the cyclically perfused rat liver. Ann. N. Y. Acad. Sci. 82, 329—337 (1959).

— — and DE WITT STETTEN: Metabolism of Insulin-J^{131}. Studies in isolated, perfused rat liver and hind-limb preparations. Diabetes 8, 307—314 (1959).

MOSCA, L.: Some effects of tolbutamide on the pancreatic islets of growing rats. Quart. J. exp. Physiol. 43, 265—269 (1958).

MOSINGER, B., and T. BRAUN: Potentiating the diabetogenic effect of alloxan by N-sulphonyl-N-butylurea (BZ 55). Experientia (Basel) 15, 317 (1959).

MOSS, D. G.: The estimation of BZ 55 and sulphonamides in blood sugar filtrates. J. clin. Path. 10, 371—372 (1957).

MOSS, J. M., and DE WITT E. DE LAWTER: Metahexamide in diabetes therapy. Ann. N. Y. Acad. Sci. 82, 614—617 (1959).

— — and J. J. CANARY: The results of the treatment with tolbutamide of 200 diabetic patients: a discussion of secondary failure. Ann. intern. Med. 50, 1407—1417 (1959).

MÜLLER, H., u. H.REINWEIN: Zur Pharmakologie des Galegins. Naunyn-Schmiedebergs Arch. exp. Path. Pharmak. 125, 212—228 (1927).

MUNRO, I. B., and D. MURRAY: Effect of carbutamide on serum-cholesterol level in diabetes mellitus. Lancet 1956 II, 1083—1084.

MURRAY, I., M. J. RIDDELL and I. WANG: Chlorpropamide a new hypoglycemic agent. Lancet 1958 II, 553—554.

— and I. WANG: Intermittent sulphonylurea therapy in the management of diabetes mellitus. Diabetes mellitus. 3. Kongr. der Internat. Diab. Feder. Düsseldorf 1958, 470—473. Stuttgart: Georg Thieme 1959.

MÜTING, D.: Über die Beeinflussung des Kohlenhydrat- und Eiweißhaushaltes Zuckerkranker durch Invenol. Ärztl. Wschr. 1957, 77—81 (1957).

NAUNYN, B.: Der Diabetes mellitus. 2. Aufl. Wien 1906.

NAYLER, W. G.: The action of salicylate, dinitrophenol and cardiac glycosides on the isolated toad heart. Austr. J. exp. Biol. med. Sci. 35, 491—498 (1957).

NEGELEIN, E.: Versuche über Glykolyse. Biochem. Z. 158, 121 (1925).

NELKEN, L.: Über den Einfluß der Guanidinvergiftung auf den Calcium- und Phosphatgehalt des Blutes. Klin. Wschr. 1923, 261.

NERENBERG, S. T.: Regranulation of beta-cells of islets of Langerhans following insulin and starvation. J. clin. Path. 23, 340 (1953).

NEUDECK, W.: Agranulocytose mit tödlichem Ausgang bei Diabetesbehandlung mit Oranil. Dtsch. Gesundh.-Wes. 12, 1326—1328 (1957).

NEUMANN, E.: Invenol in the therapy of psoriasis. Dermatologica (Basel) 117, 172—178 (1958).

NICHOLS, N.: The effect of glycogen deposition on liver phosphorous. J. clin. Invest. 34, 1710—1718 (1955).

NICOLAIER, A.: Ther. Mh. 7, 102 (1893); zit. nach M. GROSS and L. A. GREENBERG.

NIELSEN, R. L., H. E. SWANSON, D. C. TANNER and R. H. WILLIAMS: Presented at 39th Meeting of the Endocrine Society June 1957; zit. nach VOLK u. LAZARUS (1960).

— — — — and M. O'CONNELL: Effects on blood sugar of a new potent hypoglycemic compound. Arch. intern. Med. 101, 211—215 (1958).

NILSON, S.: Treatment of diabetes mellitus with a preparation containing salicylic acid, para-amino benzoic acid and ascorbic acid (Pascon). A therapeutic experiment. Acta med. scand. **165**, 273—273 (1959).

NISSEL, W., u. E. WIESEN: Behandlung des Diabetes mellitus mit Synthalin bei chirurgischen Komplikationen. Klin. Wschr. **1927**, 735.

OCHIAI, K.: On the histological changes of the organ and tissue especially of the liver and kidney caused by synthalin. J. orient. Med. **13**, 20—21 (1930).

ODELL, W. D., D. C. TANNER, D. F. STEINER and R. H. WILLIAMS: Phenethyl-amyl and isoamylbiguanide in the treatment of diabetes mellitus. Arch. intern. Med. **102**, 520 (1958).

O'DONOVAN, C. J.: Analysis of long-term experience with tolbutamide (Orinase) in the management of diabetes. Curr. therap. Res. **1**, 69—87 (1959).

OESTERREICHER, F., u. I. SNAPPER: Über die Beeinflussung des Phlorrhizindiabetes durch Synthalin. Klin. Wschr. **1927**, 1788.

OGRYZLO, M. A., and J. HARRISON: The effect of BZ 55 on pancreatic diabetes following pancreatectomy. Canad. med. Ass. J. **74**, 977—978 (1956).

ORTEL, S., u. G. MOHNIKE: Untersuchungen zur bakteriostatischen Wirkung blutzuckersenkender Substanzen und ihrer Ausscheidungsprodukte. Dtsch. med. Wschr. **1956**, 902—904.

ORTIGOSA, M. I., M. C. CARCIA-FERNANDEZ, R. R.-CANDELA y J. L. R.-CANDELA: Efecto de la tolbutamida (D 860) sobre la respiración y consumo de glucosa del cerebro y diafragma aislado de rata. Rev. ibér. Endocr. **5**, 31—37 (1957).

OTTO, H.: Behandlung jugendlicher Diabetiker mit Sulfonylharnstoff-Derivaten. Medizinische **1956**, 824—826.

— Die Zitronensäureausscheidung im Harn nach Verabfolgung von N-(4-Methyl-benzolsulfonyl)-N'-butyl-carbamid (D 860). Naturwissenschaften **44**, 12 (1957).

— Erste Erfahrungen mit Biguanid-Verbindungen in der Therapie des Diabetes mellitus. Medizinische **1958**, 1080.

— Untersuchungen mit Phenylaethylbiguanid (DBI) bei stoffwechselgesunden Menschen. In BERTRAM und MICHAEL: Internationales Biguanid-Symposium, S. 97—101. Stuttgart: G. Thieme 1960.

OTTO-BENDTFELDT, E., u. H. OTTO: Zur Frage der Spätmanifestation von Mißerfolgen der oralen Diabetesbehandlung. Arzneimittel-Forsch. **8**, 430—432 (1958).

OWEN, J. A.: A clinical comparison of tolbutamide, chlorpropamide and metahexamide in the treatment of diabetes. Metabolism **8**, 667—671 (1959).

PAGE, O. C., R. L. HARE, J. W. STEPHENS and B. HOLCOMB: Toxicity of carbutamide, report of a fatal case of bone-marrow depression and anuria. New Engl. J. Med. **256**, 74 (1957).

PAGLIARO, L.: Influenza dell'acido tioctico sul ricambio dei carboidrati, I). Boll. Soc. ital. Biol. sper. **32**, 49 (1956).

— Influenza dell'acido tioctico sul ricambio dei carboidrati II). Boll. Soc. ital. Biol. sper. **32**, 52 (1956).

PALMAS, S.: Azione della chlorpropamide in 110 casi di diabete mellito confronto con altri ipoglicemizzanti. Minerva med. (Torino) **50**, 2563—2569 (1959).

PARKER, V. H.: Analyst **74**, 646 (1949); zit. nach REID, J. (1958).

PASCHKIS, K. E., J. J. RUPP and X. JASOVSKY: Effect of cortisone, 9-alphafluorocortisol and growth hormone on the action of tolbutamide. Endocrinology **65**, 87—94 (1959).

PATEL, CH. A., and H. C. HEIM: The effect of monohydroxy benzoic acids on the respiration of rat brain homogenates. J. Amer. pharm. Ass., **43**, 251—253 (1954).

PATRICK, S. J.: Effect of hypoglycin A on liver glycogen with a method for the studies of changes in liver glycogen. J. appl. Physiol. **7**, 140—142 (1954).

— and J. A. TULLOCH: Glucose-6-phosphatase activity in human diabetics. Lancet **1957 I**, 811—812.

PEARLMAN, W.: The clinical results of the treatment of diabetes mellitus with DBI (Phenformin). Symposium on "A New Hypoglycemic Agent, Phenformin (DBI)". Houston (Texas) 1959.

PELLEGRINI, R.: Ricerche sperimentali sul un nuovo sulfamidico ad azione ipoglizemizzante. Arch. ital. Sci. farmacol. **6**, 299—304 (1956).

PENNIALL, R.: Effects of salicylic acid on aerobic respiration of rat brain preparations. Fed. Proc. **15**, 608 (1956).

PENTILÄ, I. M., and L. O. PÖLLÄNEN: Effect of insulin and tolbutamide on blood citric acid in rabbits. Scand. J. clin. Lab. Invest. **11**, 322—325 (1959).

PERKIN, F. S.: DBI in true labile or brittle "diabetes". Emphasizing influence on neuropathology. Symposium on "A New Hypoglycemic Agent, Phenformin (DBI)". Houston (Texas) 1959.

PERRINI, M., e D. RIZZI: Effetto inibitore della carbutamide su la glicogenolisi da tiroxina. Folia endocr. (Pisa) **10**, 689—694 (1957).

PETERS, G.: Insulinersatzmittel pflanzlichen Ursprungs. Dtsch. med. Wschr. **1957**, 320—322.

PETERSEN, O.: Hypoglycaemisk shock efter nadisanbehandlung. Nord. Med. **58**, 1668 (1957).

PETERSEN, P. V., and H. WEIDMANN: A study of the effect of various new synthetic compounds on the adrenal ascorbic acid. Acta pharmacol. (Kbh.) **11**, 103—110 (1955).

PETROVIC, C., CH. PILGRIM u. H. SÜDHOFF: Das Verhalten der maximalen tubulären Rückresorption für Glucose unter der Behandlung mit N_1-Sulfanilyl-N_2-n-butylcarbamid beim Hund. Naunyn-Schmiedebergs Arch. exp. Path. Pharmak. **235**, 96—102 (1959).

PETZOLD, H.: Die Wirkung von Rastinon (D 860) auf die experimentelle Fettleber der Ratte. Ärztl. Forsch. **13 (I)**, 162—167 (1959).

— u. K. STÖHR: Die Wirkung von N-(4-Amino-benzolsulfonyl)-N'-n-butylharnstoff (Oranil, Invenol) auf die Tetrachlorkohlenstoffibrose des Kaninchens. Z. Ges. inn. Med. **18**, 853 (1959).

PFAFFENBERG, R.: Über die Lungentuberkulose als Komplikation des Diabetes mellitus. S. 136—142. Leipzig: J. H. Barth Verlag 1959.

PFEFFER, K. H., K. J. FUCHS, W. MICHEL u. H. K. FOERDER: Die Wirkung von intravenös und oral verabreichten N_1-sulfanilyl-N_2-n-butylcarbamid (BZ 55) auf den Blutzucker bei Diabetikern und Stoffwechselgesunden. Ärztl. Wschr. **12**, 260—263 (1957).

— V. ZIMMER, K. J. FUCHS, H. KLUWE u. W. MICHEL: Die Behandlung der akuten und chronischen Hepatitis und ihrer Folgezustände mit Sulfonylharnstoff. Ärztl. Wschr. **1958**, 97—105.

PFEIFFER, E. F., M. PFEIFFER, H. DITSCHUNEIT and CHANG-SU AHN: Clinical and experimental studies of insulin secretion following tolbutamide and metahexamide administration. Ann. N. Y. Acad. Sci. **82**, 479—495 (1959).

— — — — Über die Bestimmung von Insulin im Blute am epididymalen Fettanhang der Ratte mit Hilfe markierter Glukose. II. Experimentelle und klinische Erfahrungen. Klin. Wschr. **1959**, 1239—1245.

— A. E. RENOLD, D. B. MARTIN, Y. DAGENAIS, J. W. MEAKIN, D. H. NELSON, G. SHOEMAKER u. G. W. THORN: Untersuchungen über die Rolle des Pankreas im Wirkungsmechanismus blutzuckersenkender Sulfonylharnstoffe. Diabetes mellitus. (III. Kongreß intern. Diabetes Federation 1958). Stuttgart 1959, 298—303.

— SCHÖFFLING u. H. STEIGERWALD: Die Ausscheidung von Nebennierenrindenhormonen während der Behandlung mit D 860. Dtsch. med. Wschr. **1956**, 838—841.

— — — H. DITSCHUNEIT u. F. HEUBEL: Die Bedeutung der einmaligen Tablettenbelastung für die Indikationsstellung der oralen Diabetestherapie. Dtsch. med. Wschr. **1957**, 1544 bis 1551.

— — — G. TRESER u. M. OTTO: Das Problem des Sekundärversagens der oralen Diabetesbehandlung. Dtsch. med. Wschr. **1957**, 1528—1531.

— H. STEIGERWALD, W. SANDRITTER, A. BÄNDER, A. MAGER, V. BECKER u. K. RETIENE: Vergleichende Untersuchungen von Morphologie und Hormongehalt des Kälberpankreas nach Sulfonylharnstoffen. Dtsch. med. Wschr. **1957**, 1568—1574.

PHEMISTER, J. C.: Thrombocytopenia and leucopenia following carbutamide. Brit. med. J. **1957 I**, 199—204.

PINES, K. L., E. LEIFER and DE WITT GOODMAN: Influence of chlorpropamide upon post pancreatectomy and spontaneous diabetes. Ann. N. Y. Acad. Sci. **74**, 997—1002 (1959).

PINTO, R. M., y R. NALLAR: Accíon del BZ 55 sobre la evolución de la preñez de la rata. Rev. argent. Endocr. **3**, 520 (1957).

PLATTNER, H. C.: Etudes sur le mode d'action des sulfonylurées dans le diabète humain. Rev. franç. Ét. clin. biol. **1957 II**, 803—807.

— Etudes sur le mode d'action des arylsulfonylurées hypoglycémiantes. Helv. med. Acta **26**, 829—859 (1959).

PLETSCHER, A.: Die Fructose, Biologie und Wirkung auf den Äthylalkohol-Spiegel. Helv. med. Acta **20**, 100—156 (1953).

— H. FAHRLÄNDER u. H. STAUB: Zum Kohlenhydratstoffwechsel. III. Fructoseumsatz bei Gesunden, Diabetikern und Leberkranken. Helv. physiol. pharmacol. Acta **9**, 46—54 (1951).

— u. K. F. GEY: Über die Wirkung blutzuckersenkender Sulfonylharnstoffe auf das isolierte Rattenzwerchfell. Experientia (Basel) **13**, 447—449 (1957).

POLLEN, R. H., R. H. BARNES, D. C. TANNER, W. H. STIMSON and R. H. WILLIAMS: Treatment of diabetes with metahexamid. Diabetes **9**, 25—30 (1960).

POMERANZE, J.: A new hypoglycemic agent. J. clin. Endocr. **17**, 1011 (1957).

— H. FUJIY and G. T. MOURATOFF: Clinical report of a new hypoglycemic agent. Proc. Soc. exp. Biol. (N. Y.) **95**, 193 (1957).

POMERANZE, J., and R. J. GADEK: Nineteen months experience with a new hypoglycemic drug. In: Diabetes mellitus. III. Kongreß d. Intern. Diab. Federation Düsseldorf 1959, S. 440. Stuttgart: G. Thieme.
— G. T. MOURATOFF, R. J. GADEK and E. J. KING: Phenethylbiguanide, a new orally given hypoglycemic agent. J. Amer. med. Ass. 171, 252—257 (1959).
POPPER, H.: Pathological findings in jaudice associated with iproniazid therapy. Amer. J. med. Ass. 168, 2235—2242 (1958).
POSSNER, W.: Betrachtungen zur Agranulozytose durch orale Antidiabetika anläßlich eines tödlich verlaufenen Falles nach Oranilmedikation. Dtsch. Gesundh.-Wes. 14, 765—770 (1959).
POZZA, G., G. GALANSINO and P. FOÀ: Insulin secretion following carbutamide injections in normal dogs. Proc. Soc. exp. Biol. (N. Y.) 93, 539—542 (1956).
— — H. HOFFIELD and P. P. FOÀ: Stimulation of insulin output by monosaccharides and monosaccharide derivatives. Amer. J. Physiol. 192, 497—500 (1958).
PRESSER, W., u. W. RITZERFELD: Untersuchungen zur bakteriostatischen Wirkung des Antidiabeticums Nadisan. Med. Klin. 1956, 1520—1523.
PRIESEL, R., u. R. WAGNER: Das Synthalin in der Behandlung der kindlichen Zuckerkrankheit. Klin. Wschr. 1927, 884.
PRINZ, R., u. A. GUTSCHKER: Agranulozytose unter Oranilbehandlung. Z. Ges. inn. Med. 12, 905—907 (1957).
PROD'HOM, S., et H. C. PLATTNER: Influence d'un sulfamidé hypoglycémiant sur la synthèse des graisses chez la souris. Arch. Sci. Geneva 10, 261—267 (1957).
— — et P. FAVARGER: Recherches sur la synthèse des graisses à partir d'acétate ou de glucose. V. Effet in vivo d'une sulfonylurée (BZ 55) chez la souris blanche et la souris obèse et hyperglycémique. Helv. physiol. pharmacol. Acta 17, 92—108 (1959).
PRÖSCHER, H.: Anwendung der Sulfonylharnstoffe in der Behandlung chirurgischer Komplikationen beim Diabetes mellitus. Berlin: VEB Verlag Volk und Gesundheit 1959.
PURNELL, R., Y. AVAI, E. PRATT, C. HLAD and H. ELRICK: Some observations on the mode of action of orinase. Metabolism 5, 778—787 (1956).
PURTSCHER, E.: Erkrankung der Sehnerven im Verlauf einer peroralen Diabetesbehandlung. Wien. klin. Wschr. 69, 340 (1957).
QUATTRIN, N., G. JACONO e A. G. BRANCACCIO: Ricerche sul metabolismo della sulfabutilurea. Minerva med. (Torino) 47, 1777—1780 (1956).
— — — Studio metabolico-farmacodinamico sulla sulfabutilurea. Minerva med. (Torino) 48, 1449—1475 (1957).
QUITZOW, G., R. SPIES u. G. WUNDRAK-WALDHEIM: Zur Frage der hepatotoxischen Wirkung chronischer Sulfonamidgaben im Rahmen der oralen Diabetestherapie. Wien. med. Wschr. 107, 464—466 (1957).
RADDING, R. S.: Metabolism of electrolytes with the use of DBI. Symposion on "A New Hypoglycemic Agent, Phenformin (DBI)". Houston (Texas) 1959.
RAFAELSEN, O. J.: Action of oral "antidiabetic" drugs on the carbohydrate metabolism of isolated rat diaphragm. In: Diabetes mellitus. III. Kongreß der International Diabetes Federation, Düsseldorf, 1959. Stuttgart: Georg Thieme 1959.
— Action of oral antidiabetic drugs on carbohydrate metabolism of isolated rat diaphragma. Metabolism 8, 195—204 (1959).
— and K. LUNDBAEK: Action of carbutamide on isolated diaphragm of alloxan-diabetic rats. Metabolism 8, 757—761 (1959).
RALLI, E. P., and A. M. TIBER: The comparative effects of synthalin and insulin on the depancreatized dog. J. Pharmacol. exp. Ther. 37, 451—461 (1929).
RAMEL, CL., et J. R. HOFSTETTER: Traitement ambulatoire des diabétiques avec un sulfamidé hypoglycémiant. Praxis 1956, 356.
RANDLE, P. J.: Anaerobic uptake of glucose in vitro by the isolated rat diaphragm. Nature (Lond.) 178, 983—984 (1956).
— and G. H. SMITH: Regulation of the uptake of glucose by the isolated rat diaphragm. Biochem. biophys. Acta 25, 442—443 (1957).
— — Regulation of glucose uptake by muscle. I. The effects of insulin, anaerobiosis and cell poisons on the uptake of glucose and release of potassium by isolated rat diaphragm. Biochem. J. 70, 490 (1958).
RATHERY, F., R. KOURILSKY et S. GIBERT: Effet de synthalin sur le glucose de sang du chien dépancréaté. C. R. Soc. Biol. (Paris) 99, 282 (1928).
— — — Effet de synthalin sur le glucose de sang du chien normal. C. R. Soc. (Paris) 99, 284 (1928).
— J. MILLOT et R. KOURILSKY: Etude des modifications histologiques dues a l'action de la synthaline. C. R. Soc. Biol. (Paris) 97, 523 (1927).
RAUSCH-STROOMANN, J. G., u. J. KRACHT: Experimentelle Untersuchungen zum Wirkungsmechanismus von Nadisan. Verh. dtsch. Ges. inn. Med. 62, 518—520 (1956).

RAUSCH-STROMANN u. H. SAUER: 17-Hydroxy-corticosteronspiegel im Plasma unter Therapie mit N_1-Sulfanilyl-N_2-N-Butylcarbamid. Klin. Wschr. 1957, 550—551.

— — Steroidhormonuntersuchungen unter Therapie mit Nadisan. Klin. Wschr. 34, 707 (1956).

READ, W. O., and J. H. FODDEN: Influence of synthalin A on glucose absorption in normal and experimental diabetic animals. Metabolism 3, 456—461 (1954).

RECANT, L., and G. L. FISCHER: Studies on the mechanism of tolbutamide hypoglycemia in animal and human subjects. Ann. N. Y. Acad. Sci. 71, 62—70 (1957).

RECKNAGEL, K.: Diabetes mellitus — BZ 55 — D 860 und Glukagon. Medizinische 1956, 1633—1639.

REICHARD, G. A., A. G. JACOBS, B. FRIEDMANN, PH. R. KIMBEL, N. J. HOCHELLA and S. WEINHOUSE: Effects of insulin and tolbutamide on production and utilization of blood sugar. Metabolism 8, 486—493 (1959); Ann. N. Y. Acad. Sci. 82, 412—419 (1959).

REID, J.: Dinitrophenol and diabetes mellitus. Brit. med. J. 2, 724—727 (1958).

— The insulin equivalence of salicylate. Brit. med. J. I, 897—900 (1959).

— A. J. DOUGALE and M. M. ANDREWS: Aspirin and diabetes. Brit. med. J. 2, 1071—1074 (1957).

REINWEIN, H.: Über die therapeutische Verwendbarkeit des Galegin bei Diabetikern. Münch. med. Wschr. 1927, 1794.

RENOLD, A. E., D. B. MARTIN, B. R. BOSHELL and G. W. THORN: Studies on the site of action of the arylsulfonylureas in man. Ann. N. Y. Acad. Sci. 71, 71—80 (1957).

— A. I. WINEGRAD, E. R. FROESCH and G. W. THORN: Studies on the action of certain sulfonylurea derivatives. Metabolism 5, 757—767 (1956).

— G. R. ZAHND, B. JEANRENAUD and B. R. BOSHELL: Some effects of tolbutamide and chlorpropamide in vitro. Ann. N. Y. Acad. Sci. 74, 490—498 (1959).

RICHTER, H.: Über die Blutzuckersenkung durch N-(4-Aminobenzolsulphonyl-)-N′-n-butylharnstoff und N-(4-Methylbenzolsulphonyl)-N′-n-butylharnstoff nach Leberausschaltung. Naturwissenschaften 45, 165 (1958).

RICKETTS, H. T., H. L. WILDBERGER and H. SCHMID: Long-term studies of the sulfonylureas in totally depancreatized dogs. Ann. N. Y. Acad. Sci. 71, 170—176 (1957).

RIDOLFO, A. S., and W. R. KIRTLEY: Clinical experiences with carbutamide, an orally given hypoglycemic agent. J. Amer. med. Ass. 160, 1285 (1956).

ROBBERS, H., u. F. SPECK: Die Nadisanbehandlung des Diabetes mellitus. Dtsch. med. Wschr. 1956, 1278.

R.-CANDELA, J. L., y R. R.-CANDELA: Acción de la carbutamida (BZ 55) sobre el efecto in sulínico del plasma. Rev. ibér. Endocr. 4, 413—415 (1957).

— and C. LOPEZ-QUIJADA: Influence "in vitro" of tolbutamide on the glucose up-take and glycogen synthesis of the epididymal fat. Med. exp. 2, 40—41 (1960).

RODRIGUEZ-MIÑÓN, J. L., y J. C. DE OYA: Sobre el mecanismo de acción de los derivados sulfamidicos hipoglucemicos. Rev. clin. esp. 66, 303—305 (1957).

RONDANINI, G. B.: Purpora emorragica bollosa da carbutamide. Minerva med. (Torino) 49, 1480—1481 (1958).

ROOT, M. A.: Pharmacology of carbutamide (p-aminophenylsulfonylbutylcarbamide). J. Pharmacol. 119, 468—478 (1957).

— Effect of carbutamide on the insulin content of the dog pancreas. Diabetes 6, 12—16 (1957).

— Diskussionsbemerkung zu J. A. SCHNEIDER u. Mitarb. Ann. N. Y. Acad. Sci. 74, 427 (1959); Ann. N. Y. Acad. Sci. 74, 441—442 (1959).

— R. C. ANDERSON and J. S. WELLES: Toxicology and pharmacology of metahexamide. Metabolism 8, 565—576 (1959).

— M. V. SIGAL and R. C. ANDERSON: Pharmacology of 1-(p-chlorobenzenesulfonyl)-3-n-propylurea (chlorpropamide). Diabetes 8, 7—13 (1959).

ROPP DE, R. S., J. C. VAN METER, E. C. DE RENZO, K. W. McKERNS, C. PIDACKS, P. H. BELL, E. F. ULLMANN, S. R. SAFIR, W. J. FANSHAWE and S. B. DAVIS: The structure and biological activities of hypoglycin. J. Amer. chem. Soc. 80, 1004 (1958).

ROSENKRANZ, A.: Die Beeinflussung des Diabetes mellitus durch Biguanid (DBI) im Kindesalter. Wien. med. Wschr. 1959, 1034—1039.

RÖTTGER, P. H.: Untersuchungen an der Rattenleber über die chronische und akute Thioacetamidvergiftung und ihre Beeinflussung durch Prednison und Rastinon. Dissertation, Freiburg i. Br. 1959.

ROWE, G. G., G. M. MAXWELL, C. CASTINO, D. A. EMANUEL, J. F. BROWN and B. SCHUSTER: Hemodynamic effects of salicylate. Circulation 14, 991 (1956).

RUIZ, C. L., L. L. SILVA and L. LIBENSON: Contribución al estudio sobre la composición química de la insulina. Estudio de algunos cuerpos sintéticos sulfurados con acción hipoglucemiante. Rev. Soc. argent. Biol. 6, 134—141 (1930).

RUNGE, W.: Die Wirkung des Synthalin A auf das Inselorgan des Meerschweinchens. Klin. Wschr. 1954, 748.

Runge, W., u. H. Heinrich: Über eine selektive Mitosehemmung und -schädigung bei jungen Ratten durch Synthalin A. Experientia (Basel) 11, 489 (1955).

Ruschig, H., G. Korger, W. Aumüller, H. Wagner, R. Weyer, A. Bänder u. J. Scholz: Neue peroral wirksame blutzuckersenkende Substanzen. Arzneimittel-Forsch. 8, 448—454 (1958).

— — — — — — — Über neue peroral wirksame blutzuckersenkende Substanzen. Med. u. Chem. 6, 61—118 (1958).

Sachsse, B.: Akute Belastungen mit D 860 im Hinblick auf die orale Diabetestherapie. Ärztl. Wschr. 1957, 870—871.

— Untersuchungen der Leberfunktion bei Diabetikern nach langdauernder Sulfonyl-Harnstoff-Therapie. Ärztl. Wschr. 1958, 886—887.

Sandritter, W., U. Becker, D. Müller u. E. F. Pfeiffer: Histochemische Untersuchungen zur Frage der Funktion der B-Zellen der Langerhansschen Inseln nach Stimulierung mit D 860. Endokrinologie 37, 193—217 (1959).

Sauer, H., u. G. Landbeck: Allergische Thrombocytopenie bei Sulfonylharnstofftherapie des Diabetes mellitus. Münch. med. Wschr. 1958, 1629.

Sauerbrei, H. U.: Zur oralen Behandlung des Diabetes mellitus im Kindesalter. Kinderärztl. Prax. 25, 2—7 (1957).

Savagnone, L.: Sulfamidi e ricambio idrocarbonato influenza della somministrazione di sulfamidi sul tasso glicemico in condizioni normali e patologiche. Settim. med. 29, 1005 (1941).

Sayers, G., M. A. Sayers, H. C. Lewis and C. N. H. Long: Effect of adrenotropic homone on ascorbic acid and cholesterol content of the adrenal. Proc. Soc. exp. Biol. (N. Y.) 55, 238—239 (1944).

Schadt, D. C., and D. C. Purnell: Salicylate intoxication in an adult. A. M. A. Arch. int. Med. 102, 213—216 (1958).

Schambye, P.: On the action of BZ 55 and D 860 in pancreatectomized dogs. Diabetes 6, 146—150 (1957).

— Etude physiologique et toxicologique de quelques substances hypoglycémiantes sur chiens normaux et dépancréatés. Ann. Endocr. (Paris) 18, 174—183 (1957).

— and F. Tarding: Changes induced by insulin and tolbutamide in the glucose output of the liver. Ann. N. Y. Acad. Sci. 74, 557—566 (1959).

Schilling, I.: Über die orale Behandlung des Diabetes mellitus mit Biguaniden. I. und II. Mitteilung. Z. ges. inn. Med. 14, 705 (1959); 14, 753 (1959).

Schirosa, G., e L. Pagliaro: L'acido tioctico nella terapia degli stati iperglicemici. Rif. med. 71, 32 (1957).

— — e G. Furitano: Sul meccanismo dell' azione ipoglicemizzante dell' acido tioctico. Boll. Soc. ital. Biol. sper. 32, 725 (1956).

Schliack, V., u. I. Schilling: Zur Therapie tuberkulöser Diabetiker mit blutzuckersenkenden Harnstoffderivaten I, II u. III. Schriftenreihe zur Z. ges. inn. Med. (Leipzig) 11, 7—41 (1959).

Schmidt, C. H., H. B. Hughes and C. C. Smith: On the pharmacology of N_1-parachlorophenyl-N_5-isopropylbiguanide (paludrine). J. Pharmacol. exp. Ther. 90, 233 (1947).

Schmidt, R.: Über glykämische und glykosurische Dyskrasien. Med. Klin. 1924, 511—516.

— Klinik des „sthenischen" Überdruckdiabetes. Klin. Wschr. 1930, 1969—1974.

Schmid, R., u. R. Blobel: Zur Frage der Beeinflussung der A-Zellen der Langerhansschen Inseln durch das Antidiabeticum D 860. Endokrinologie 34, 155—161 (1957).

Schnall, Ch., and J. S. Wiener: Nephrosis occurring during tolbutamide administration. J. Amer. med. Ass. 167, 214—215 (1958).

Schneeweiss, J., W. Gassmann u. A. Buding: Klinische Erfahrungen mit dem peroralen Antidiabeticum Invenol. Ärztl. Wschr. 1956, 266.

Schneider, J. A., E. D. Salgado, D. Jaeger and Ch. Delahunt: The pharmacology of chlorpropamide. Ann. N. Y. Acad. Sci. 74, 427—442 (1959).

Schöffling, K.: Diskussion zu Creutzfeldt, W. u. St. Schlagintweit. Dtsch. med. Wschr. 1957, 1541.

— E. F. Pfeiffer, H. Steigerwald, I. Bachrach u. U. Becker: Die Nebenwirkungen der langfristigen D 860-Behandlung. Dtsch. med. Wschr. 1957, 1537—1539.

— — G. Treser, H. Ditschuneit, H. Steigerwald u. M. Otto: Erfahrungen bei der ambulanten Einstellung und Dauerbehandlung von 758 Zuckerkranken mit D 860. Dtsch. med. Wschr. 1957, 1515—1518.

Schöler, H. F. L., and J. H. Gaarenstroom: The effect of BZ 55 on the pancreatic islets. Acta endocr. (Kbh.) 29, 147—159 (1958).

Scholz, J., u. A. Bänder: Pharmakologie des D 860. Dtsch. med. Wschr. 1956, 825—826.

Schreus, H. Th., u. H. Ippen: Photoallergie, hervorgerufen durch ein orales Antidiabeticum. Dtsch. med. Wschr. 1958, 98.

Schricker, K. T.: Ergebnisse der peroralen Therapie des Diabetes mellitus. Med. Klin. 1958, 57—59.

Searle, G. L., G. E. Mortimore, R. E. Buckley and W. A. Reilly: Plasma-glucose turnover in humans as studies with C^{14}-glucose. Influence of insulin and tolbutamide. Diabetes 8, 167—173 (1959).
— R. D. Palmer and W. A. Reilly: Influence of insulin and tolbutamide on glucose oxidation in man. Metabolism 9, 88—90 (1960).
Segal, S., T. F. Frawley and J. Foley: A comparison of tolbutamide and insulin on infused pentoses. A study in man. Diabetes 6, 422—425 (1957).
— A. Blair and A. Weinberg: In vitro effects of salicylate on carbohydrate metabolism. Metabolism 9, 1033—1046 (1960).
Seidler, I., W. Endres, R. Seus, M. Furthmüller, F. Martini, Th. Dorfmüller u. G. Stötter: Erfahrungen mit zweijähriger Behandlung mit Rastinon. Dtsch. med. Wschr. 1957, 1518—1523.
Seltzer, H. S., and W. L. Smith: "Plasma-insulin activity" in human diabetes during hypoglycemic response to tolbutamide and indole-3-acetic acid. Proc. Soc. exp. Biol. (N. Y.) 100, 171—174 (1959).
— and W. L. Smith: Plasma insulin activity after glucose. Diabetes 8, 417—424 (1959).
Seydl, G., u. H. Schulleri: Zur Behandlung des Diabetes mellitus mit Biguanid. Med. Klin. 1959, 1081.
Shannon, I. A., S. Farber u. L. Troast: The measurement of glucose T_m in the normal dog Amer. Physiol. 133, 752(1941).
Shapiro, L. S.: Chemical properties of DBI and other hypoglycemic biguanides. Symposium on "A New Hypoglycemic Agent, Phenformin (DBI)". Houston (Texas) 1959.
Shepherd jr., H. G., and J. H. McDonald: Effect of Phenethylbiguanide on serum inorganic phosphate. Proc. Soc. exp. Biol. (N. Y.) 102, 390—392 (1959).
— — The binding affinity of purified plasma proteins for phenethyldiguanide, an oral hypoglycemic compound. (In press).
Sherif, M. A. F., M. B. Razzak and A. M. Hassaballah: Comparative study of some imidazoline derivatives and dihydrogenated ergot alkaloids on blood sugar and gastric acidity. Arch. int. Pharmacodyn. 110, 1—9 (1957).
Shoemaker, W. C., R. Mahler and J. Ashmore: The effect of insulin on hepatic glucose metabolism in the unaesthetized dog. Metabolism 8, 491—511 (1959).
— — — D. E. Pugh and A. B. Hastings: The hepatic glucose response to insulin in the unaesthetized dog. J. biol. Chem. 234, 1631—1633 (1959).
Signorelli, S.: Tolerance for alcohol in patients on chlorpropamide. Ann. N. Y. Acad. Sci. 74, 900—903 (1959).
— e P. Posa: La nostra esperienza sull' impiego terapeutico di una nuova sulfanilurea: N-propil-N-(p-cloro-benzensulfonil)urea-P 607, per via orale nel diabete mellito. Minerva med. (Torino) 50, 2535—2542 (1959).
Silver, A. A., and H. Nagel: The effects of chronic administration of tolbutamide (orinase) in aged diabetics. Maryland med. J. 6, 690 (1957).
— H. Wishinsky, R. F. Caplan and C. Monk: Laboratory and clinical observations with a new sulfonylurea. Ann. N. Y. Acad. Sci. 82, 624—631 (1959).
Simmonnet, H., et G. Tanret: Sur les propriétés hypoglycémiantes du sulfate de galégine. Bull. Soc. chim. biol. 9, 908 (1927).
Simoes, M. S., and W. Osswald: Chlorpromazine protection against alloxan diabetes. Metabolism 4, 333—336 (1955).
Simola, P. E.: Über die Wirkung des Synthalins im Tierorganismus. Hoppe-Seylers Z. physiol. Chem. 168, 274 (1927).
Singer, H.: Über Aspirin. Beitrag zur Kenntnis der Salicylwirkung. Pflügers Arch. ges. Physiol. 84, 527—546 (1901).
Singh, I., and P. N. Bardhan: Tolbutamide in the treatment of angina pectoris. Lancet 1959 II, 1141—1142.
Siperstein, M. D.: Inter-relationships of glucose and lipid metabolism. Amer. J. med. 26, 685—702 (1959).
Siperstein, M., and L. L. Madison: The stimulatory effect of DBI on oxidation of glucose via the hexose monophosphate shunt. (To be published); zit. bei Madison u. Unger (1960).
Sirek, A., and O. V. Sirek: The action of BZ 55 in dogs. I. Observations on depancreatized and houssay dogs. Canad. med. Ass. J. 74, 960—962 (1956).
— — and Ch. Best: The toxic effect of carbutamide (BZ 55) in diabetic dogs. Diabetes 6, 151—153 (1957).
— — Y. Hanus, F. C. Monkhouse and Ch. H. Best: Effect of prolonged administration of tolbutamide in depancreatized dogs. Diabetes 8, 284—288 (1959).
— — J. Logothetopolous and Ch. H. Best: Histologic studies in tolbutamide-treated dogs. Metabolism 8, 577—584 (1959).

Skillman, T. G., F. A. Kruger and G. J. Hamwi: Metabolic and endocrine studies with phenetylbiguanide (DBI). Diabetes 8, 274—278 (1959).
— — L. G. Peterson and G. J. Hamwi: Clinical studies with DBI. Clin. Res. 6, 253 (1958).
Slotta, K. H., u. R. Tschesche: Über Biguanide. II. Die Blutzucker-senkende Wirkung der Biguanide. Ber. dtsch. chem. Gesellsch. 62 B, 1398—1405 (1929).
Smith, M. J. H.: The effect of salicylate on the glycosuria and hyperglycemia induced by cortisone in the normal rat. Biochem. J. 52, 649—652 (1952).
— The effect of salicylate on liver glycogen in the rat. Biochem. J. 57, 349—352 (1954).
— The effect of salicylate on liver glycogen, blood glucose and the passage of a barium meal in the rat. Proc. of the Bioch. Society. Biochem. J. 57, VII (1954).
— The effects of salicylate and adrenocortical preparations added in vitro upon glycogen content of liver slices. Biochem. J. 59, 52—55 (1955).
— The effect of Na-salicylate on blood glucose in the rat. Brit. J. Pharmacol. 10, 110—112 (1955).
— and S. W. Jeffrey: The effects of salicylate on oxygen consumption and carbohydrate metabolism in the isolated rat diaphragm. Biochem. J. 63, 524—528 (1956).
— B. W. Meade and J. Bornstein: The effect of salicylate on glycosuria blood glucose and liver glycogen of the alloxan-diabetic rat. Biochem. J. 51, 18—20 (1952).
Smith, P. K.: Certain aspects of the pharmacology of the salicylates. Pharmacol. Rev. 1, 353 bis 382 (1949).
Sobel, G. W., J. Rodriguez-Inigo, J. V. Morton and R. Levine: Studies on the action of the sulfonylureas in liverless dogs. Metabolism 7, 222—226 (1958).
Sokal, J. E., and E. J. Sarcione: Effect of epinephrine on glycogen stores. Amer. J. Physiol. 196, 1253—1257 (1959).
Söling, H. D. u. W. Creutzfeldt: Tierexperimentelle Untersuchungen zur Pharmakologie und zum Wirkungsmechanismus von N_1-β-Phenylaethylbiguanid und N_1-n-Butylbiguanid. In Bertram u. Michael „Internationales Biguanid-Symposium". Stuttgart: G. Thieme 1960, p. 17—28.
— E. Rauh u. W. Creutzfeldt: Die Wirkung von N_1-n-Butylbiguanid auf den chronischen Alloxandiabetes der Ratte. In preparation.
— H. D. Jarre u. L. Schmidt: Über die Wirkung von Salicylat und Khellin auf den Blutzucker normaler und alloxandiabetischer Ratten. Zschr. f. exp. Med. 1961 in press.
— H. Werchau, G. Arens u. W. Creutzfeldt: Der Einfluß von Methylenblau auf die Blutzuckersenkung durch DBI und N_1-n-Butylbiguanid. In preparation.
— H. Werchau u. W. Creutzfeldt: Klinische und experimentelle Untersuchungen zur Wirkungsweise von N_1-n-Butylbiguanid. In preparation.
Soskin, S., R. Levine and O. Hechter: The relation between the phosphate changes in blood and muscle following dextrose, insulin and epinephrine administration. Amer. J. Physiol. 134, 40—46 (1941).
Spanár, E., V. Baláz u. O. Adamec: Klinische Studien über die Wirkungsweise der peroralen Antidiabetica. Z. ges. inn. Med. 14, 476—485 (1959).
Späth, E., u. S. Prokopp: Über das Galegin. Ber. dtsch. chem. Gesell. 57, 474—480 (1924).
Spingler, H.: Über eine Möglichkeit zur colorimetrischen Bestimmung von N-(4-Methyl-benzol-sulfonyl) N'-Butyl-Harnstoff im Serum. Klin. Wschr. 35, 533—535 (1957).
Sproull, D. H.: The glycogenolytic action of Na-salicylate. Brit. J. Pharmacol. 9, 121—124 (1954).
Stahl, J., et M. Dorner: Activité insulinique et glucagonique d'extraits de pancréas provenant de chiens traités par du BZ 55. Ann. Endocr. (Paris) 18, 258—259 (1957).
Stahl, R., u. K. Bahn: Unsere Erfahrungen mit Synthalin. Dtsch. med. Wschr. 1927, 1687—1689.
Starkenstein, E.: Über die pharmakologische Wirkung kalziumfällender Säuren und der Magnesiumsalze. Naunyn-Schmiedebergs Arch. exp. Path. Pharmak. 77, 45—82 (1914).
Staub, H.: Experimentelle Untersuchungen über Synthalinwirkung. Z. klin. Med. 108, 607—658 (1928).
— u. A. Jezler: Zum Synthalinmechanismus. Z. klin. Med. 112, 1—18 (1929).
— u. O. Küng: Zum Synthalin-Mechanismus. Klin. Wschr. 1928, 1365.
Steele, R.: Use of C^{14}-glucose to measure hepatic glucose production following an intravenous glucose load or after injection of insulin. Metabolism 8, 512—519 (1959).
— Influences of glucose loading and of injected insulin on hepatic glucose output. Ann. N. Y. Acad. Sci. 82, 420—430 (1959).
Steigerwald, H., E. Böhle, K. Schöffling u. E. F. Pfeiffer: Das Verhalten des Inter-mediärstoffwechsels unter Belastungen mit Insulin und D 860 bei Stoffwechselgesunden und Diabetikern. Dtsch. med. Wschr. 1957, 1554—1556.
— E. F. Pfeiffer, K. Schöffling u. H. Ditschuneit: Bemerkenswerte klinische Beobachtungen unter D 860. Dtsch. med. Wschr. 1957, 1541—1542.
— K. Schöffling, E. F. Pfeiffer u. K. Meyer: Klinische Kontrolluntersuchungen nach Dauerbehandlung mit D 860. Dtsch. med. Wschr. 1957, 1525—1526.

STEIGERWALDT, F.: Perorale Therapie des Diabetes mellitus. Therapiewoche 7, 151—154 (1957).
— Klinische Anwendung und Indikationsbreite des n-Butyl-biguanids (W 37). In BERTRAM und
MICHAEL: Internationales Biguanid-Symposium, S. 117—121. Stuttgart: G. Thieme 1960.
STEINER, D. F., and R. H. WILLIAMS: Respiratory inhibition and hypoglycemia by biguanides
and decamethylenediguanidine. Biochim. biophys. Acta 30, 325—340 (1958).
— — Actions of phenethylbiguanide and related compunds. Diabetes 8, 154—157 (1959).
— — The effect of biguanide compounds upon respiratory enzymes. Diabetes (in press).
STERLING, K., and R. S. CHODOS: Radiothyroxine turnover studies in myxedema, thyreo-
toxicosis and hypermetabolism without endocrine disease. J. clin. Invest. 35, 806 (1956).
STERNE, J.: Du nouveau dans les antidiabétiques, la N-N-diméthylaminoguanyl-guanidine.
Maroc. méd. 1957, 1295 (Décembre).
— L'action hypoglycémiante de la N. N. diméthylaminoguanyl-guanidine. Thérapie 1958, 13.
— Traitement du diabète sucré par la N. N. Dimethyl Guanil Guanidine (LA. 6023, gluco-
phage). Thérapie 1959, 625—630.
— et D. DUVAL: Effets hypoglycémiantes de la N-N-dimethyldiguanide. In Diabetes mellitus:
III. Kongreß der International Federation Düsseldorf 1959, S. 443. Stuttgart: Georg
Thieme Verlag 1959.
STERZING, L.: Über eine generalisierte epidermolytische Reaktion bei der Behandlung des
Diabetes mellitus mit BZ 55. Dtsch. med. Wschr. 1958, 100.
STETTEN DE WITT: Comments on the fate of and responses to insulin in the liver. Metabolism 8,
559—564 (1959).
STEWART, G. A.: Effets du BZ 55 et du D 860 sur certaines activités des hormones du lobe
postérieur de l'hypophyse et de l'hexoestrol. Ann. Endocr. (Paris) 18, 196—203 (1957).
— Effets du BZ 55 et du D 860 sur des animaux de laboratoire normaux ou rendus diabétiques
par l'administration d'alloxane. Ann. (Paris) Endocr. 18, 230—245 (1957).
STEWART, R. C., E. U. PIAZZA, H. HYMAN and D. HURWITZ: Chlorporpamide therapy of
diabetes. New Engl. J. Med. 261, 427—430 (1959).
STICH, W., R. MARX u. M. EHRHART: Hämatologie des Diabetes mellitus und Rastinontherapie.
Dtsch. med. Wschr. 1957, 1533—1537.
STÖTTER, G.: Indikationen und Ergebnisse der oralen Diabetesbehandlung III. Dtsch. med.
Wschr. 1958, 1256—1260.
— Neue Gesichtspunkte der Pharmakotherapie des Diabetes mit Sulfonylharnstoffen. Münch.
med. Wschr. 1958, 1069—1073.
— u. W. CREUTZFELDT: Die Harnzuckerausscheidung unter Cortison bzw. Prednison und
D 860. Dtsch. med. Wschr. 1956, 840—841.
— G. MOHNIKE, W. CREUTZFELDT, R. SEUS, ST. SCHLAGINTWEIT u. H. ULRICH: Belastungs-
versuche mit Glukose, Adrenalin und Glukagon bei Stoffwechselgesunden und Diabetikern
unter D 860. Dtsch. med. Wschr. 1956, 835—837.
STOWERS, J. M., L. W. CONSTABLE and R. B. HUNTER: A clinical and pharmacological compari-
son of chlorpropamide and other sulfonylureas. Ann. N. Y. Acad. Sci. 74, 689—695 (1959).
— R. F. MAHLER and R. B. HUNTER: Pharmacology and mode of action of the sulphonylureas
in man. Lancet 1958 I, 278—283.
STRÄSSLE, R., u. A. PLETSCHER: Über Hemmung von Insulinase durch Sulfonylharnstoffe.
Klin. Wschr. 1957, 719—722.
STRATMANN, F. W.: Über Spätversager bei der peroralen Diabetestherapie and ihre kombi-
nierte Behandlung. Med. Klin. 1957, 589—591.
STRAUSS, H.: Zur Frage der Synthalinwirkung bei Diabetikern. Med. Klin. 1927, 117.
STRAUZENBERG, S. E., u. H. HALLER: Beitrag zum Wirkungsmechanismus der blutzucker-
senkenden Sulfonylharnstoffe. Dtsch. med. Wschr. 1959, 1097—1103.
— — Klinische Indikationen und Kontraindikationen für die perorale Behandlung der Diabe-
tiker mit Sulfonylharnstoffpräparaten. Z. ges. inn. Med. 14, 528 (1959).
— — u. H. MEYER: Beitrag zum Problem der Versagerfälle bei der peroralen Diabetestherapie.
Münch. med. Wschr. 1958, 1535—1540.
STUHLFAUTH, K., H. MEHNERT, G. SCHÄFER u. G. KALIAMPETSOS: Untersuchungen zum Wirkungsmechanismus der Sulfonylharnstoffe. Klin. Wschr. 1960, 825—826.
SÜDHOF, H, S. ALTENBURG u. E. SANDER: Zur Frage der D 860-Eliminationsgeschwindigkeit
aus dem Serum beim Diabetiker. Klin. Wschr. 1958, 585.
— W. EGER, S. ALTENBURG u. G. SCHUMACHER: Blutzuckersenkung durch orale Antidiabetica
und Verhalten des N-(4-Methyl-benzolsulfonyl)-N'-butylharnstoffes im Serum in Ab-
hängigkeit von der Leberfunktion. Arzneimittel-Forsch. 8, 438—442 (1958).
SUGAR, S. J. N.: Use of the sulfonylureas in diabetes mellitus. Ann. N. Y. Acad. Sci. 71,
256—263 (1957).
— L. J. THOMAS and S. TATLIER: Use of chlorpropamide in diabetes mellitus in usual diabetic
patients and in primary and secondary tolbutamido failures. Ann. N. Y. Acad. Sci. 74,
625—631 (1959).

SUMM, H. D.: Untersuchungen über die Aktivität von Stoffwechselenzymen bei Lactation, Diabetes mellitus und Behandlung mit oralen antidiabetischen Mitteln. Dissertation, Freiburg i. Br. 1958.
— W. CREUTZFELDT u. K. WALLENFELS: Über den Einfluß von N-(4-Methylbenzolsulfonyl)-N'-butylharnstoff (D 860) und Insulin auf die $^{14}CO_2$-Fixierung im Leberglykogen. Klin. Wschr. **1960**, 85—87.
SÜTTERLE, H.: Tierexperimentelle Untersuchungen zur Differenzierung der Insulinwirkung von der Wirkung eines blutzuckersenkenden Sulfonylharnstoffes. Dissertation Freiburg i. Br. 1957.
SWENSSON, Å.: Contributions to the knowledge of the effect of exogenous insulin on the glycogen storage of normal animals. Acta physiol. scand. 11, Suppl. 33, 1—158 (1945).
SZCEKLIK, E.: Über die toxischen Nebenwirkungen des Synthalins. Wien. klin. Wschr. **1927**, 1075.
SZÜCS, S., and A. TISZAI: Effect of carbutamide on blood levels of glucose, potassium and inorganic phosphate. Diabetes 7, 288—292 (1958).
TAKEDA, M., K. NAKANO and K. WAKABAYASHI: Effect of mesoxalate upon the carbohydrate figures of liver in normal and alloxan diabetic rabbits. Endocr. jap. 2, 171—174 (1955).
TAPLEY, D. F.: Magnesium balance in myxedematous patients treated with triidothyronine. Bull. Johns Hopk. Hosp. 96, 274 (1956).
TARAIL, R., and T. E. BENNETT: Hypoglycemic activity of tris buffer in man and dog. Proc. Soc. exp. Biol. (N. Y.) 102, 208—209 (1959).
TARDING, F., and P. SCHAMBYE: The action of sulfonylureas and insulin on the glucose output from the liver of normal dogs. Endokrinologie 36, 222—228 (1958).
TENNEY, S. M., and R. M. MILLER: The respiratory and circulatory actions of salicylate. Amer. J. Med. 19, 498—508 (1955).
TISZAI, A., u. S. SZÜCS: Akute Wirkung von BZ 55 auf den Blutzucker, Kalium- und anorganischen Phosphorspiegel des Serums an pankreatektomisierten Hunden. Z. ges. inn. Med. 13, 314—316 (1958).
TOLOMELLI, E., e L. BACCI: Attività terapeutica nel diabete mellito di un nuovo ipoglicemizzante orale (clorpropamide). Minerva med. (Torino) 50, 2543—2546 (1959).
TONIELLI, J., R. LUCINI e R. CAPANNA: Contributo allo studio dell'agranulocitosi immunilogica; su due casi di agranulocitosi anafilattica medicamentosa da prodotto antidiabetico. G. Clin. med. 38, 917—924 (1957).
TOOLAN, TH. J., and R. L. WAGNER: The physical properties of chlorpropamide and its determination in human serum. Ann. N. Y. Acad. Sci. 74, 449—458.
TORNOW, A. M., M. R. ZINKE, PH. GREENBERG and C. M. LEEVY: Hypoglycemic effects of 1-(p-chlorobenzene-sulfonyl)-3-n-propylurea. Diabetes 8, 1—6 (1959).
TRANQUADA, R. E., CH. R. KLEEMAN and J. S. BROWN: The acute effects of DBI on human hepatic intermediary metabolism. Clin. Res. 7, 110 (1959).
— — — Clinical trials with phenethyldiguanide in selected patients. Amer. J. med. Sci. 238, 187—191 (1959).
— — — Some effects of Phenethylbiguanide on human hepatic metabolism as measured by hepatic vein catheterization. Diabetes 9, 207—214 (1960).
TRINDER, P.: Rapid determination of salicylate in biological fluids. Biochem. J. 57, 301 (1954).
TUCHMANN-DUPLESSIS, H., et L. MERCIER-PAROT: Sur l'action tératogène de l'amino-phénurobutane (BZ 55) chez la ratte. C. R. Soc. Biol. (Paris) 152, 460—463 (1958).
— — Sur l'action tératogène d'un sulfamide hypoglycémiant. Etude expérimentale chez la ratte. J. Physiol. (Paris) 51, 65—83 (1959).
— — Influence de divers sulfamides hypoglycémiants sur le développment de l'embryon. Etude expérimentale chez le rat. Bull. Acad. nat. Méd. (Paris) 143, 238—241 (1959).
TULLOCH, J. A.: A multiplicity of reactions to carbutamide (BZ 55) therapy. Diabetes 7, 316—319 (1958).
TYBERGHEIN, J., and R. H. WILLIAMS: Relationship of glucagon to the mode of action of oral antidiabetic compounds. Clin. Res. Proc. 4, 124 (1956).
TYBERGHEIN, J. M., Y. D. HALSEY and R. H. WILLIAMS: Action of butyl-tolylsulfonylurea on liver glycogenolysis. Proc. Soc. exp. Biol. (N. Y.) 92, 322—324 (1956).
— and R. H. WILLIAMS: Metabolic effects of phenethyldiguanide: A new hypoglycemic compound. Proc. Soc. exp. Biol. (N. Y.) 96, 29 (1957).
UEXKÜLL, TH, v.: Die orale Behandlung des Diabetes mellitus mit Sulfonylharnstoffderivaten. Ther. d. Gegenw. 97, 300—308 (1958).
UHRY, P., G. MARCEL, M. DUIZEND, R. VARIN, M. COHEN et TEXIER: Résultats statistiques sur le traitement du diabète sucré par les hypoglycémiants de synthèse. Bull. Soc. méd. Hôp. Paris 73, 630—638 (1957).
UMBER, F.: Zur Synthalinbehandlung der Zuckerkranken. Dtsch. med. Wschr. **1927**, 1121.

UNDERHILL, F. D., and N. R. BLATHERWICK: Studies in carbohydrate metabolism. VI. The influence of thyreoparathyroidectomy upon the sugar content of the blood and the glycogen content of the liver. J. biol. Chem. 18, 87 (1914).
— — Studies in carbohydrate metabolism. VII. The influence of subcutaneous injections of dextrose and of calciumlactate upon the blood sugar content and upon tetany after thyreoparathyroidectomy. J. biol. Chem. 19, 119 (1914).
UNGAR, G.: Pharmacology and toxicology of phenethylbiguanide (DBI). Symposium on "A New Hypoglycemic Agent, Phenformin (DBI)". Houston (Texas) 1959.
— Diskussionsbemerkung. Diabetes 9, 179 (1960).
— L. FREEDMAN and S. L. SHAPIRO: Pharmacological studies of a new hypoglycemic drug. Proc. Soc. exp. Biol. (N. Y.) 95, 190 (1957).
— S. PSYCHOYOS and H. A. HALL: Action of phenethylbiguanide, a hypoglycemic agent, on tricarboxylic acid cycle. Metabolism 9, 36 (1960).
UNGER, H.: Zur Frage der Wirksamkeit der Nikotinsäure auf den Kohlenhydratstoffwechsel. Z. ges. inn. Med. 14, 924—926 (1959).
UNGER, R. H., and L. L. MADISON: Comparison of response to intravenously administered sodium tolbutamide in mild diabetic and non diabetic subjects. J. clin. Invest. 37, 627—630 (1958).
— — A new diagnostic procedure for mild diabetes mellitus. Evaluation of an intravenous tolbutamide response test. Diabetes 7, 455—461 (1958).
— — and N. W. CARTER: Relative effectiveness of newer oral agents in the regulation of diabetic patients imperfectly controlled by tolbutamide studied with the frame work of a tentative subclassification of the disease. Ann. N. Y. Acad. Sci. 82, 570—584 (1959).
VALLANCE-OWEN, J., G. F. JOPLIN and R. FRASER: Tolbutamide control of diabetes mellitus, clinical responsiveness and insulin reserve. Lancet 1959 I, 584—586.
VARELA, B., J. A. COLLAZO et P. RUBINO: Toxicité expérimentale d'un dérivé polyméthylé de la guanidine. C. R. Soc. Biol. (Paris) 99, 1444 (1928).
VARELA FUENTES, B., R. CANZANI et J. MILSTEIN: Agranulocytose aigue avec insuffisance rénale aigue, létale, pendant une dermatose provoquée par la drogue antidiabétique le BZ 55. Arch. Mal. Appar. dig. 46, 305 (1957).
VAUGHAN, M.: In vitro studies on the action of sulfonamide hypoglycemic agents. Science 123, 885 (1956).
— Studies on the mechanism of action of orinase (tolbutamide). Diabetes 6, 16—18 (1957).
VOELKEL, A.: Erste Erfahrungen mit einer Insulin-Nadisan-Kombination zur Hypoglykämie-behandlung der Psychosen. Klin. Wschr. 1956, 210—211.
— J. CH. DRESLER u. CH. MOTHES: Die kombinierte Hypoglykämie-Behandlung der Psychosen mit Insulin und blutzuckersenkenden Substanzen. Nervenarzt 28, 220—221 (1957).
VOLK, B. W., M. G. GOLDNER, S. WEISENFELD and S. S. LAZARUS: Functional and histological studies concerning the action of sulfonylureas. Ann. N. Y. Acad. Sci. 71, 141—151 (1957).
— — Histologic and histochemical observations in the rabbit after Phenethylbiguanide. Diabetes 9, 174—177 (1960).
— and S. S. LAZARUS: Pathogenesis of orinase-induced betacell degranulation. Diabetes 7, 125—128 (1958).
— — Significance of effectiveness of combined insulin-orinase treatment in maturity-onset diabetes. Amer. J. med. Sci. 237, 1—7 (1959).
— SH. WEISENFELD, S. S. LAZARUS and M. G. GOLDNER: Mechanisms of action of the hypoglycemia-producing sulfonylurea derivatives. Metabolism 5, 894—903 (1956).
VONKENNEL, J., u. J. KIMMIG: Versuche und Untersuchungen mit neuen Sulfonamiden. Klin. Wschr. 1941, 2—8.
VUYLSTEKE, CH. A., et C. DEDUVE: Zit. nach DEDUVE, C. et J. BERTHET. "Le Glucagon". Colloque d'Endocrinologie Paris 1957, S. 345. Paris: Masson 1957.
WADDELL, W. R.: Effect of tolbutamide on serum cholesterol levels in hypercholesterilemic patients. Proc. Soc. exp. Biol. (N. Y.) 98, 280 (1958).
WAIFE, S. O., L. O. BRENNER and C. M. THOMPSON: The insulin tolerance test in cirrhosis of the liver. Gastroenterology 17, 236 (1951).
WALDMANN, K.: Agranulocytose nach BZ 55. Med. Klin. 1957, 1794—1796.
WALKER, G., W. L. B. LEESE and J. D. N. NABARRO: Hypoglycaemic sulphonamides in treatment of diabetes. Brit. med. J. 1956, 4990, 451—452.
— J. D. H. SLATER, E. K. WESTLAKE and J. D. N. NABARRO: Clinical experience with tolbutamide. Brit. med. J. 1957 II, 323.
WALKER, J. B.: Chlorpropamide. Lancet 1958 II, 641.
WALKER, R. S.: The long-term use of carbutamide (BZ 55) in the treatment of diabetes mellitus. Acta endocr. (Kbh.) 31, 261—266 (1959).
— Preliminary observations on phenethylbiguanide. Brit. med. J. 1959, 405—406.

WALKER, R. S., and A. L. LINTON: Phenethylbiguanide: A dangerous sideeffect. Brit. med. J. **1959**, 1005—1006.

WALLENFELS, K., W. BURCHARD u. H. SUND: Einfluß von Sulfonylharnstoffderivaten auf die Dissoziation von Zinkinsulin und Glutaminsäuredehydrogenase. To be published.

— W. CREUTZFELDT u. H. D. SUMM: Die Enzyme des Kohlenhydratstoffwechsels in Leberpunktaten von Normalpersonen und Diabetikern. Diabetes mellitus. 3. Kongr. der internat. Diab. Feder. Düsseldorf 1958, S. 330—336. Stuttgart: Georg Thieme 1959.

— u. H. D. SUMM: Hemmung und Aktivierung von DPN-abhängigen Zinkenzymen durch blutzuckersenkende Sulfonylharnstoffverbindungen. Klin. Wschr. **1957**, 849—851.

— — u. W. CREUTZFELDT: Enzymatische Untersuchungen zum Wirkungsmechanismus der blutzuckersenkenden Medikamente. Dtsch. med. Wschr. **1957**, 1581—1585.

WALTNER jr., K., B. TANOS and E. KELEMEN: Increase of venous oxygen saturation after a high salicylate dose in human adults. Acta med. Acad. Sci. hung. **12**, 147—151 (1958).

WATANABE, C. K.: Studies in the metabolic changes induced by administration of guanidine bases. I. Influence of injected guanidine hydrochloride upon blood sugar content. J. biol. Chem. **33**, 253 (1918).

— Studies in the metabolic changes induced by the administration of guanidine bases. V. The change of phosphate and calcium content in serum in guanidine tetany and the relation between the calcium content and sugar in the blood. J. biol. Chem. **36**, 531 (1918).

WEAVER, J. A., T. E. PROUT and G. W. SCOTT: Role of insulin in acute hypoglycemic action of tolbutamide. Brit. med. J. **1958** I, 425—429.

WEBER, G., and A. CANTERO: Effect of orinase on hepatic enzymes involved in glucose-6-phosphate utilization. Metabolism **7**, 333—337 (1958).

WEHLING, H.: Klinischer Bericht über 450 mit dem oralen Antidiabeticum Rastinon (D 860) behandelte Diabetiker. Münch. med. Wschr. **98**, 1699 (1956).

WELLER, CH., A. MACAULAY, M. LINDER and J. D. TRACY: Clinical evaluation of metahexamide in the treatment of patients with diabetes mellitus. Metabolism 8, 672—675 (1959).

WELLER, P.: Klinische Beobachtungen zur Spätresistenz auf orale Antidiabetica. Z. ges. inn. Med. **13**, 564—568 (1958).

WELLS, R., and T. BOCK: Oral therapy for diabetes with tuberculosis. Brit. med. J. **1958**, 220.

WENDEROTH, H., u. F. BALZEREIT: Zwei Agranulozytosefälle nach Sulfonamidtherapie des Diabetes. Med. Klin. **1958**, 1560—1561.

WENGER, V.: Zur Wirkungsweise peroraler Antidiabetica: Sulfonylharnstoff und Hypophysen-Nebennierenrinden-System. Helv. med. Acta **24**, 91—99 (1957).

WEST, K. M., and PH. C. JOHNSON: The comparative pharmacology of tolbutamide, Carbutamide, chlorpropamide and metahexamide in man. Metabolism 8, 596—605 (1959).

— and ST. R. MCCAMPBELL: Relative potencies of chlorpropamide and tolbutamide in man. Ann. N. Y. Acad. Sci. **74**, 473—477 (1959).

WHITE, P., and L. P. KRALL: Prolonged use of the biguanides in diabetic children. Symposion on "A New Hypoglycemic Agent, Phenformin (DBI)". Houston (Texas), 1959.

WICK, A. N., B. BRITTON and R. GRABOWSKI: The action of a sulfonylurea hypoglycemic agent (orinase) in extrahepatic tissues. Metabolism 5, 739—743 (1956).

— and E. LARSON: Studies with phenethylbiguanide — a hypoglycemic agent. Clin. Res. **6**, 91 (1958).

WICK, A. N., E. R. LARSON and G. S. SERIF: A site of action of phenetylbiguanide — a hypoglycemic compound. J. biol. Chem. **233**, 296 (1958).

WICK, A. N., and C. J. STEWART: Tissue distribution of administered DBI and its relationship to DBI action. Clin. Res. Proc. **7**, 111 (1959).

— — and G. S. SERIF: Tissue distribution of C^{14}-labeled beta-phenethyl-biguanide. Diabetes **9**, 163—166 (1960).

WIELAND, O.: Störungen der biochemischen Regulation von Kohlenhydrat- und Fettstoffwechsel beim Diabetes. Diabetes mellitus: III. Kongr. der Internationalen Diabetes Federation Düsseldorf Juli 1958, 20—26. Stuttgart: Georg Thieme 1959.

WILD, H., u. H. W. LINDEN: Klinische Beobachtungen über Schädigungen des peripheren Nervensystems und der Leber bei Diabetikern unter der Behandlung mit Sulfanilylharnstoff. Dtsch. med. J. **10**, 286—292 (1959).

WILDBERGER, H. L., and H. T. RICKETTS: The effect of tolbutamide on glucose and nitrogen metabolism in the totally depancreatized dog. J. Lab. clin. Med. **52**, 958—959 (1958).

WILDHACK, R.: Zur Bewertung der akuten Belastung mit oralen Antidiabetica. Klin. Wschr. **1959**, 198—201.

WILKINSON, S.: Structure of hypoglycin A. Chem. and Ind. **1958**, 17—18.

WILLE, K.: Vergleichende Untersuchungen mit intravenöser Glukose- und Tolbutamidbelastung bei Stoffwechselgesunden und Diabetikern mit und ohne Lebercirrhosen. Med. Dissertation Freiburg i. Br. 1961.

WILLIAMS, R. H.: Diskussionsbemerkung: Symposion on the hypoglycemic agents. Metabolism 8, 557 (1959).
— D. C. TANNER and W. D. ODELL: Hypoglycemic action of phenethyl-, Amyl- and isoamyl-diguanide. Diabetes 7, 87 (1958).
— and B. W. TUCKER: Hypoglycemic actions of tolbutamide and carbutamide. Metabolism 5, 801—806 (1956).
— J. M. TYBERGHEIN, P. M. HYDE and R. L. NIELSEN: Studies related to the hypoglycemic action of phenethyldiguanide. Metabolism 6, 311 (1957).
WILLIAMSON, R. T.: On the treatment of glykosuria and diabetes mellitus with sodium salicylate. Brit. med. J. 1, 760—762 (1901).
WILSON, J. W.: Protective action of sulfa drugs against injury to liver of mouse by CCl_4. Fed. Proc. 11, 433—434 (1952).
— E. H. LEDUC and L. E. ARNOLD: Protective action of sulfa drugs against CCl_4-poisoning in mice. Fed. Proc. 9, 349 (1950).
WINTERS, R. W., and M. F. MORRILL: Carbohydrate metabolism in experimental salicylism. Proc. Soc. exp. Biol. (N. Y.) 88, 409—411 (1955).
WITTENHAGEN, G.: Qualitativer Eiweißnachweis im Harn bei Anwesenheit des Ausscheidungs-produktes von D 860. Dtsch. med. Wschr. 1957, 254.
— u. G. MOHNIKE: Über das Ausscheidungsprodukt von D 860. Dtsch. med. Wschr. 1956, 887.
— — u. W. LANGENBECK: Beiträge zu Abbau und Ausscheidung von N-(4-Methyl-benzol-sulfonyl)-N'-butylharnstoff (D 860). Hoppe-Seylers Z. physiol. Chem. 316, 157—163 (1959).
WOLFF, F. W., G. A. STEWART and M. F. CROWLEY: Trial of an oral hypoglycemic agent in diabetes. Brit. med. J. 1956 II, 440—445.
WOLFF, H., u. D. RINGLEB: Histochemische Untersuchungen über das Inselzink. Z. exp. Med. 124, 236—256 (1954); 126, 390—416 (1955).
WRENSHALL, G. A.: Reports on studies with carbutamide and tolbutamide done at the Charles H. Best institute, university of Toronto. Ann. N. Y. Acad. Sci. 71, 164—169 (1957).
— ST. B. ANDRUS and J. MAYER: High levels of pancreatic insulin coexistent with hyper-plasia and degranulation of beta-cells in mice with the hereditary obese-hyperglycemic syndrome. Endocrinology 56, 335—340 (1955).
— and C. H. BEST: Extractable insulin of the pancreas and effectiveness of oral hypoglycemic sulfonylureas in the treatment of diabetes in man — a comparison. Canad. med. Ass. J. 74, 968—972 (1956).
— A. BOGOCH and R. C. RITCHIE: Extractable insulin of pancreas, correlation with patho-logical and clinical findings in diabetic and nondiabetic cases. Diabetes 1, 87 (1952).
— J. COLLINS-WILLIAMS and W. S. HARTROFT: Incidence, control and regression of diabetic symptoms in the alloxan treated rat. Amer. J. Physiol. 156, 100—116 (1949).
— and J. D. HAMILTON: Sex differences in the amount of insulin extractable from diabetic human pancreas. Ann. N. Y. Acad. Sci. 71, 154—163 (1957).
— W. ST. HARTROFT and C. H. BEST: Insulin extractable from the pancreas and islet cell histology. Comparative studies in spontaneous diabetes in dogs and human subjects. Diabetes 3, 444—452 (1954).
— and G. HETENYI: Successive measured injections of tracer as a method for determining characteristics of accumulation and turnover in higher animals with access limited to blood: tests in hydrodynamic systems and initial observations on insulin action in dogs. Metabolism 8, 531—543 (1959).
YALOW, R. S., H. BLACK, M. VILLAZON and S. A. BERSON: Comparison of plasma insulin levels following administration of tulbutamide and glucose. Diabetes 9, 356—362 (1960).
ZACCO, M., M. LEONARDI e U. NERINI: Inibizione dell' alanina transaminasi con i derivati ipoglicemizzanti della sulfonilurea. Minerva med. (Torino) 49, 1537—1538 (1958).
ZAROWITZ, H., and B. EIS: The role of a tolbutamide tolerance test in the detection of the mild diabetic state: a preliminary report. Ann. N. Y. Acad. Sci. 74, 662—666 (1959).
ZAWACKI, F., u. F. JUNG: Über neue blutzuckerwirksame Verbindungen. Klin. Wschr. 1957, 363—364.
ZEFFREN, L., and S. SHERRY: Effects of prolonged tolbutamide therapy on hepatic function and serum cholester ol of adult diabetic patients. Metabolism 6, 504—508 (1957).
ZUNZ, E., et J. LA BARRE: Action de la decamethylene-diguanidine sur la secretion interne du pancreas. Arch. int. Pharmacodyn. 34, 442—463 (1928).
ZÜRN, H.: Die Einwirkung von Phenylbutazon (Butalidon, Butazolidin) auf den Kohlen-hydratstoffwechsel bei Diabetikern. Z. ges. inn. Med. 14, 897—901 (1959).
ZWANG, H., u. M. JACUBEIT: Über die Beeinflussung des Blutzuckerspiegels durch Pyribenz-amin (Benzyl-pyridyl-dimethyl-äthylen-diamin). Biochem. Z. 323, 355—362 (1952).